Atlas of Surgical Treatment of Inflammatory Bowel Disease

Tomas M. Heimann
Editor

Atlas of Surgical Treatment of Inflammatory Bowel Disease

Springer

Editor
Tomas M. Heimann
Department of Surgery
Icahn School of Medicine at Mount Sinai
New York, USA

ISBN 978-3-031-62430-8 ISBN 978-3-031-62431-5 (eBook)
https://doi.org/10.1007/978-3-031-62431-5

This Springer imprint is published by the registered company Springer Nature Switzerland AG
The registered company address is: Gewerbestrasse 11, 6330 Cham, Switzerland

The authors would like to dedicate this Atlas to Dr. Arthur H. Aufses, Jr., MD. Dr. Aufses, an excellent teacher and master surgeon, was the chairman of the Department of Surgery at the Mount Sinai Medical Center for most of our surgical residency and the following 20 years. Mount Sinai is regarded as a world-renowned center for the treatment of Inflammatory Bowel Disease and Dr. Aufses, an outstanding IBD surgeon, was instrumental in maintaining this reputation. One of his greatest achievements was the creation of an outstanding department of surgery which is now named after him. Without his foresight and guidance, this Atlas would not have been possible.

Foreword

Basic science and the contribution on the possibility of an infectious cause, causes of Inflammatory Bowel disease at the Mt Sinai hospital and its affiliates.

When the first report of what is now known as Crohn's disease was communicated from the Mt Sinai Hospital in 1932 [1], the authors commented on its similarity to intestinal tuberculosis and made diligent efforts to identify a possible infectious association. They were unable to do so. In a preceding report from Scotland in 1913 [2], the surgeon reported on identical cases to the Mt Sinai ones, once again commenting on the similarity to intestinal tuberculosis. There was a diligent attempt to identify a known infectious cause. It too was unsuccessful. Interestingly, Dalziel commented on the pathological similarity to a disease in cattle [3] caused by *Mycobacterium avium* subspecies *paratuberculosis* (MAP). This is now referred to as Johne's disease.

Over the ensuing decades, multiple attempts have been made to identify a possible infectious etiology of Inflammatory Bowel Disease, of which Crohn's is a major component. The results are, at best, equivocal [4].

The Veterans Affairs Medical Center in Bronx, an academic affiliate of The Mt Sinai Hospital, housed the laboratory of Roslyn S. Yalow. In 1977, she became the second woman to win the Nobel Prize in Medicine, for the development of the technique of Radio-Immuno assay. She welcomed young investigators into her laboratory and encouraged "non-directed" research. Following a surgical residency at Mt Sinai Hospital, I joined the Surgical Department at the VA and, with the encouragement of Dr Yalow, in 1982 I established a basic science laboratory at the VA.

My brother Adrian was an Inflammatory Bowel Disease surgeon at Mt Sinai. On clinical grounds, he had suggested that there might be two forms of Crohn's disease, which he called "perforating" and "non-perforating" [5]. A Dutch medical student came to do an elective with my brother. He had no agenda. I suggested that he attempt to replicate a study showing the different cytokine responses in the two forms of leprosy: tuberculoid and lepromatous [6]. Using surgical specimens provided by Adrian, we showed a different cytokine expression in the two forms of Crohn's disease [7]. Subsequently, we identified the RNA of MAP in all Crohn's samples as well as patients with Ulcerative Colitis [8]. From this the hypothesis evolved that all of IBD was a disparate manifestation of an MAP infectious spectrum of gut pathology [9].

Anti-MAP antibiotic studies in Crohn's disease have been inconclusive [4]. We suggest that the etiological role of MAP in IBD has been missed because, unrecognized, MAP is being treated with "anti-inflammatory" and "immune-modulating" pharmaceutical agents [10, 11], whose actual primary mechanism of action are as anti-MAP antibiotics [12–14]. Others subsequently confirmed our observations [15–17].

Hence, until appropriate anti-MAP antibiotic studies are performed in CD, the possible zoonotic MAP/CD enigma will remain unresolved.

References

1. Crohn BB, Ginzberg L, Oppenheimer GD. Regional Ileitis. J Amer Med Assoc. 1932;99:1323–8.
2. Dalziel TK. Chronic intestinal enteritis. Br Med J. 1913;ii:1068–70.
3. Johne HA, Frothingham L. Ein eigenthumlicher fall von tuberculose beim rind (A particular case of tuberculosis in a cow). Dtsch Zeitschr Tiermed, Vergl Pathol. 1895;21:438–54.
4. Peyrin-Biroulet L, Neut C, Colombel JF. Antimycobacterial therapy in Crohn's disease: game over? Gastroenterology. 2007;132:2594–8.
5. Greenstein AJ, Lachman P, Sachar DB, et al. Perforating and non-perforating indications for repeated operations in Crohn's disease: evidence for two clinical forms. Gut. 1988;29:588–92.
6. Yamamura M, Uyemura K, Deans RJ, et al. Defining protective responses to pathogens: cytokine profiles in leprosy lesions. Science. 1991;254:277–9.
7. Gilberts EC, Greenstein AJ, Katsel P, Harpaz N, Greenstein RJ. Molecular evidence for two forms of Crohn disease. Proc Natl Acad Sci U S A. 1994;91:12721–4.
8. Mishina D, Katsel P, Brown ST, Gilberts EC, Greenstein RJ. On the etiology of Crohn disease. Proc Natl Acad Sci U S A. 1996;93:9816–20.
9. Greenstein RJ. Is Crohn's disease caused by a mycobacterium? Comparisons with leprosy, tuberculosis, and Johne's disease. Lancet Infect Dis. 2003;3:507–14.
10. Greenstein RJ, Cameron DW, Brown ST. "Add-on" is scientifically more accurate than "Placebo control" in multiple Inflammatory Bowel Disease (IBD) trials. J Crohn's Colitis. 2014;8:1334–5.
11. Greenstein RJ, Cameron DW, Brown ST. Yet another flawed "placebo controlled" study in Crohn's disease? Foodborne Pathog Dis. 2015;12:812.
12. Greenstein RJ, Su L, Haroutunian V, Shahidi A, Brown ST. On the action of methotrexate and 6-mercaptopurine on M. avium subspecies paratuberculosis. PLoS One. 2007;2:e161.
13. Greenstein RJ, Su L, Juste RA, Brown ST. On the action of cyclosporine A, rapamycin and tacrolimus on M. avium including subspecies paratuberculosis. PLoS One. 2008;3:e2496.
14. Greenstein RJ, Su L, Shahidi A, Brown ST. On the action of 5-amino-salicylic acid and sulfapyridine on M. avium including subspecies paratuberculosis. PLoS One. 2007;2:e516.

15. Shin SJ, Collins MT. Thiopurine drugs azathioprine and 6-mercaptopurine inhibit Mycobacterium paratuberculosis growth in vitro. Antimicrob Agents Chemother. 2008;52:418–26.
16. Krishnan MY, Manning EJ, Collins MT. Effects of interactions of antibacterial drugs with each other and with 6-mercaptopurine on in vitro growth of Mycobacterium avium subspecies paratuberculosis. J Antimicrob Chemother. 2009;64:1018–23.
17. Zhang S, Fu J, Dogan B, Scherl EJ, Simpson KW. 5-Aminosalicylic acid down-regulates the growth and virulence of Escherichia coli associated with IBD and colorectal cancer, and upregulates host anti-inflammatory activity. J Antibiot (Tokyo). 2018;71(11):950–61.

Robert J. Greenstein

Department of Surgery
James J. Peters Veterans
Administration Hospital,
Bronx, NY, USA

Contents

Contributors

Robert J. Greenstein Department of Surgery, James J. Peters Veterans Administration Hospital, Bronx, NY, USA

Tomas M. Heimann Department of Surgery, Icahn School of Medicine at Mount Sinai, New York, NY, USA

Robert J. Kurtz Department of Surgery, Icahn School of Medicine at Mount Sinai, New York, NY, USA

Part I

Crohn's Disease

IBD Surgery at Mount Sinai

1

Tomas M. Heimann and Robert J. Kurtz

Crohn's disease was first described at Mount Sinai in 1932 by Drs. Crohn, Oppenheimer, and Ginsburg (Figs. 1.1 and 1.2) [1]. Subsequently, Mount Sinai became arguably the world center for the treatment of complex gastrointestinal disease. When Dr. Kurtz and I arrived at Mount Sinai as surgical interns in the early 1970s, the first generation of gastroenterologists and surgeons such as Crohn and Garlock (Fig. 1.3) were no longer practicing.

Dr. Crohn was retired and Dr. Garlock, an extraordinary surgeon, had died of a ruptured aortic aneurysm. Dr. Ginsburg was still operating, and we had the opportunity to scrub with him. He always told us that Crohn's disease should have been called Ginsburg's disease because he did all the surgery described in the manuscript.

The surgical training program at Mount Sinai was intense. It was a pyramidal system where only the best residents became Chief Resident and graduated. We worked every other night for 6 years; to get a weekend off, you had to stay in the hospital from Thursday at 6 am until Saturday around 1 pm when M + M conference was finally over, and they let you go. Yes, it was a tough residency. I always compared it to the Marine Corps except that this basic training was much longer, but when you completed the program, you were fully and well trained in all areas of surgery including GI, vascular, head and neck, and thoracic surgery. We lived for the big cases and sometimes the attending surgeon, unable to scrub, allowed us to do the case by ourselves. I remember doing an aorto-bifemoral bypass by myself because the attending surgeon was busy and unable to come down to the OR. An aorto-bifemoral bypass is a highly complex vascular surgery and he trusted me enough to let me do it by myself. Furthermore, I knew that I could do it without any hesitation. That would never happen today. Our teachers were competent and experienced surgeons, most of whom were trained by the previous generation of surgical giants. There were also medical giants at Mount Sinai in those days. The medical service chair was Dr. Solomon

T. M. Heimann (✉) · R. J. Kurtz
Department of Surgery, Icahn School of Medicine at Mount Sinai, New York, NY, USA
e-mail: Tomas.Heimann@mountsinai.org; Robert.Kurtz@mountsinai.org

T. M. Heimann (ed.), *Atlas of Surgical Treatment of Inflammatory Bowel Disease*, https://doi.org/10.1007/978-3-031-62431-5_1

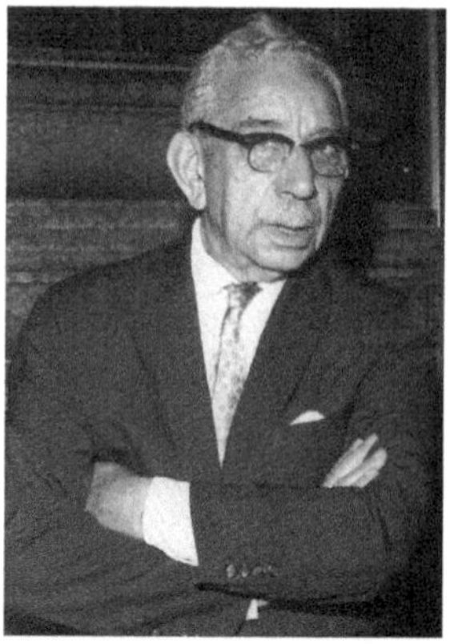

Fig. 1.1 Dr. Burrill Crohn

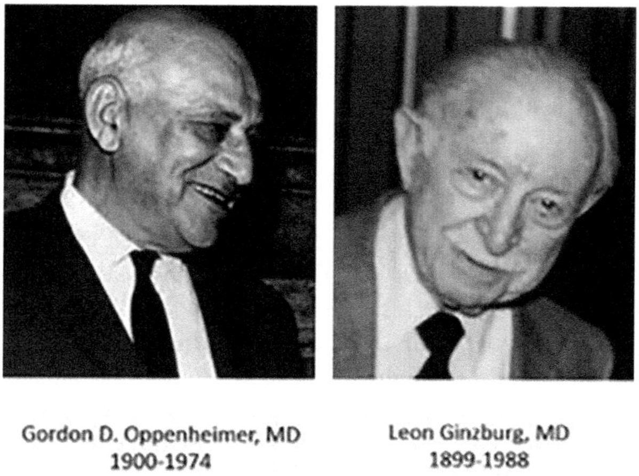

Fig. 1.2 Dr. Gordon D. Oppenheimer and Dr. Leon Ginsburg

Berson, the co-developer together with Rosalyn Yalow [2] of radioimmunoassay for which she received the Nobel Prize (Fig. 1.4). Unfortunately, Dr. Berson had died of a ruptured cerebral aneurysm and could not be present to receive the Nobel Prize.

I had the opportunity to rotate through the medical service as an intern. Dr. Berson was a hands-on chief. At 6 am every morning, the chief medical resident had to present the admissions from the previous night to him and be able to quote the latest literature for the recommended treatment. Dr. Berson was extremely intelligent but also very friendly to the house staff. It is said that he loved to play chess and could do so without the chess board, moving the pieces in his head, and he also liked to play multiple opponents at the same time.

Surgery in the 1970s was at the cusp of revolutionary advances. Amongst these advances were the imaging revolution with the advent of CT and MRI scanners, flexible endoscopy, intravenous hyperalimentation, and later minimally invasive surgery and use of staplers. Yes, this was the beginning of the golden age of gastrointestinal surgery. You can easily see from the cases presented in this Atlas the complexity of the cases we did every day and their successful outcomes.

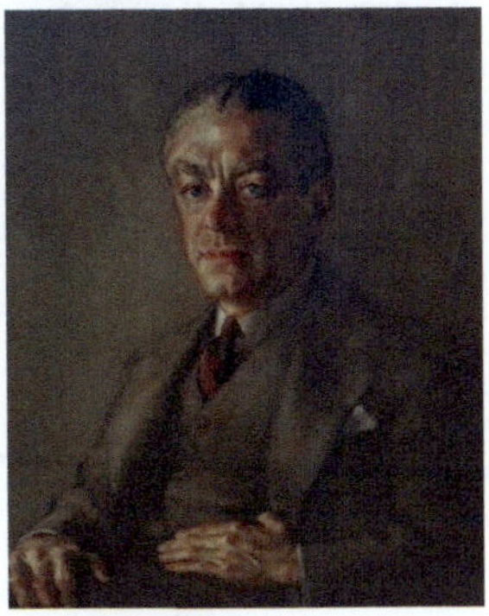

Fig. 1.3 Dr. John Garlock

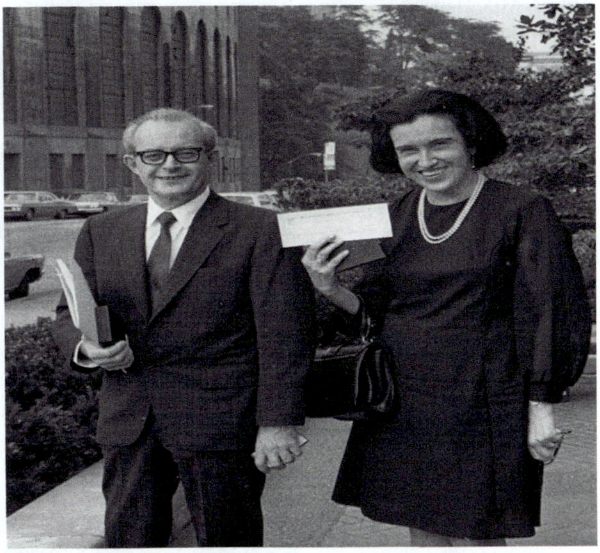

Fig. 1.4 Drs. Solomon Berson and Rosalyn Yalow

We would like to say a few words regarding the development of the ileoanal pull through operation. Dr. Ravitch (Fig. 1.5) described the operation while in Baltimore at Johns Hopkins [3] and then became chief of surgery at Mount Sinai in the 1950s. He did a few of these operations while at Mount Sinai. They were straight pull throughs without a reservoir or a protective ileostomy. After 3 years at Mount Sinai, Dr. Ravitch returned to Baltimore and for over 20 years this operation was no longer done at Mount Sinai for ulcerative colitis. In 1975, I was the third-year resident rotating through pediatric surgery when Dr. A. Robert Beck, a pediatric surgeon, told me that he had an 11-year-old patient from Puerto Rico with Familial Adenomatous Polyposis for whom he wanted to do an ileoanal pull through. I scrubbed with him and the chief resident Dr. Robert Kulak. The patient ultimately did well and went back home [4].

After completing my residency, I was hired by Dr. Arthur Aufses to do research in Inflammatory Bowel Disease and join the colorectal service. It was the

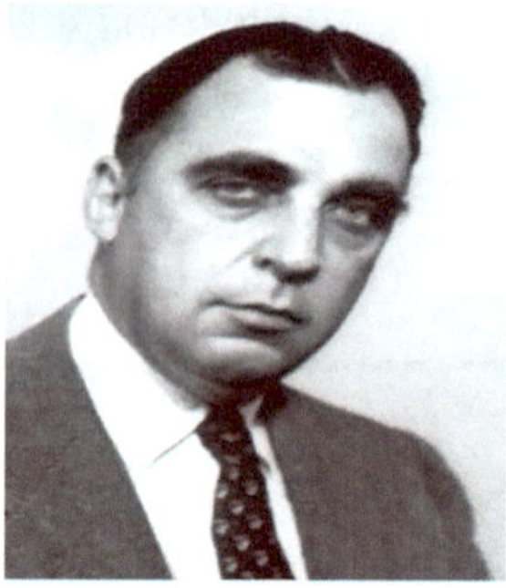

Fig. 1.5 Dr. Mark Ravitch

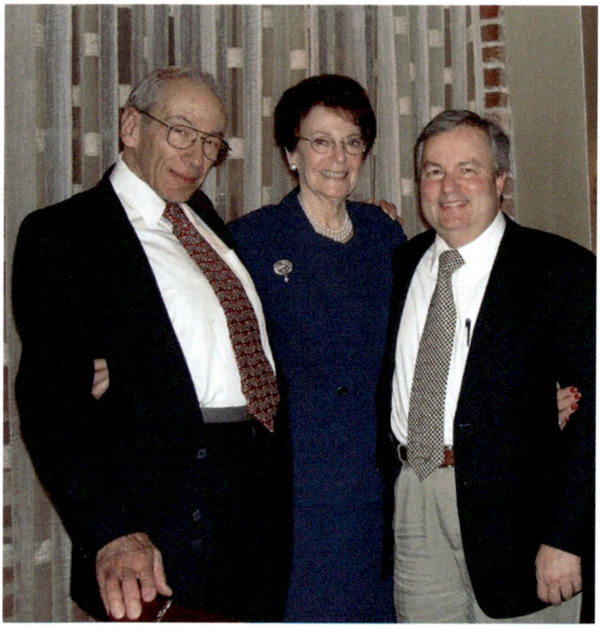

Fig. 1.6 Dr. Arthur Aufses, Mrs. Harriet Aufses, and Dr. Tomas Heimann

opportunity of a lifetime. Dr. Kurtz was also hired to stay on as a surgical attending on the colorectal service. His background in electrical engineering was invaluable for the understanding of the new surgical technology being developed for the operating room (Fig. 1.6).

In 1978, Dr. David Dreiling (Fig. 1.7) was the Associate Chair of Surgery and we told him we had a patient with ulcerative colitis who needed surgery. He recommended we do an ileoanal pull through. We did that case in two teams with Dr. Adrian Greenstein, a junior attending surgeon at that time. Later Dr. Utsunomya [5] described the J-pouch and temporary ileostomies were added making recovery from this operation less difficult. For the next several years, from the late 1970s to the early 1980s, Dr. Kurtz, Dr. Greenstein, and I performed the early ileoanal pull through operations at Mount Sinai [6]. These operations required two teams working simultaneously with a high complexity level (Fig. 1.8).

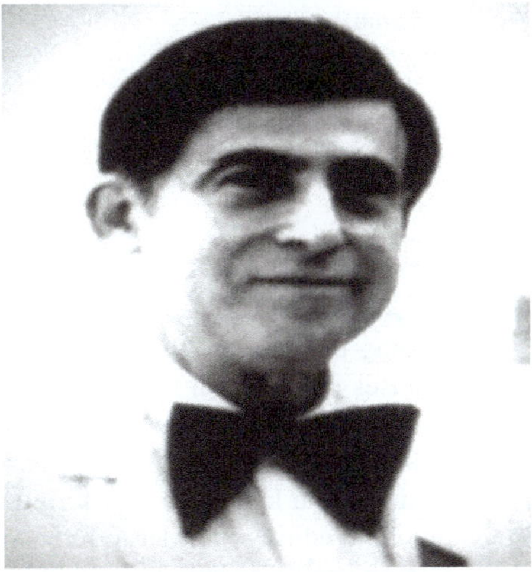

Fig. 1.7 Dr. David Dreiling

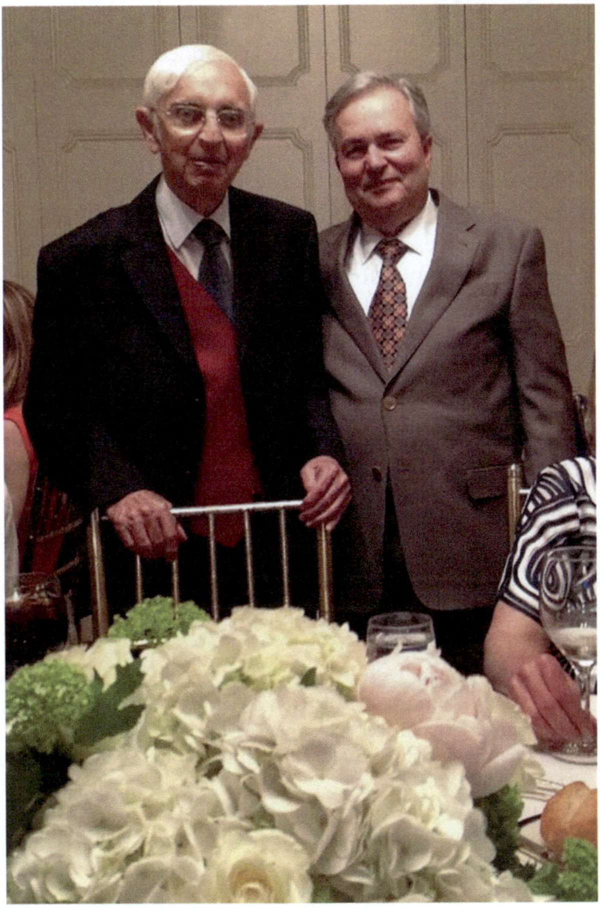

Fig. 1.8 Dr. Adrian Greenstein and Dr. Tomas Heimann

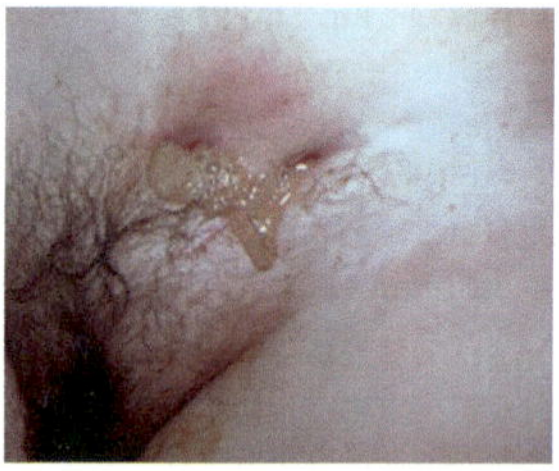

Fig. 1.9 Fistulizing Crohn's disease

Regarding the cases in this Atlas, they are a collection of Inflammatory Bowel Disease cases operated on by the authors. The photographs of the resected specimens were taken in the operating room at the completion of the case with a Lester Dyne camera with special close-up lenses and flash deflector. The pictures were then digitized on a DVD and transferred to the Atlas. The background was cleaned up using photo editing in order to remove stains and blood. The image of the surgical specimen itself was only minimally edited.

Regarding the description of the cases, we placed most emphasis on the surgical aspect of the patients and tried to add follow-up data when available. The medical treatment of Crohn's disease and ulcerative colitis continues to evolve, and we removed specific references to medical treatment, other than steroids and cyclosporine, since we felt that it would not be helpful to add therapy that has evolved over the years.

Inflammatory bowel disease is a fascinating, complex and interesting medical condition that is increasing in incidence throughout the globe. After nearly one century since its description at Mount Sinai, we still don't know the etiology. The fact is that there are two forms of the disease: one is the stricturing type and the other is the fistulizing type. The fistulizing disease in particular is debilitating, recurs sooner, and needs more frequent surgery (Fig. 1.9).

We asked Dr. Robert Greenstein [7] to write the foreword to this Atlas. He has studied the etiology of Crohn's disease for decades and worked in Dr. Yalow's laboratory for many years. I hope that you will enjoy reading this Atlas as much as we did putting it together.

References

1. Crohn BB, Ginzburg L, Oppenheimer GD. Regional ileitis: a pathologic and clinical entity. JAMA. 1932;99(16):1323–9.
2. Yalow RS. A probe for fine structure of biologic systems. Nobel Lecture, 8 December, 1977 Veterans Administration Hospital, Bronx, New York, NY and The Mount Sinai School of Medicine, City University of New York, New York, NY.
3. Ravitch MM, Sabiston DC Jr. Anal ileostomy with preservation of the sphincter. Surg Gynec Obst. 1947;84:1095–9.
4. Heimann T, Beck AR, Greenstein AJ. Familial polyposis coli: management by total colectomy with preservation of continence. Arch Surg. 1978;113(1104):1106.

5. Utsunomiya J, Iwama T, Imajo M, et al. Total colectomy, mucosal proctectomy, and ileonal anastomosis. Dis Colon Rectum. 1980;23:459–66.
6. Heimann T, Gelernt I, Bauer J, Salky B, Bleicher M, Beck AR, Kreel I. Mucosal proctectomy without reservoir. Am J Surg. 1983;145(674):677.
7. Greenstein RJ. Is Crohn's disease caused by a mycobacterium? Comparisons with leprosy, tuberculosis, and Johne's disease. Lancet Infect Dis. 2003;3:507–14.

Jejunoileitis

2

Tomas M. Heimann and Robert J. Kurtz

Patients with jejunoileitis comprise about 40% of the population with Crohn's disease. Resection is indicated for those with intestinal obstruction, fistula, and abscess. Patients with extensive disease and symptoms of obstruction may benefit from strictureplasty in order to avoid multiple resections of long segments of intestine, which may produce short bowel syndrome. The results of strictureplasty are equivalent to those of intestinal resection as far as potential for recurrence of symptoms. Very rarely the cause of the problem may be a small bowel adenocarcinoma. These tumors may be difficult to identify and biopsy of the stricture should be sent routinely for histologic examination. All patients with jejunoileitis requiring surgery are given prophylactic medication following surgery in order to suppress the recurrence potential of Crohn's disease.

Patients with jejunoileitis and fistula often present with entero-enteric or mesenteric fistulas. The most common entero-enteric fistulas are ileocolic, usually to the cecum or ascending colon, and may be asymptomatic. Another common location is ileosigmoid fistula. The colon is not always diseased at the site of these fistulas, and often a limited resection or even repair of the fistula is possible with resection of the diseased ileal segment.

Colonoscopy prior to surgery is the best diagnostic test to determine the extent of colonic disease. Mesenteric fistulas are also common, and these may present as a mesenteric or retroperitoneal abscess. Significant abscesses are best treated with CT-guided drainage and antibiotics followed by surgical resection of the diseased bowel several days later.

T. M. Heimann (✉) · R. J. Kurtz
Department of Surgery, Icahn School of Medicine at Mount Sinai, New York, NY, USA
e-mail: Tomas.Heimann@mountsinai.org; Robert.Kurtz@mountsinai.org

T. M. Heimann (ed.), *Atlas of Surgical Treatment of Inflammatory Bowel Disease*, https://doi.org/10.1007/978-3-031-62431-5_2

2.1 Ileitis, Obstruction, and Mesenteric Phlegmon

Clinical Presentation A 24-year-old male with long-standing history of Crohn's disease who presents with partial intestinal obstruction and severe right lower quadrant pain and tenderness.

Diagnostic Studies CT scan showed a phlegmon in the right lower quadrant with disease in the terminal ileum and proximal dilatation. Preoperative colonoscopy showed a normal colon (see Fig. 2.1b, c).

Surgical Treatment He was initially treated with nasogastric suction and intravenous antibiotics. He subsequently underwent an ileocolic resection with ileo ascending anastomosis (see Fig. 2.1a).

Pathology Active ileitis with ulcerations, stricture, and chronic serositis. Epithelioid granulomas were present. Multiple penetrating sinus tracts were seen. The margins of resection and colon were normal.

Follow-Up The patient did well and was discharged on the seventh postoperative day. He is well 1 year later.

Comment This patient had a fairly long segment of ileitis almost 30 cm in length with a surrounding phlegmon and an early enterocutaneous fistula. Since he had extensive disease at an early age and signs of both obstruction and perforation, he is at high risk for early recurrence and multiple reoperations. This case illustrates the fact that not all patients can easily be divided into perforating or obstructing disease categories, and some patients have features of both (Fig. 2.1).

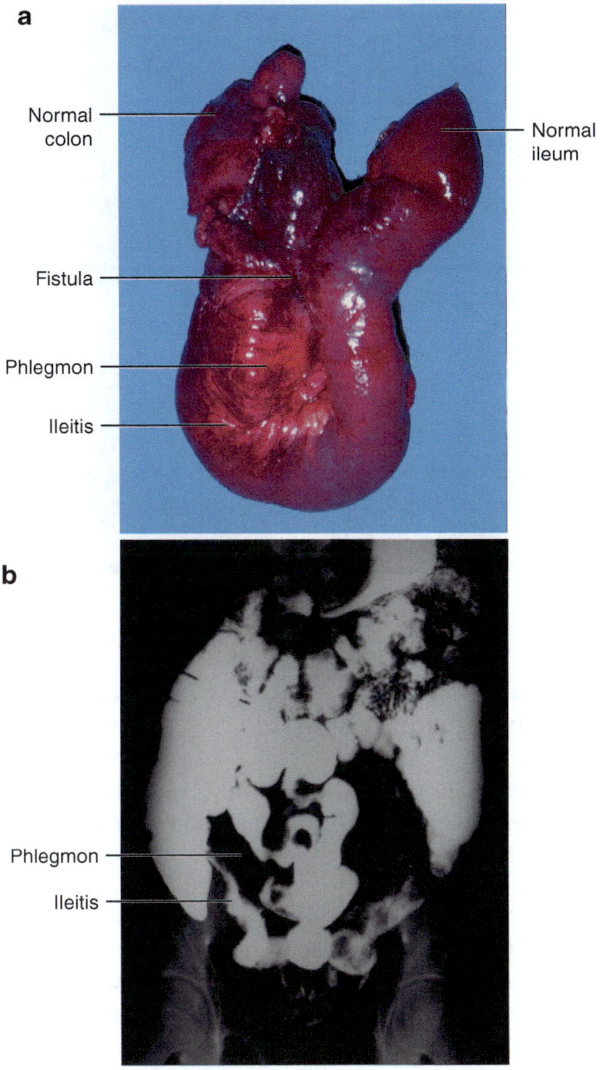

Fig. 2.1 Ileitis, obstruction, and mesenteric phlegmon

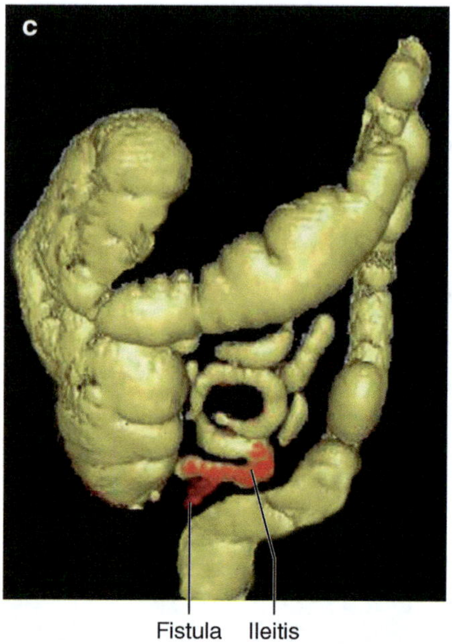

Fig. 2.1 (continued)

2.2 Ileitis with Ileosigmoid Fistula

Clinical Presentation A 26-year-old male with Crohn's disease for 14 years with previous history of perianal fistulas. He now comes in with 20 lb weight loss, recurrent abdominal pain, and fever.

Diagnostic Studies CT scan of the abdomen showed a mass in the right lower quadrant with dilatation of the right ureter. Small bowel series showed a diseased terminal ileum, adherent to the sigmoid colon. Colonoscopy showed that the sigmoid colon was normal except for localized secondary inflammation at the fistula site. The rest of the colon was unremarkable (see Fig. 2.2b-d).

Surgical Treatment This patient was treated with intravenous antibiotics and parenteral nutrition for 1 week and subsequently underwent ileocolic resection with closure of ileosigmoid fistula. No abscess was found, although there was extensive inflammation surrounding the diseased ileum, which also involved the right ureter (see Fig. 2.2a).

Pathology Active Crohn's ileitis with transmural inflammation and severe serositis. Epithelioid granulomas are present. Proximal margin of resection and colon are normal.

Follow-Up Postoperative recovery was uneventful. He was placed on mesalamine following surgery and is doing well 4 years later.

Comment This patient developed weight loss due to the extensive narrowing of the diseased terminal ileum. The fistula from the ileum to normal colon requires ileocolic resection, while the opening in the colon without evidence of Crohn's colitis can be treated with primary closure. It is important to have a preoperative colonoscopy to evaluate the colon, since intraoperative examination of the serosal surface is unreliable. Dilatation of the right ureter is frequently seen with ileitis and usually resolves after ileocolic resection. Early onset of disease as in this patient is usually an indication of increased severity, and early recurrence potential therefore postoperative prophylaxis is imperative (Fig. 2.2).

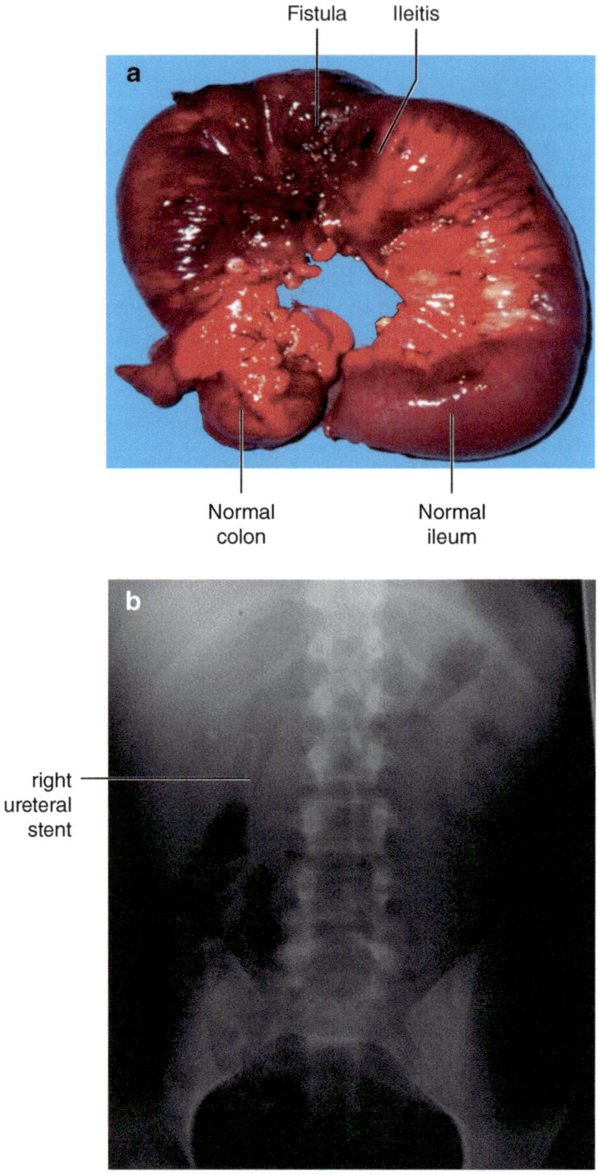

Fig. 2.2 Ileitis with ileosigmoid fistula

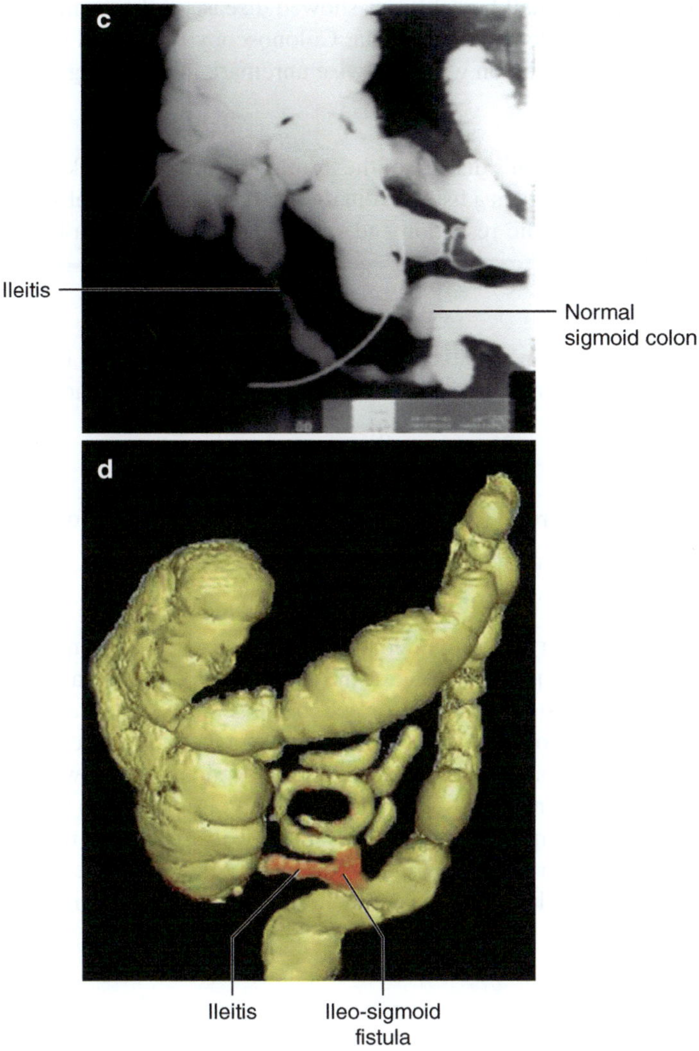

Fig. 2.2 (continued)

2.3 Ileitis with Ileosigmoid Fistula

Clinical Presentation A 30-year-old man with long-standing history of Crohn's disease. Patient comes in with severe weight loss and malnutrition due to inability to eat. He has severe colicky abdominal pain, which has not improved with medical treatment. On physical exam, there was right lower quadrant tenderness and a pelvic mass on rectal exam.

Diagnostic Studies Small bowel series showed disease in the terminal ileum with severe narrowing and ileosigmoid fistula. Colonoscopy confirmed the presence of the sigmoid fistula. The colon was otherwise unremarkable (see Fig. 2.3b, c).

Surgical Findings Crohn's disease of the terminal ileum with marked stricture and proximal dilatation. There is a fistula from diseased ileum to normal sigmoid colon. He underwent an ileocolic resection and sigmoid resection with a loop ileostomy (see Fig. 2.3a).

Pathology Active Crohn's ileitis with inflammatory stricture and ileosigmoid fistula. The sigmoid colon is free of intrinsic disease. The ileal margin and cecum are normal.

Follow-Up He recovered well following surgery; the loop ileostomy was closed 3 months later after his weight returned to normal.

Comment This patient had a significant degree of malnutrition from the severity of Crohn's disease. He required 1 week of intravenous hyperalimentation before surgery, and the loop ileostomy was performed, because of the risk that in his precarious nutritional condition, the anastomosis may not heal. Had he been in better physical condition, a double resection would have been performed without the need to defunctionalize the anastomosis. Fistulas from diseased ileum to normal sigmoid colon are relatively common and usually respond well to surgical resection. Small fistulas to normal colon may sometimes require only ileocolic resection with excision of the fistula and closure of the defect in the sigmoid colon (Fig. 2.3).

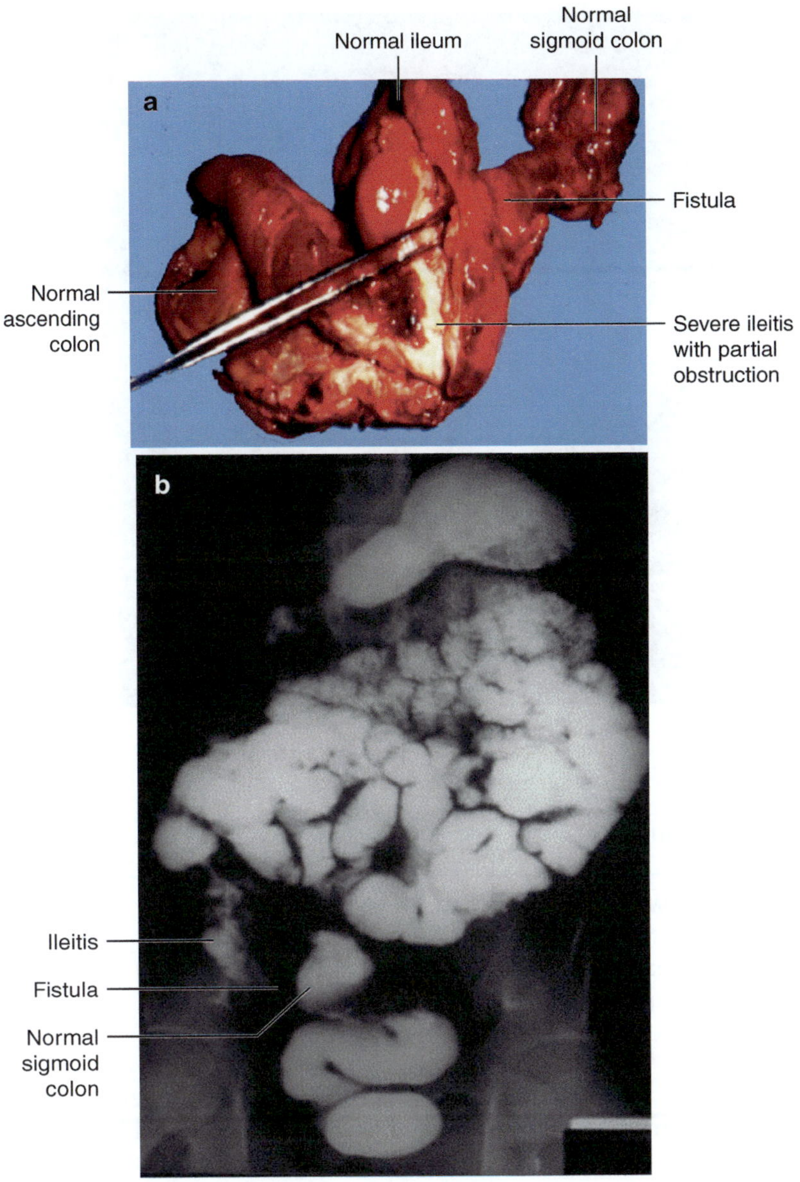

Fig. 2.3 Ileitis with ileosigmoid fistula

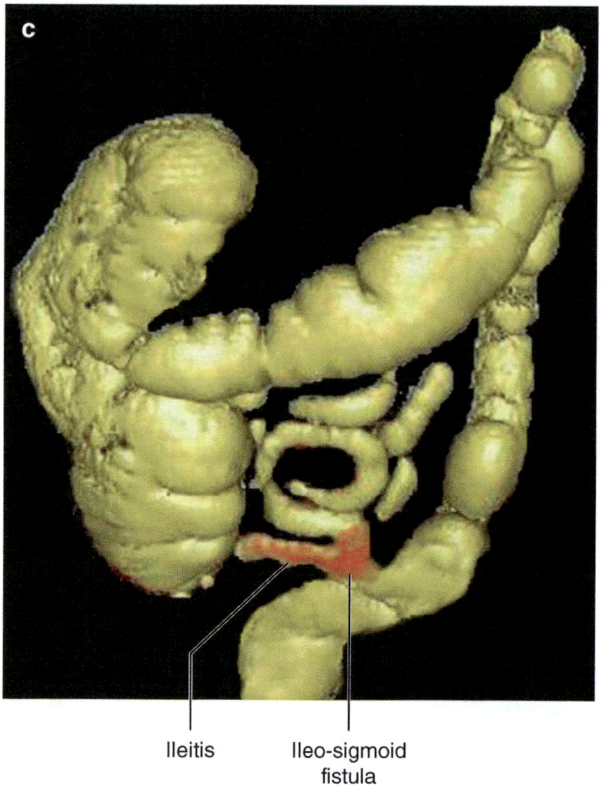

Fig. 2.3 (continued)

2.4 Ileitis with Abscess and Ileocolic Fistula

History A 37-year-old woman with Crohn's disease present for 1 year. She developed right lower quadrant pain and fever 3 weeks ago.

Clinical Course After admission, she was treated with intravenous antibiotics without improvement. A CT scan showed an abscess in the right lower quadrant, which was drained under CT guidance. Following drainage, the patient remained on intravenous antibiotics and improved. Cultures grew *E. coli*. One week later, she underwent laparotomy (see Fig. 2.4c, d).

Surgical Findings At surgery, 20 cm of terminal ileum was inflamed with a fistula to the transverse colon. A small residual abscess was present behind the ascending colon extending into the psoas muscle. A right hemicolectomy was performed with ileotransverse anastomosis (see Fig. 2.4a, b).

Pathology Crohn's ileitis with fistula secondarily involving the transverse colon. Epithelioid granulomas are present. The margins appear normal, but there is mild mucosal inflammation at the proximal margin.

Follow-Up This patient had an uneventful recovery following surgery.

Comment Preliminary abscess drainage under CT guidance and treatment with antibiotics may convert a complicated contaminated operation into a simpler procedure with minimal or no contamination. This patient had a fistula from the diseased ileum to the psoas muscle and another to the right transverse colon, which was intrinsically normal. Both were resected and the anastomosis was performed to normal colon. The presence of mild microscopic inflammation at the proximal margin has been shown to have no correlation with timing of recurrence of symptoms. This patient has remained asymptomatic on medical prophylactic therapy (Fig. 2.4).

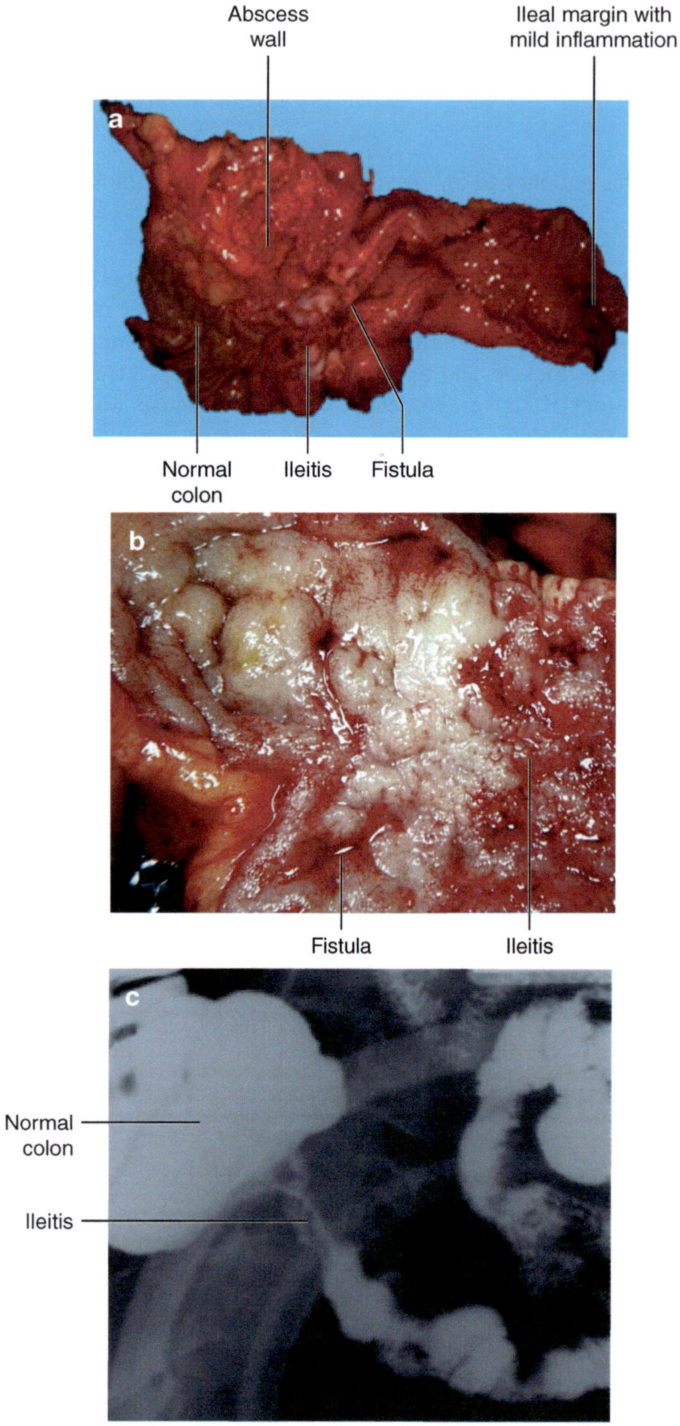

Fig. 2.4 Ileitis with abscess and ileocolic fistula

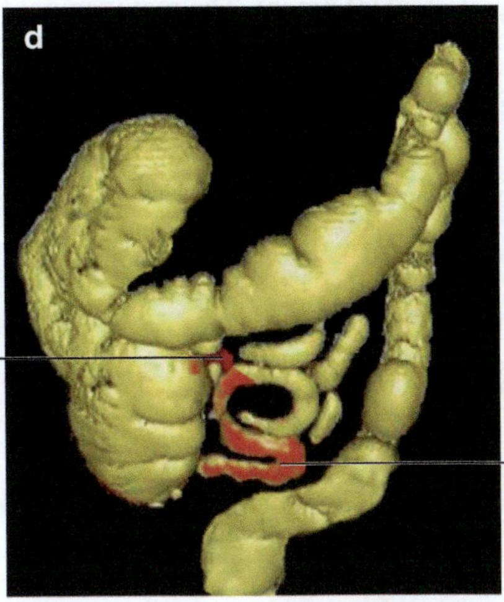

Fig. 2.4 (continued)

2.5 Ileitis with Ileocolic Fistula

Clinical Presentation A 32-year-old woman with a long-standing history of Crohn's disease. She developed a rectovaginal fistula after a vaginal delivery of her first child 4 years ago. She now comes in with severe abdominal pain and fever shortly after a premature delivery of her second child.

Diagnostic Studies Physical exam showed abdominal distention consistent with intestinal obstruction. Obstructive series showed small bowel distention, and she failed to improve with nasogastric suction (see Fig. 2.5b, d).

Surgical Treatment At surgery, she was found to have severe Crohn's disease of the terminal ileum and adhesive intestinal obstruction at a site just proximal to the involved ileum. She was treated with a Brooke ileostomy. Four months later, she underwent an ileocolic resection with ileotransverse anastomosis (see Fig. 2.5a).

Pathology Crohn's ileitis with ileocolic fistula. No granulomas are present. The colon and proximal margin are normal.

Follow-Up This patient recovered well after both operations. She is doing well 3 years after the second procedure. The rectovaginal fistula was repaired at the time of her second delivery and remains healed (see Fig. 2.5c).

Comment This patient shows some of the problems associated with pregnancy with Crohn's disease. She developed a rectovaginal fistula after perineal trauma from the first delivery. The second pregnancy was complicated by an early delivery precipitated by exacerbation of her Crohn's disease resulting in intestinal obstruction requiring surgical treatment. The rectovaginal fistula was repaired at the second delivery and remains healed. She is well but has occasional episodes of incontinence due to sphincteric damage demonstrated in the endorectal ultrasound study (see Fig. 2.5d).

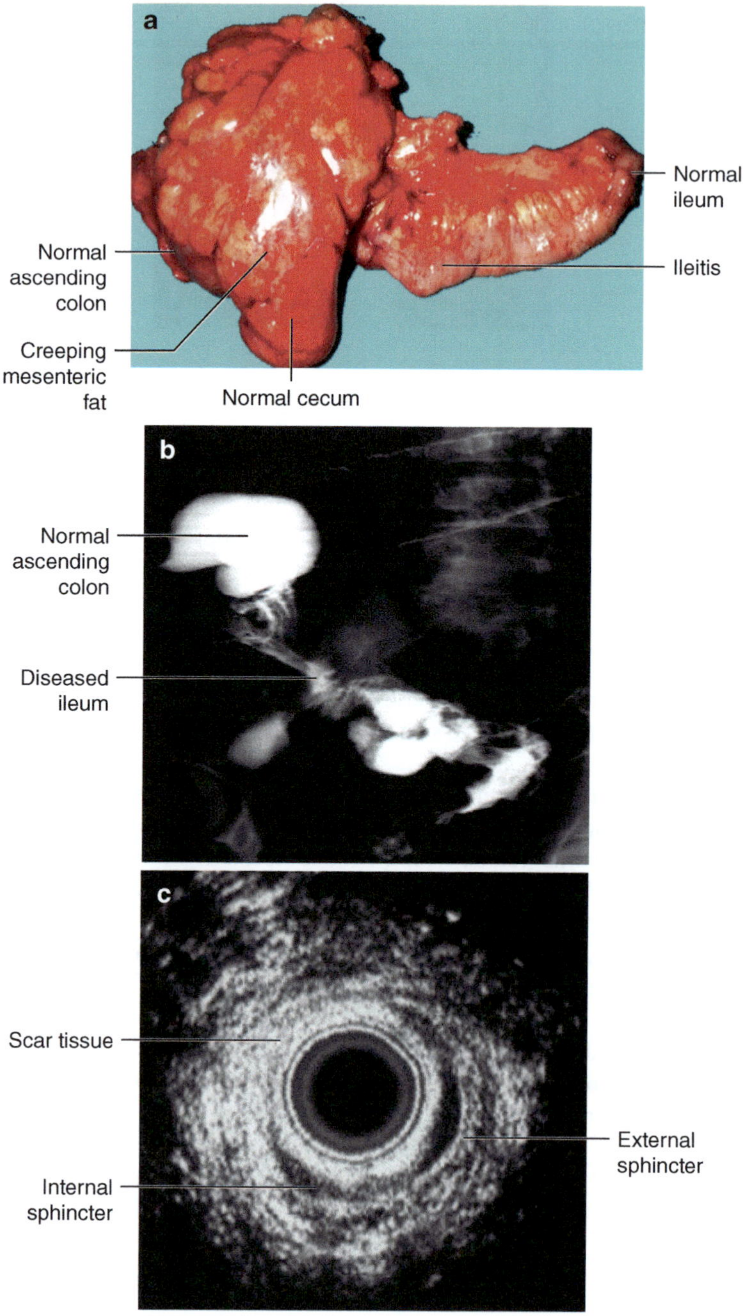

Fig. 2.5 Ileitis with ileocolic fistula

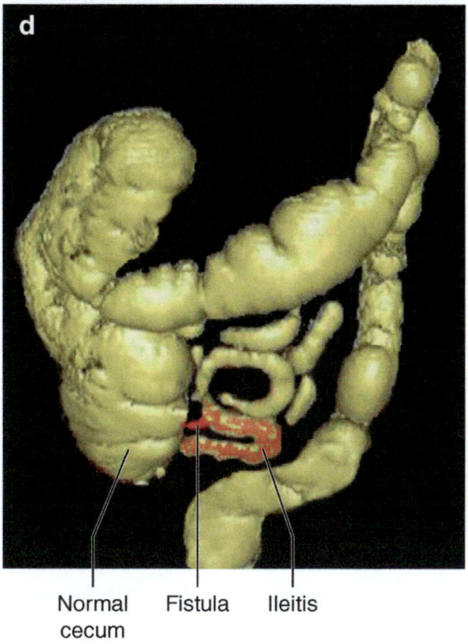

Fig. 2.5 (continued)

2.6 Ileitis with Retroperitoneal Abscess

Clinical Presentation A 23-year-old woman with Crohn's disease for 5 years presenting initially with an abscess in the right lower quadrant which was treated with drainage and a loop ileostomy.

Diagnostic Studies Colonoscopy revealed a normal colon; CT scan of the abdomen and pelvis showed some residual collection in the right lower quadrant and thickened terminal ileum consistent with Crohn's disease (see Fig. 2.6c, d).

Surgical Findings She had a chronic draining sinus in the right lower quadrant and a small residual abscess in the psoas muscle. The terminal ileum showed severe inflammation with a stricture. She underwent an ileocolic resection with drainage of the abscess and ileostomy (see Fig. 2.6a, b).

Pathology Ileitis with inflammatory stricture and ileocecal fistula. The colon is normal. No granulomas are seen.

Follow-Up She recovered well following resection but required readmission 1 month later for percutaneous drainage of a recurrent abscess in the right lower quadrant. She subsequently did well, and after being asymptomatic for several months, she returned for restoration of intestinal continuity with an ileocolic anastomosis.

Comment This patient presented with a retroperitoneal abscess and severe inflammation in the ileocecal area. The initial treatment of surgical drainage and loop ileostomy provided only temporary improvement. Even after ileocolic resection with second drainage of the abscess and ileostomy, she still required readmission for intravenous antibiotics and percutaneous drainage of this persistent abscess. She is finally doing well and has regained most of her weight. Since the remaining colon and small bowel is normal, she has done well following restoration of intestinal continuity (Fig. 2.6).

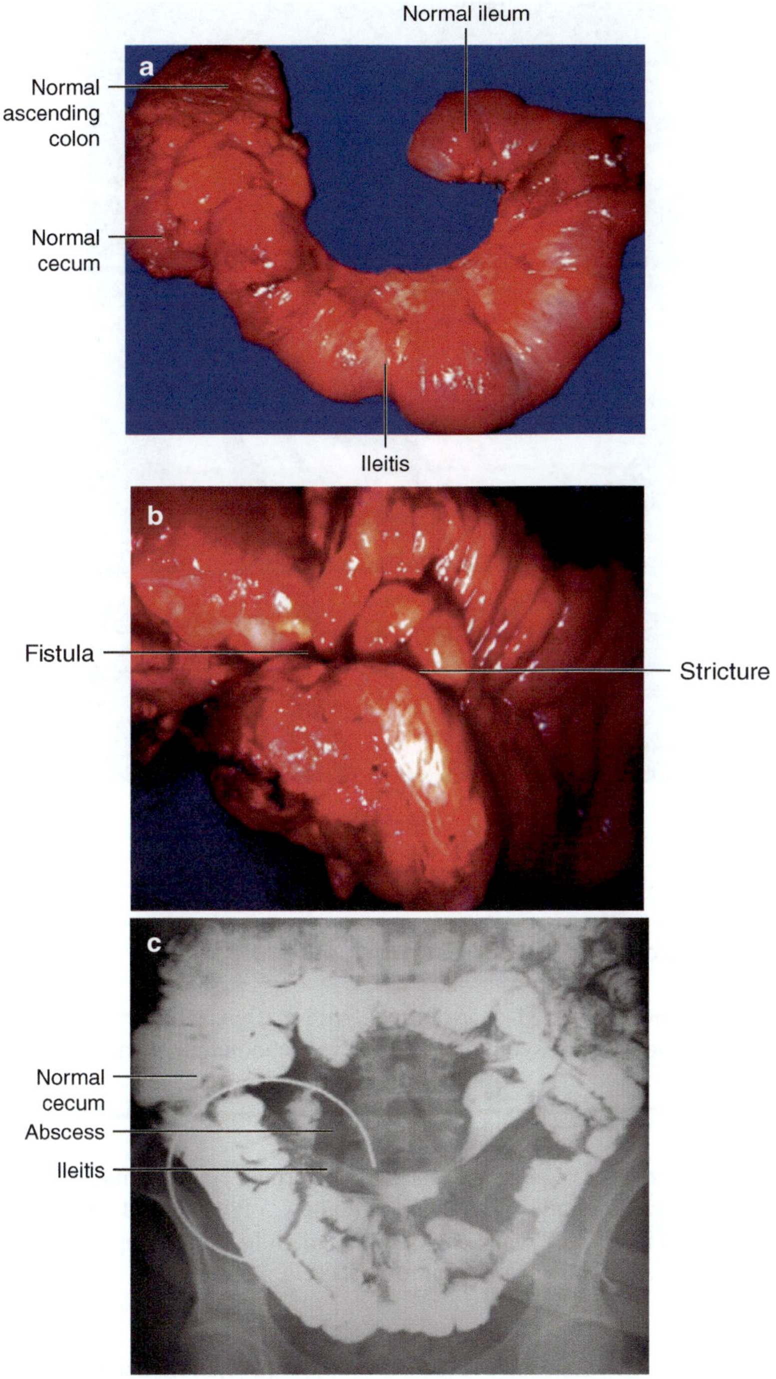

Fig. 2.6 Ileitis with retroperitoneal abscess

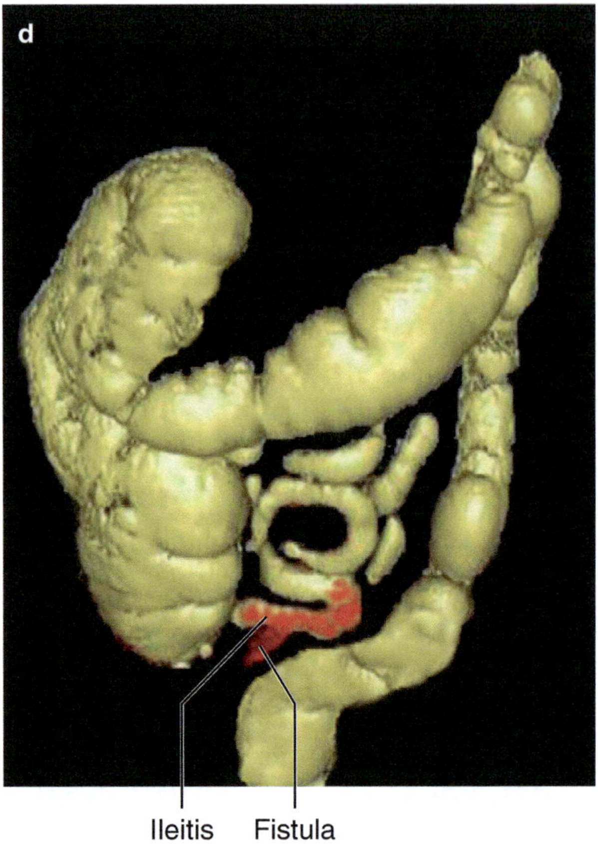

Fig. 2.6 (continued)

2.7 Jejunoileitis with Mesenteric Abscess

Clinical Presentation A 31-year-old man with a 10-year history of Crohn's disease. Recent increase in symptoms with fever, abdominal pain, distention, and weight loss.

Diagnostic Studies Colonoscopy showed a normal colon. Small bowel series revealed extensive jejunoileitis with approximately 5 ft of normal jejunum and 2 ft of normal distal ileum. CT scan showed a phlegmon in the left upper quadrant with several loops of small bowel adherent to it (see Fig. 2.7c–e).

Surgical Treatment Extensive resection of involved jejunum and ileum, drainage of mesenteric abscess, and jejunoileal anastomosis (see Fig. 2.7a, b).

Pathology Active Crohn's enteritis with transmural inflammation, penetrating sinus tracts, and mesenteric abscess. No granulomas were found, and the margins of resection are uninvolved.

Follow-Up He recovered well following surgery. He was discharged on a low residue diet with small frequent meals and intravenous hyperalimentation. After 3 months, the patient regained his weight, the intravenous hyperalimentation was discontinued, and he remains well 3 years later. He presently has about 7 ft of remaining small intestine and the entire colon is normal.

Comment This patient had extensive involvement of the small intestine. There were only 5 ft of normal jejunum and a very short segment of terminal ileum that was spared. Since this patient presented with a mesenteric abscess, an extensive resection was necessary. However, he has done extremely well. After a period of intravenous hyperalimentation, he is able to maintain his weight and has adapted well to the remaining 7 ft of small bowel. The presence of a normal colon is critical in these patients, since it decreases fluid loss and allows for better intestinal adaptation (Fig. 2.7).

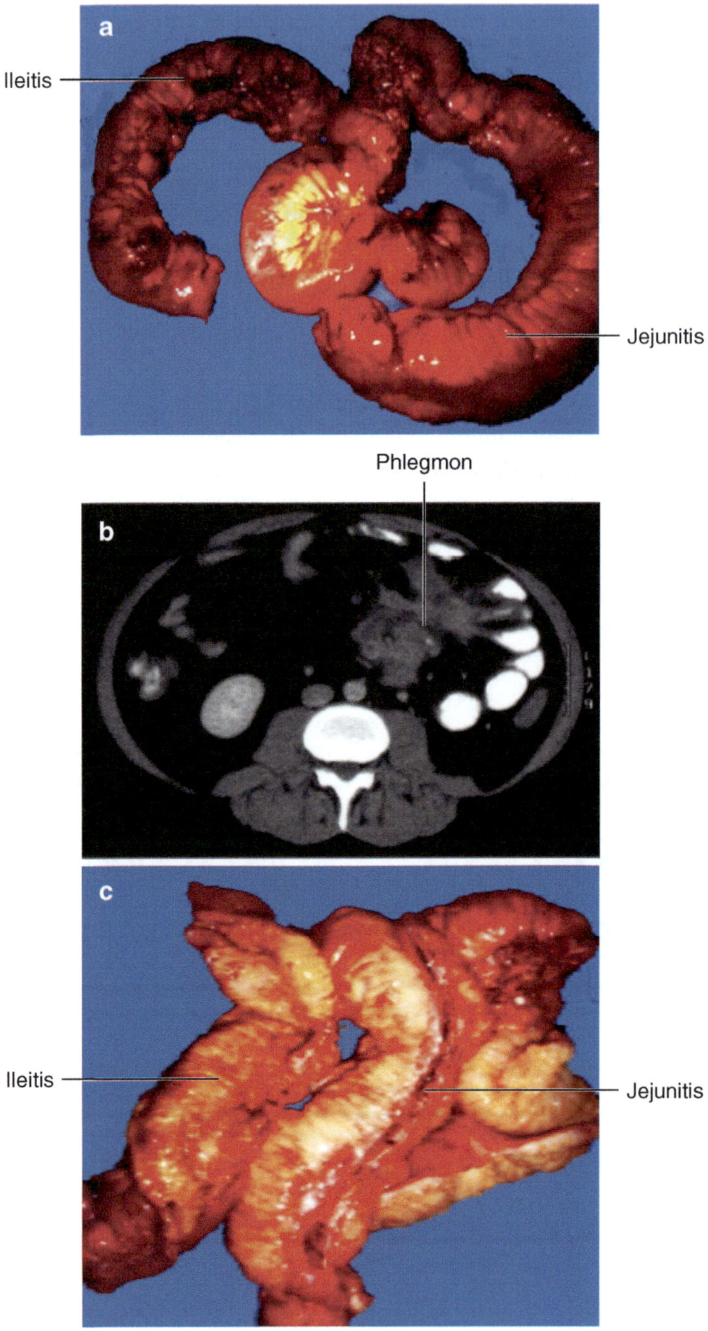

Fig. 2.7 Jejunoileitis with mesenteric abscess

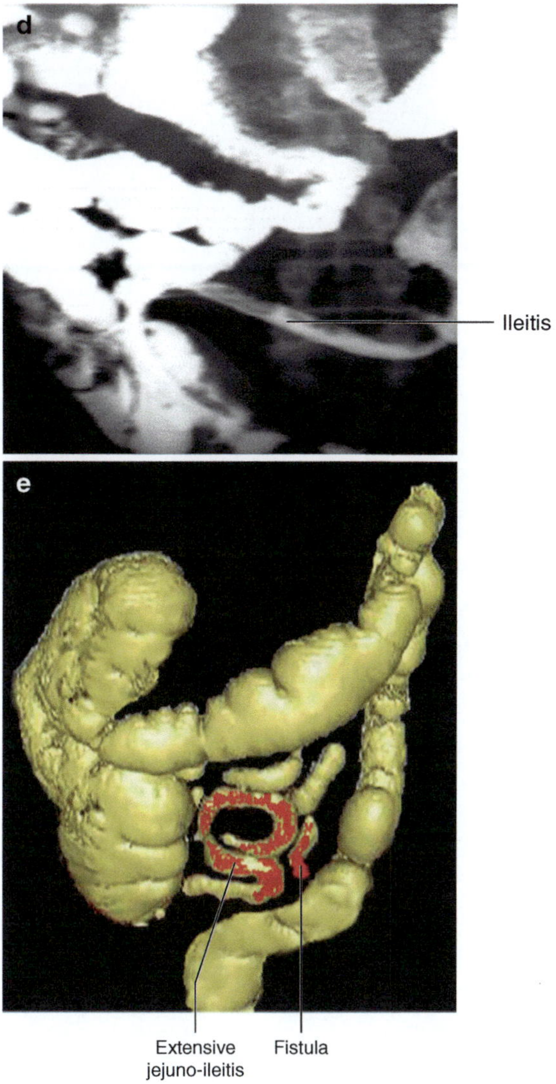

Fig. 2.7 (continued)

Further Reading

Greenstein AJ, Sachar DB, Mann D, Lachman P, Heimann TM, Aufses AH Jr. Spontaneous free perforation and perforated abscess in 30 patients with Crohn's disease. Ann Surg. 1987;205:72–6.

Heimann T, Gelernt I, Schanzer H, Sachar DB, Greenstein A, Aufses AH Jr. Surgical treatment, skin test reactivity, and lymphocytes in inflammatory bowel disease. Am J Surg. 1983;145:199–201.

3 Jejunoileitis with Obstruction

Tomas M. Heimann and Robert J. Kurtz

Obstruction is a common feature of Crohn's disease. Although the most common location is found in the terminal ileum, it can also occur more proximally as seen in several of the patients being presented. It is also frequently seen in association with fistulas usually from the diseased small bowel to the mesentery or another loop of small or large bowel. The division of Crohn's disease into obstructive versus fistulizing disease is somewhat arbitrary and is based mostly on the predominant symptom. Treatment of obstructive symptoms is usually by resection; although in cases with extensive disease or multiple previous resections, strictureplasty is a good alternative since it allows for bowel preservation.

3.1 Ileitis with Obstruction

Clinical Presentation A 69-year-old woman with 10-year history of Crohn's disease now presenting with recurrent cramps, abdominal distention, and 12 lb weight loss.

Diagnostic Studies Small bowel series showed severe narrowing of the terminal ileum and marked proximal dilatation. Colonoscopy 2 years ago showed a normal colon (see Fig. 3.1c, d, e).

Surgical Treatment This patient underwent an ileocolic resection with removal of 60 cm of diseased terminal ileum. Several loops of distal ileum were adherent and severely inflamed with marked narrowing of the lumen (see Fig. 3.1a, b).

Pathology Crohn's ileitis with mucosal ulcerations and transmural chronic inflammation with severe stricture. No granulomas are seen. The colon and margins of resection are normal.

T. M. Heimann (✉) · R. J. Kurtz
Department of Surgery, Icahn School of Medicine at Mount Sinai, New York, NY, USA
e-mail: Tomas.Heimann@mountsinai.org; Robert.Kurtz@mountsinai.org

T. M. Heimann (ed.), *Atlas of Surgical Treatment of Inflammatory Bowel Disease*, https://doi.org/10.1007/978-3-031-62431-5_3

Follow-Up She had an uneventful recovery after surgery and was discharged after 7 days. One year after surgery, she has gained her weight back but still has frequent loose bowel movements.

Comment This patient had chronic intestinal obstruction with massive proximal small bowel dilatation. These findings are often seen in patients with Crohn's disease with long-standing obstructive symptoms. Initially, patients with chronic obstruction are able to compensate by changing their dietary habits to low residue or semi-liquid diet and smaller meals. Eventually as the stricture progresses, their nutritional status deteriorates and surgery becomes unavoidable. Following resection of the stricture, the small bowel diameter gradually returns to normal and the weight of the patient also eventually improves (Fig. 3.1).

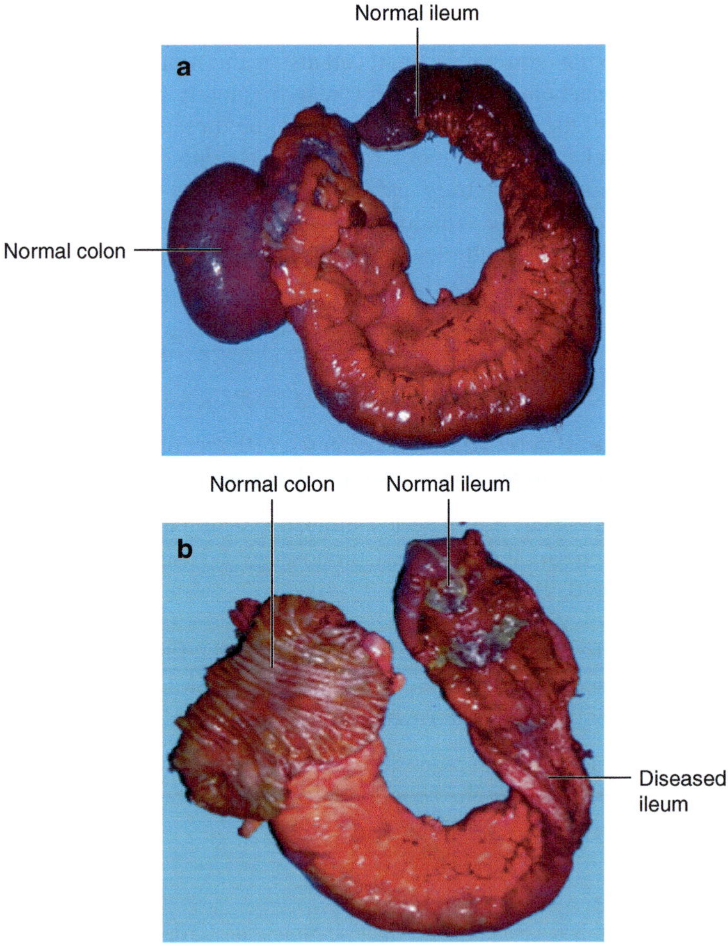

Fig. 3.1 (**a**–**e**) Ileitis with obstruction

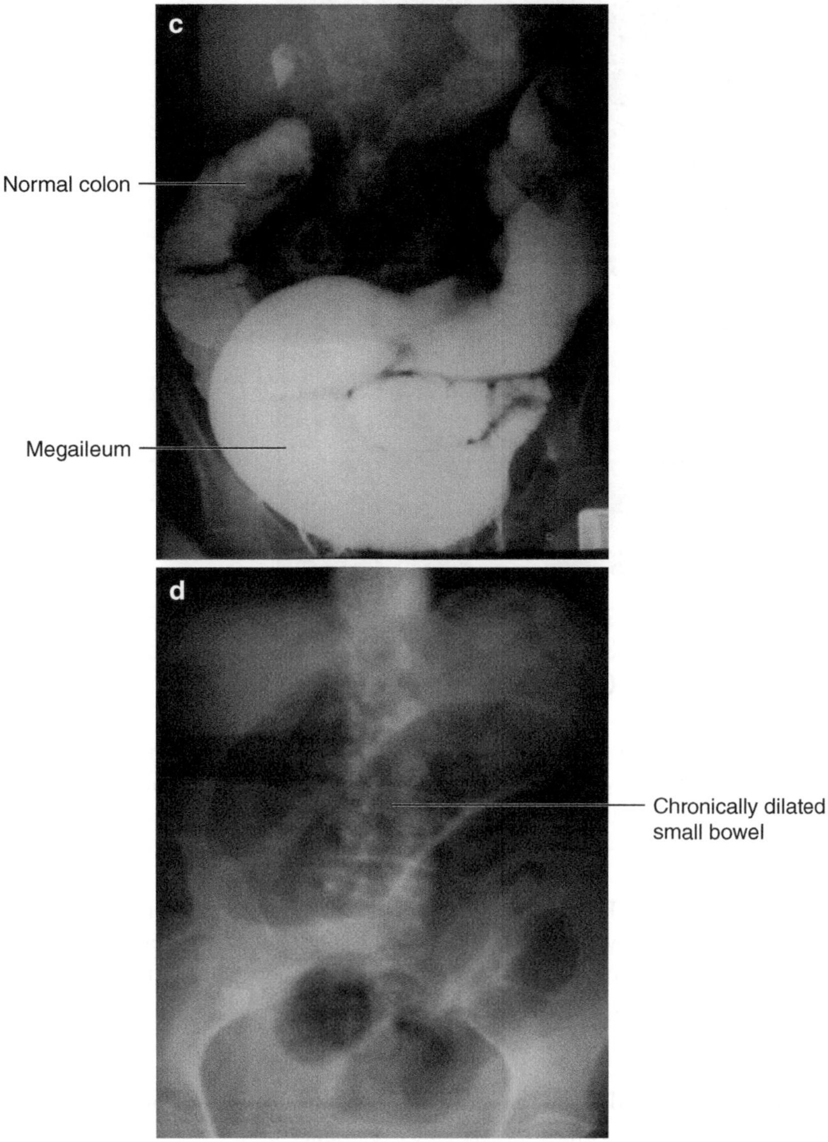

Fig. 3.1 (continued)

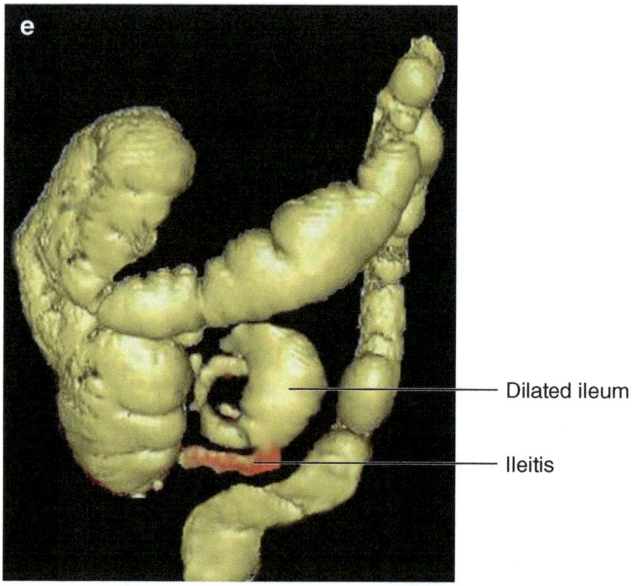

Fig. 3.1 (continued)

3.2 Ileitis with Obstruction and Fistula

Clinical Presentation A 57-year-old woman with Crohn's disease for 35 years. Patient now comes in with increasing symptoms of obstruction manifested by colicky abdominal pain, abdominal distention, and weight loss.

Diagnostic Studies On physical exam, her abdomen is moderately distended. Small bowel series shows severely dilated small bowel with a stricture in the terminal ileum and an ileocolic fistula from the diseased ileum to the transverse colon. The colon is normal on colonoscopy (see Fig. 3.2c, d).

Surgical Treatment Ileocolic resection with removal of the cecum and ascending colon and ileotransverse anastomosis (see Fig. 3.2a, b).

Pathology Active Crohn's ileitis with transmural chronic inflammation, inflammatory stricture, and ileocolic fistula. There are no granulomas. The proximal margin and colonic segment are uninvolved.

Follow-Up She had an uneventful recovery and is doing well 3 years later.

Comment This is an example of chronic Crohn's disease with gradual progression of symptoms. The chronic obstructive process allows for massive small bowel dilatation with minimal symptoms. Eventually the stricture becomes nearly pinpoint in diameter and surgical treatment becomes necessary. Occasionally acute obstruction is precipitated by the formation of fecaliths or ingestion of non-digestible pits or vegetable fiber. Following surgery, the diameter of the bowel eventually returns to normal. Patients with long-standing history of Crohn's disease before requiring surgery are more likely to have a long asymptomatic period after surgery (Fig. 3.2).

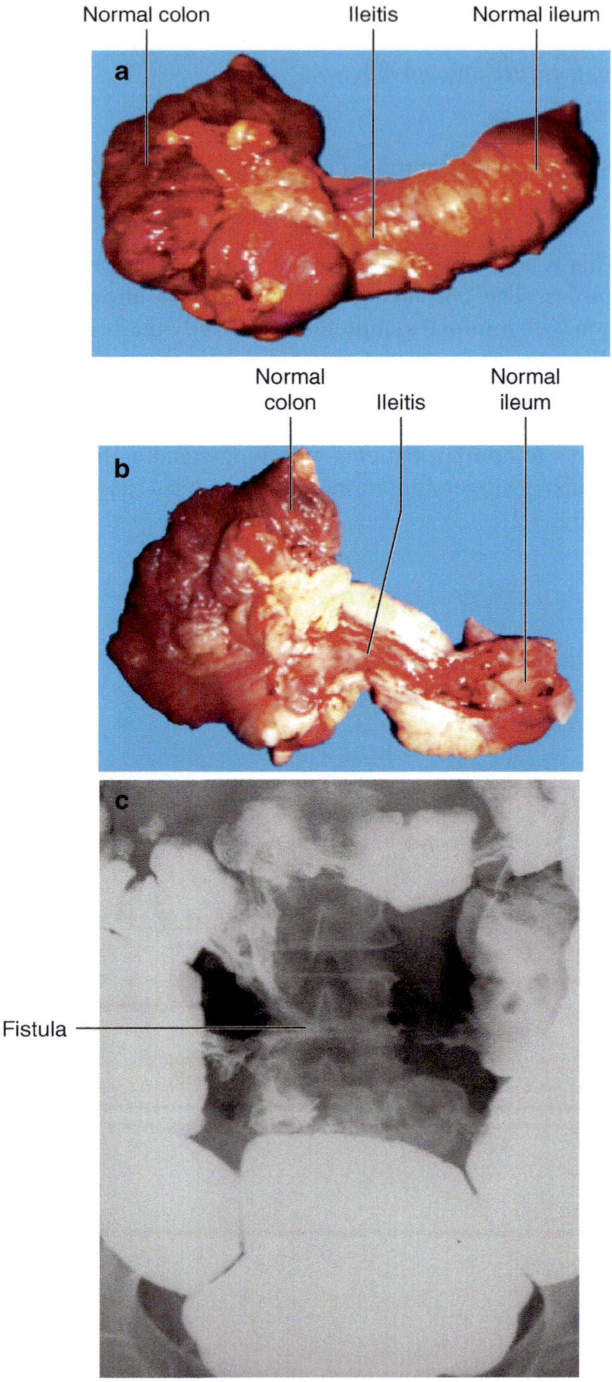

Fig. 3.2 (**a**–**d**) Ileitis with obstruction and fistula

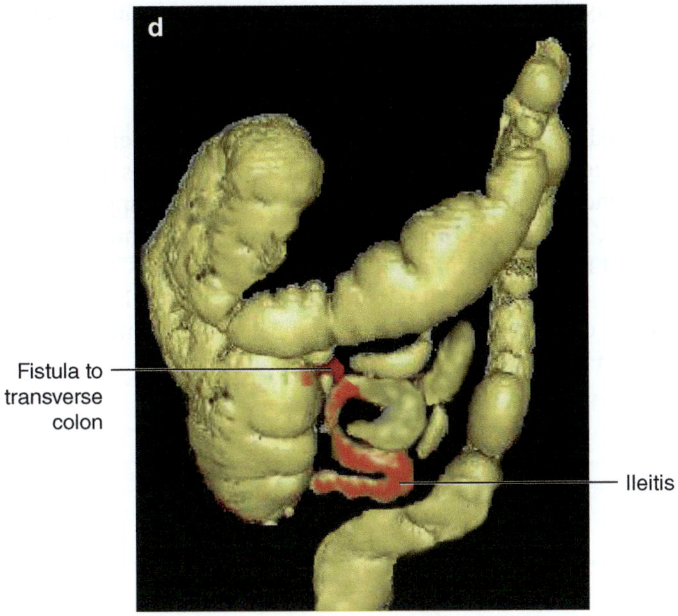

Fig. 3.2 (continued)

3.3 Ileitis with Bleeding and Stricture

Clinical Presentation A 48-year-old woman with Crohn's ileitis and rectovaginal fistula who presented with severe anemia due to chronic intestinal bleeding.

Diagnostic Studies Colonoscopy showed a normal colon with a large rectovaginal fistula. Upper gastrointestinal endoscopy was unremarkable. The endorectal ulreasound images show damage to the sphincter muscles at the site of the rectovaginal fistula. Small bowel series showed Crohn's disease of the distal ileum (see Fig. 3.3d, e, f).

Surgical Treatment This patient underwent an ileocolic resection with Brooke ileostomy. The rectovaginal fistula was repaired 3 months later (see Fig. 3.3a, b, c).

Pathology Active Crohn's ileitis with inflammatory stricture and transmural chronic inflammation. The proximal margin and colonic segment are uninvolved.

Follow-Up She had an uneventful recovery following both operations. The hemoglobin is now stable and the fistula is healed. An endorectal sonogram before repair of the rectovaginal fistula revealed scarring of the internal and external sphincter muscles anteriorly. The ileostomy was closed 1 year later, and the patient is mostly continent with occasional seepage when having loose bowel movements.

Comment Bleeding is an uncommon presentation for patients with Crohn's disease. When it occurs, it is the result of erosion of a blood vessel in an ulcerated area usually on the mesenteric side of the bowel. Medical therapy for this problem is often ineffective, and surgical resection is necessary to remove the bleeding site. The rectovaginal fistula is common in women with perianal Crohn's disease. When there is a solitary fistula, surgical repair may be successful. In patients with severe perianal disease, often proctectomy with permanent ileostomy is the only solution to this problem (Fig. 3.3).

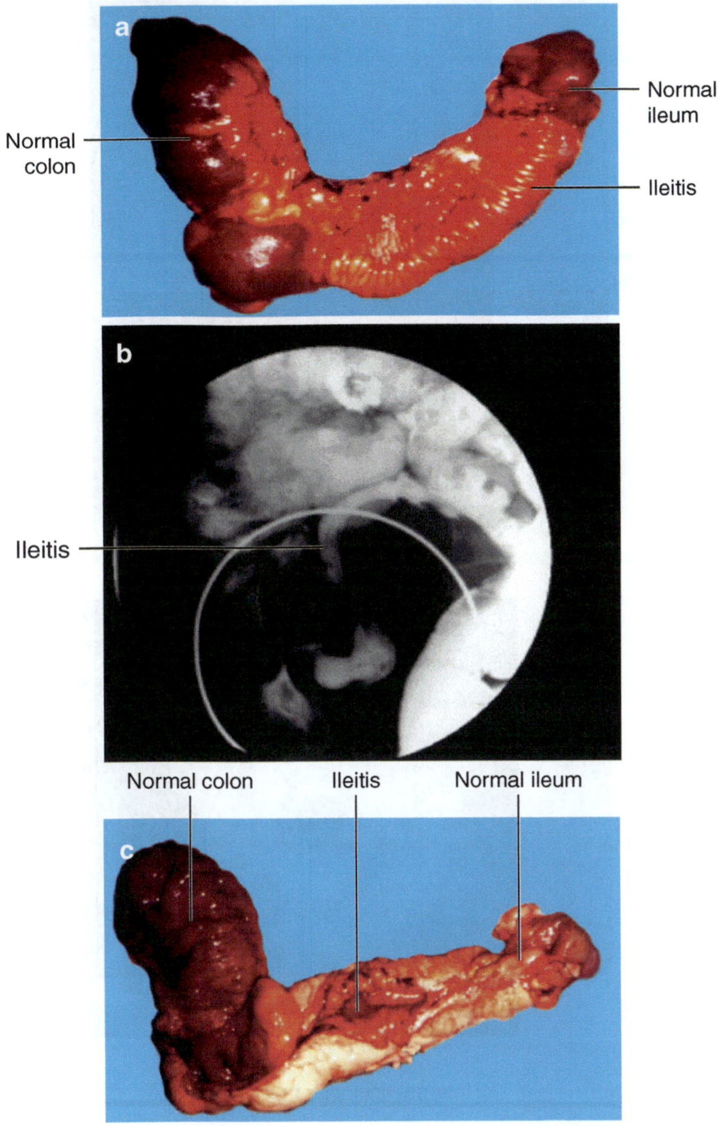

Fig. 3.3 (**a**–**e**) Ileitis with bleeding and stricture

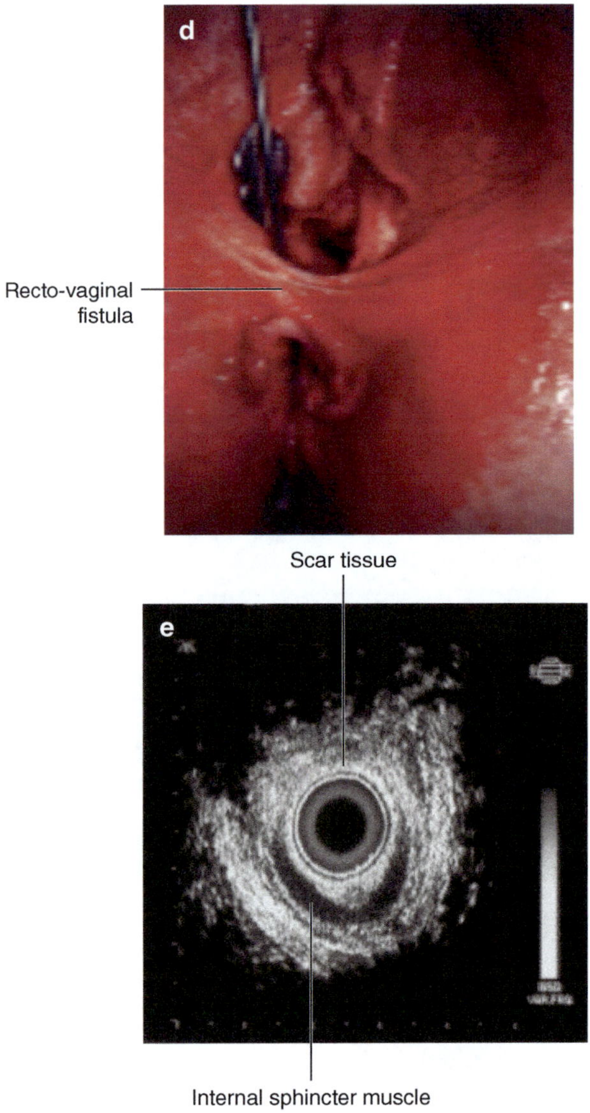

Fig. 3.3 (continued)

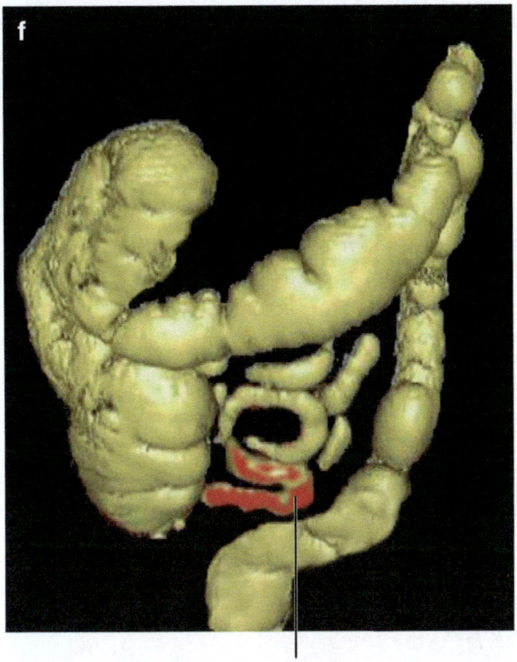

Fig. 3.3 (continued)

3.4 Ileitis, Chronic Obstruction, and Fistula

Clinical Presentation A 43-year-old woman with Crohn's disease for 22 years. She now presents with abdominal distention, bloating, colicky abdominal pain, and weight loss.

Diagnostic Studies Colonoscopy showed a normal colon. Small bowel study showed a stricture at the terminal ileum with severe proximal dilatation (see Fig. 3.4c, d, e).

Surgical Findings Severe small bowel distention starting in the distal jejunum. The terminal ileum showed a stricture with dense adhesions to the sigmoid colon consistent with an ileosigmoid fistula. She underwent an ileocolic and sigmoid resection with two end-end anastomoses (see Fig. 3.4a, b).

Pathology Crohn's ileitis with stenosis and obstructive dilatation. Ulceration and transmural inflammation are present. The sigmoid colon has focal inflammation with a fistula tract. The resection margins are normal, and no granulomas are seen.

Follow-Up She had an uneventful recovery after surgery. Return of intestinal function was slow, and she was discharged on the 14th postoperative day. The abdominal distention has gradually resolved as the small bowel diameter returned to normal. She is well 2 years later.

Comment Massive small bowel dilatation is the result of chronic intestinal obstruction. In this patient, the obstructive symptoms go back to 4 years before surgery. The diameter of the small bowel in this case was so large that 100 mm staplers were required to transect it. There is also muscular hypertrophy and edema, making the use of thick tissue staplers necessary. In some extreme cases, the serum albumin may be near 1.0 g/dL due to chronic starvation, and intravenous nutrition prior to and after surgery is advisable (Fig. 3.4).

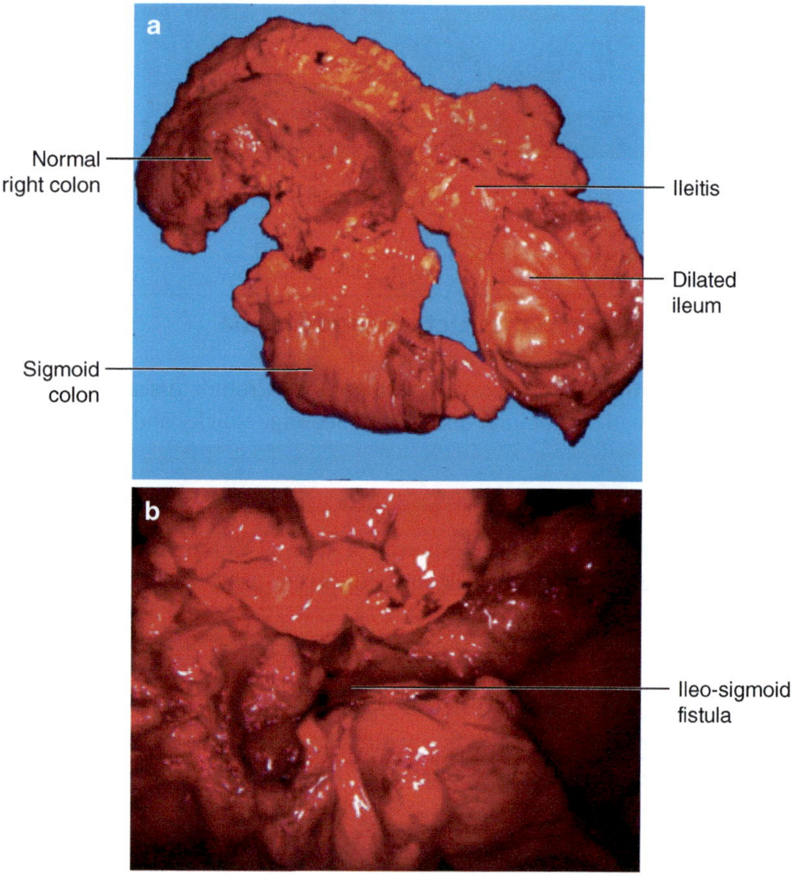

Fig. 3.4 (a–e) Ileitis with chronic obstruction and fistula

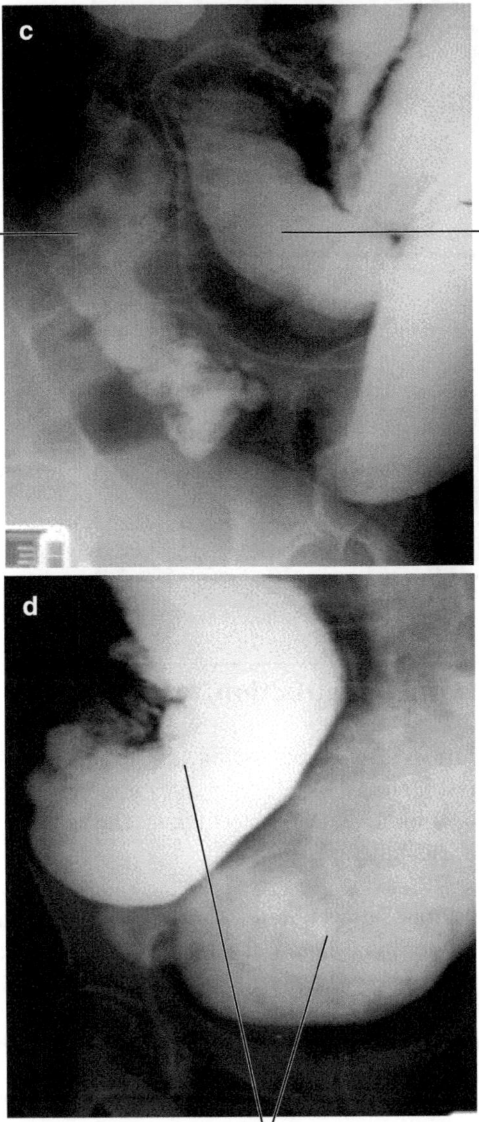

Fig. 3.4 (continued)

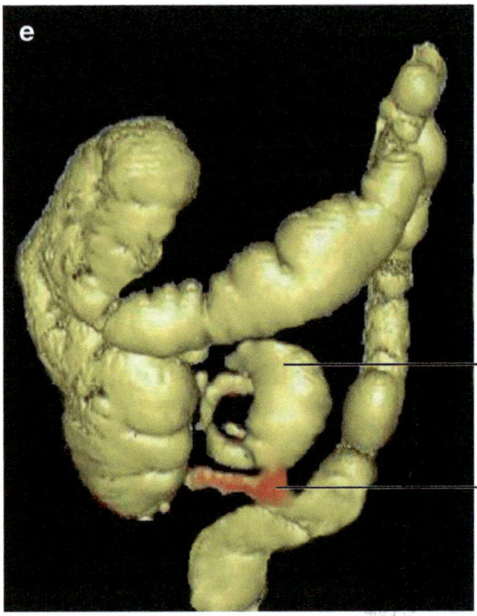

Fig. 3.4 (continued)

3.5 Ileitis, Chronic Obstruction, and Fistula

Clinical Presentation A 22-year-old male with Crohn's disease for at least 3 years who presents with symptoms of chronic intestinal obstruction. His symptoms include chronic abdominal distention, cramps, and 25 lb weight loss. He is not responding to medical therapy.

Diagnostic Studies Small bowel series showed massive dilatation of the ileum with a stricture in the terminal ileum and several short fistulas extending into the mesentery. Colonoscopy showed a normal colon (see Fig. 3.5c, d, e).

Surgical Treatment He underwent an ileocolic resection with anastomosis to the ascending colon (see Fig. 3.5a, b).

Pathology Active Crohn's ileitis with obstructive dilatation, ulcerations, inflammatory stricture, and chronic fissures. Epithelioid granulomas are present. The margins of resection and the colon are uninvolved.

Follow-Up He had an uneventful recovery following surgery. The anastomosis healed well; he has 2–4 bowel movements daily and regained his weight.

Comment This is an example of chronic intestinal obstruction resulting in massive small bowel dilatation. At this stage, medical treatment is no longer effective, and resection of the strictured segment becomes necessary. The massively dilated bowel also shows hypertrophy of the wall, making stapled anastomosis difficult to perform. The largest thick tissue staplers are required to transect the bowel safely, and the staple lines should be oversewn for extra security. Following surgery, there is gradual return of the bowel to a more normal diameter. Although earlier surgery before massive dilatation develops is safer, it is not uncommon for patients to wait until this stage due to anxiety regarding surgical treatment (Fig. 3.5).

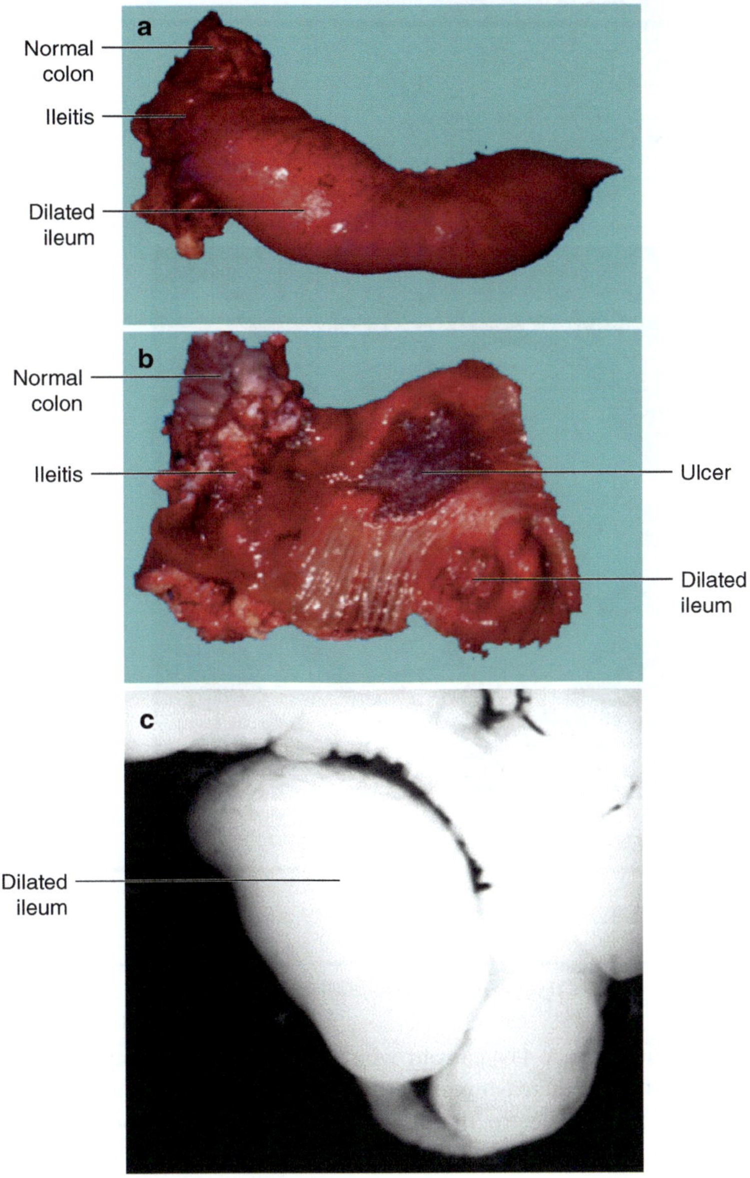

Fig. 3.5 (**a**–**e**) Ileitis with chronic obstruction and fistula

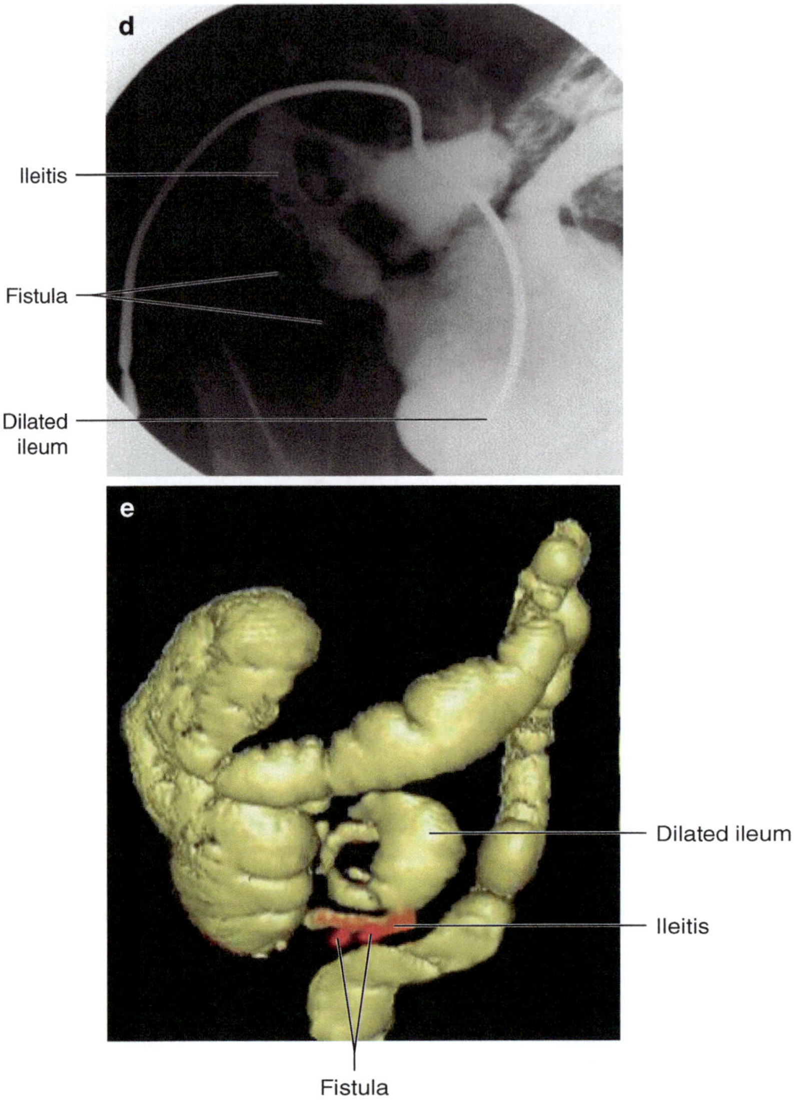

Fig. 3.5 (continued)

3.6 Ileitis with Obstruction

Clinical Presentation A 41-year-old woman with Crohn's disease for 24 years. She now presents with increasing tenderness in the right lower quadrant and a palpable mass. She also has obstructive symptoms with colicky abdominal pain, which has not improved with increased doses of steroids.

Diagnostic Studies Small bowel series showed Crohn's disease in the terminal ileum with some proximal dilatation of the small bowel. Colonoscopy was normal (see Fig. 3.6c, d, e).

Surgical Findings Disease in the terminal ileum with narrowing of the lumen and proximal dilatation. She underwent an ileocolic resection with ileo-ascending anastomosis (see Fig. 3.6a, b).

Pathology Active Crohn's ileitis with inflammatory stenosis. The proximal margin and colonic segment are unremarkable. No granulomas are found.

Follow-Up She had an uneventful recovery after surgery. She is doing well 5 years later.

Comment This patient had a long-standing history of cicatrizing Crohn's disease of the terminal ileum. She finally required surgery due to severe narrowing of the lumen causing increasing obstructive symptoms. Since she had slow progression of disease following diagnosis combined with short segment disease and no evidence of fistulas, she has an excellent prognosis. Nevertheless, prophylaxis is indicated in order to decrease the risk of early recurrence of symptoms (Fig. 3.6).

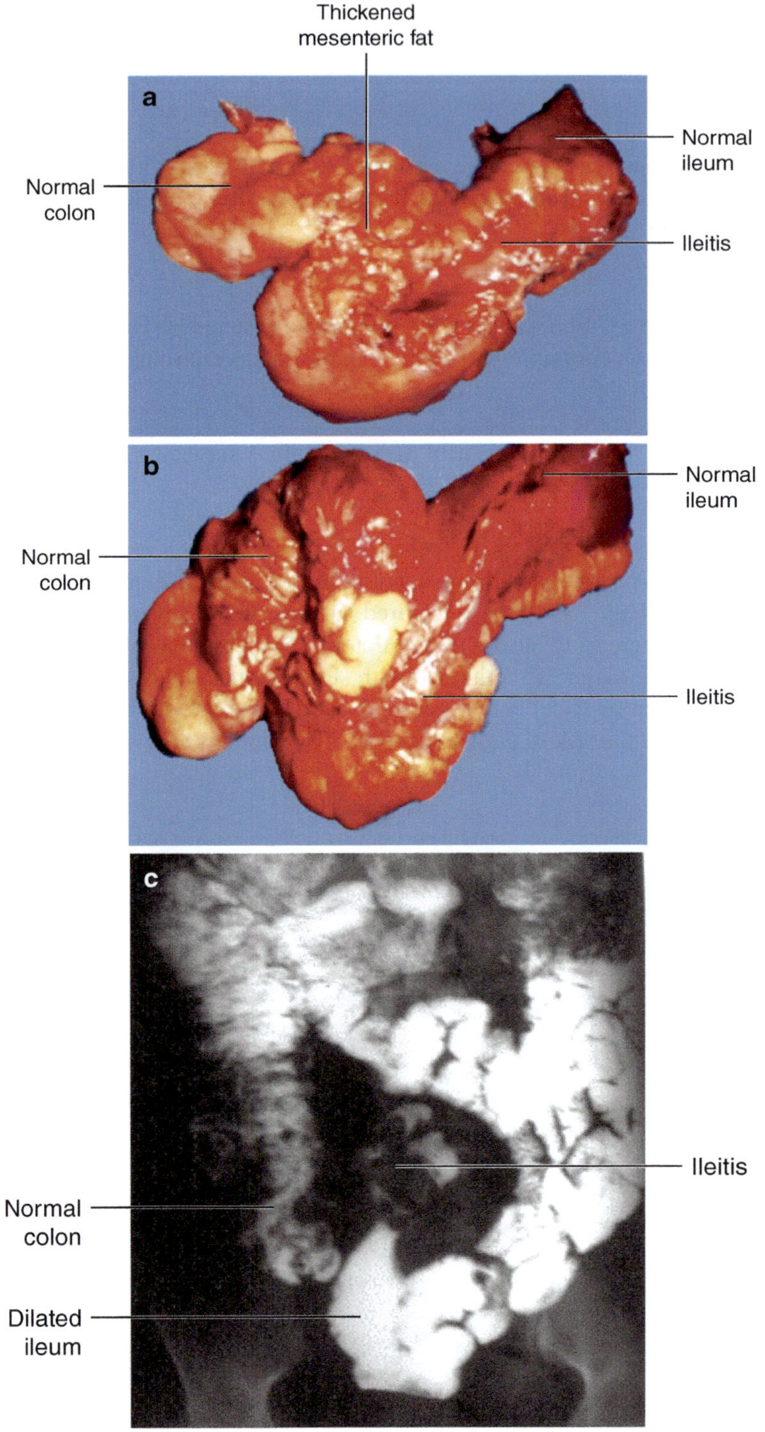

Fig. 3.6 (**a**–**e**) Ileitis with obstruction

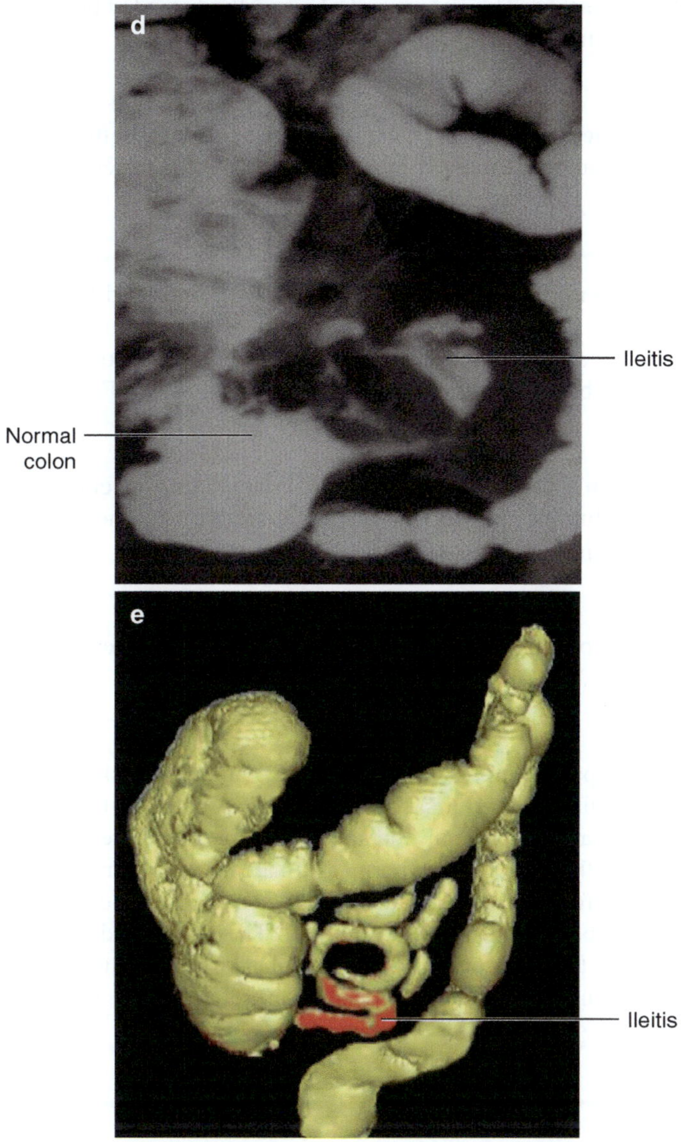

Fig. 3.6 (continued)

3.7 Extensive Jejunoileitis with Obstruction

History A 27-year-old male with Crohn's disease for 10 years. His current symptoms are 28 lb weight loss and colicky abdominal pain after eating. He is being treated medically without improvement.

Physical Examination The abdomen is chronically distended but soft. No masses are palpable, and there is no tenderness.

Diagnostic Studies A 45 cm segment of severe narrowing in the mid small bowel with proximal dilatation followed by a skip area and 20 cm segment of disease in the terminal ileum (see Fig. 3.7a, b).

Surgical Treatment This patient was found to have marked dilatation of the jejunum with a 45 cm segment of distal jejunum with severe stricture. A second area of disease involving a 20 cm segment of terminal ileum was also present. He underwent a mid small bowel resection and ileocolic resection (see Fig. 3.7c, d).

Pathology Crohn's disease with transmural inflammation, ulcerations, and inflammatory polyps. Multiple epithelioid granulomas are present. The disease is confined to the small intestine.

Follow-Up This patient had an uneventful recovery after surgery and remains well 4 years later.

Comment This patient represents a typical example of intestinal adaptation to a chronic Crohn's disease stricture. The long narrow segment in the mid small bowel is preceded by marked proximal dilatation. A second stricture was present in the terminal ileum with an intervening normal skip area. The proximal segment was too long for a strictureplasty, and about 65 cm of small intestine was resected. The remaining small bowel and colon are normal. The patient did well after surgery. Since he required two anastomosis, he is at higher risk for recurrent disease. If further surgery is necessary, strictureplasty is preferable to intestinal resection (Fig. 3.7).

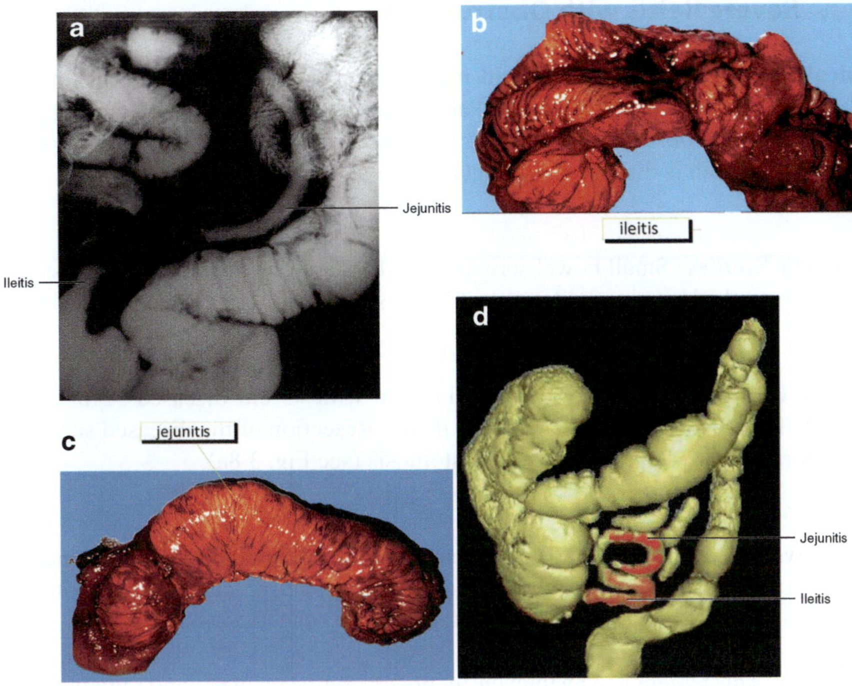

Fig. 3.7 (**a**–**d**) Extensive jejunoileitis with obstruction

3.8 Severe Ileitis with Obstruction

Clinical Presentation A 52-year-old male patient with long-standing history of Crohn's disease treated with steroids. Patient has recently developed recurrent episodes of intestinal obstruction requiring multiple hospital admissions. On physical exam, his abdomen is distended without any masses or tenderness.

Diagnostic Studies Small bowel series showed a 45 cm segment of diseased small bowel with marked proximal dilatation. Colonoscopy was normal (see Fig. 3.8b, c).

Surgical Treatment Chronic jejunal dilatation with 45 cm diseased segment of proximal ileum. Normal colon and distal ileum. Resection of the diseased segment was performed with stapled end-end anastomosis (see Fig. 3.8a).

Pathology Active Crohn's enteritis with transmural chronic inflammation, longitudinal ulcerations, inflammatory stricture, penetrating sinus tracts, and granulomas.

Follow-Up This patient had an uneventful postoperative recovery and remains well 4 years later.

Comment This patient had proximal ileal disease manifested by intestinal obstruction with marked dilatation of the proximal small intestine. Although the symptoms had been present for some time, eventually he became unresponsive to medical treatment and was unable to eat. The terminal ileum and colon were normal in this patient, although he did have an anal stricture and hypertrophied skin tags. He did well after small bowel resection with stapled anastomosis. The 100 mm linear stapler was used to transect the markedly dilated small bowel (Fig. 3.8).

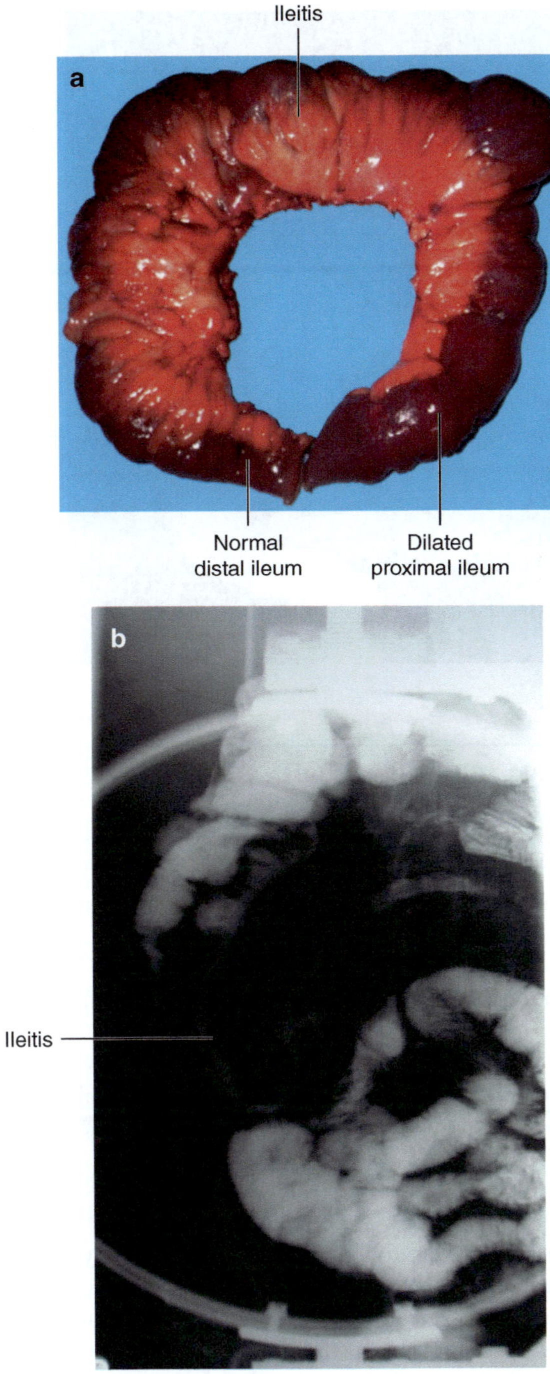

Fig. 3.8 (**a**–**c**) Severe ileitis with obstruction

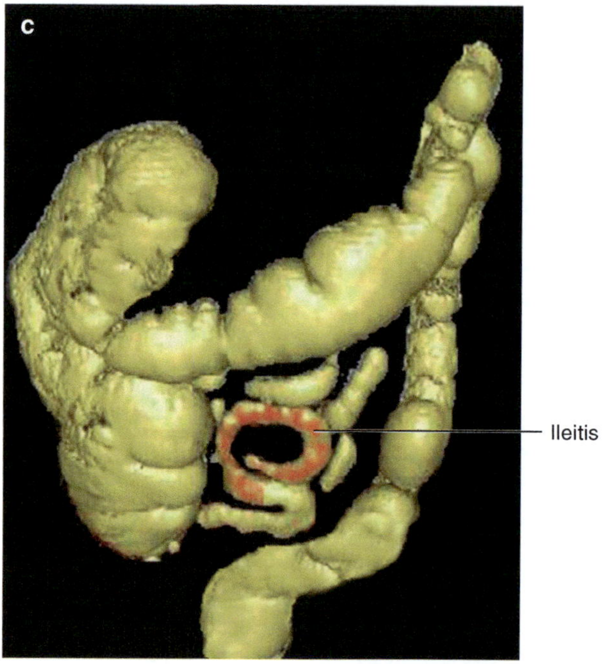

Fig. 3.8 (continued)

3.9 Extensive Jejunoileitis with Obstruction

History A 35-year-old male with long-standing history of Crohn's disease. He underwent multiple strictureplasties 4 years ago for obstructive symptoms. He now returns with recurrent abdominal distention, colicky abdominal pain, and weight loss.

Physical Examination Abdominal distention present, no masses palpable.

Diagnostic Studies Small bowel study showed dilated jejunum with transition point in the mid ileum and collapsed distal small bowel. The colon was normal on colonoscopy (see Fig. 3.9c, d).

Surgical Treatment He was found to have approximately 5 ft of dilated small bowel from the ligament of Treitz to the site of the previous strictureplasties. Several areas of severe narrowing were present followed by a segment of terminal ileum that was unremarkable. Resection of a 1-ft segment of small bowel with the multiple strictures was carried out with functional end-end anastomosis (see Fig. 3.9a, b).

Pathology Crohn's ileitis with mucosal ulceration, transmural inflammation, and strictures. Epithelioid granulomas are present. One margin has inactive disease.

Follow-Up He did well after resection and was discharged on the 9th postoperative day. This patient has extensive disease in the small bowel, which progressed rapidly since his previous operation. His potential for further problems with recurrent disease is high.

Comment Strictureplasty is often used for treatment of obstructive symptoms in patients with multiple strictures because it allows preservation of the bowel. Re-stricture is uncommon and often recurrent disease requiring further surgery develops in other areas away from the strictureplasties. In this case, the recurrent stricture causing the obstruction was at the site of the distal strictureplasty. Resection was required in order to be able to perform a safe anastomosis in an undisturbed segment of small bowel. This patient has about 6 ft of small bowel, and his entire colon is normal. He is able to maintain a normal weight without the need for nutritional supplements (Fig. 3.9).

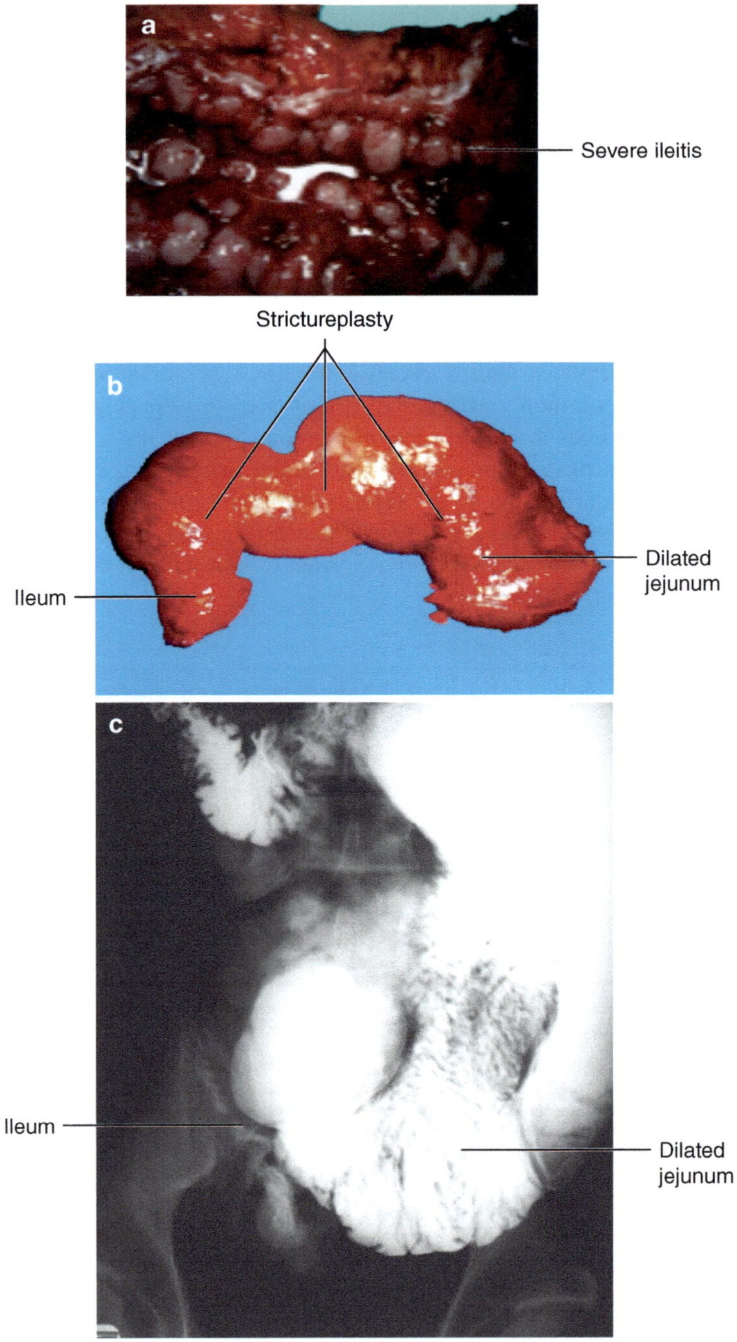

Fig. 3.9 (**a–d**) Extensive jejunoileitis with obstruction

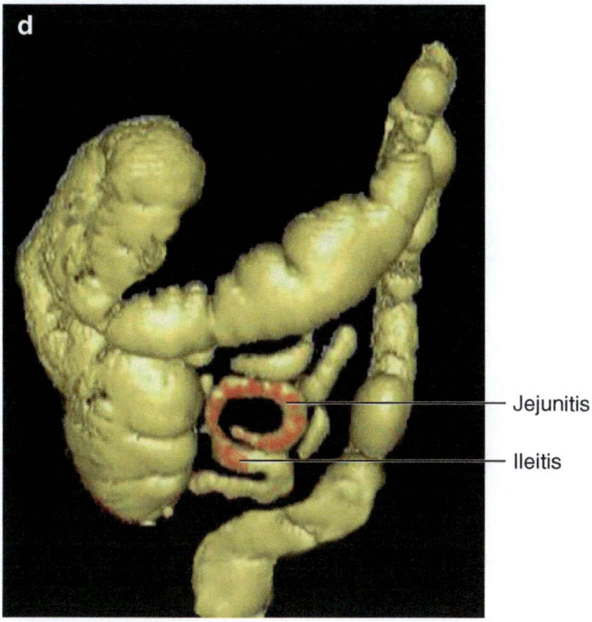

Fig. 3.9 (continued)

Further Reading

Heimann TM, Aufses AH Jr. Surgical complications and skin test reactivity in patients with inflammatory bowel disease. Arch Surg. 1984;119:885–7.

Heimann TM, Greenstein AJ, Mechanic L, Aufses AH Jr. Early complications following surgical treatment for Crohn's disease. Ann Surg. 1985;201:494–8.

Ileocolitis with Fistula

4

Tomas M. Heimann and Robert J. Kurtz

Patients with ileocolitis can be divided into two major categories. About half of the patients will present with obstructive symptoms due to strictures either in the colon or ileum. The rest have disease that manifests itself mainly by the presence of fistulas. Some of these fistulas may be entero-enteric or enterovesical. Often the fistulas drain into the intestinal mesentery or retroperitoneum, and these patients present with chronic pain, fever, and weight loss. Many patients with fistulas have chronic phlegmons, which have a thick wall and some purulent content. Most of these phlegmons can be resected with the segment of diseased bowel. Patients presenting with an acute abscess containing a large amount of purulent material benefit from CT-guided drainage and antibiotics prior to surgical resection. Fortunately, free perforation rarely occurs in patients with Crohn's disease. Colonic strictures are especially troublesome when they do not allow for colonic surveillance and occasionally may be caused by a carcinoma. The presence of these strictures is a common indication for surgery.

Ileocolitis with fistula often presents as a retroperitoneal or pelvic abscess. Right lower quadrant abscesses are most common since the disease is often confined to the terminal ileum and cecum. Fistulas between the ileum and cecum or sigmoid colon are also common but less likely to cause significant symptoms. Enteroenteric fistulas are not always obvious on preoperative studies and must be recognized at the time of surgery. When the bowel at one end of the fistula is intrinsically normal, the opening into normal bowel may be excised and repaired. When both loops are diseased, a double resection becomes necessary. Preoperative colonoscopy is by far the best method to assess the state of the colon prior to surgery for Crohn's disease.

T. M. Heimann (✉) · R. J. Kurtz
Department of Surgery, Icahn School of Medicine at Mount Sinai, New York, NY, USA
e-mail: Tomas.Heimann@mountsinai.org; Robert.Kurtz@mountsinai.org

T. M. Heimann (ed.), *Atlas of Surgical Treatment of Inflammatory Bowel Disease*, https://doi.org/10.1007/978-3-031-62431-5_4

4.1 Ileocolitis with Retroperitoneal Fistula

Clinical Presentation A 19-year-old male with 3-year history of Crohn's disease now presenting with low grade fever, night sweats, weight loss, and increasing back pain. On physical exam, a 15 cm mass is palpable in the right lower quadrant.

Diagnostic Studies Small bowel series shows diseased terminal ileum with a surrounding inflammatory mass and a retroperitoneal fistula. Colonoscopy showed mild inflammation of the cecum (see Fig. 4.1c, d).

Surgical Treatment At operation, diseased terminal ileum and cecum were found with a retroperitoneal fistula and inflammatory mass. The mass was adherent to the proximal transverse colon, and a right hemicolectomy was performed. The cultures obtained at surgery grew *E. coli* (see Fig. 4.1a, b).

Pathology Crohn's ileocolitis with ulcerations, inflammatory polyps, penetrating fistulas, and acute and chronic serositis. The resection margins were normal.

Follow-Up The patient is doing well 4 years after surgery.

Comment This patient is an example of a chronic retroperitoneal fistula, which is surrounded by a phlegmon. Although there is a communication with the bowel and cultures grew *E. coli*, there is no significant collection of pus, presumably because it drains back into the bowel. The patient usually presents with chronic symptoms such as back pain and weight loss, associated with night sweats and fever. Surgical resection removes the diseased bowel and the retroperitoneal mass with immediate improvement of symptoms. Unfortunately, the age of the patient as well as the presence of fistulas puts him in a high-risk category for early recurrence of symptoms following surgery (Fig. 4.1).

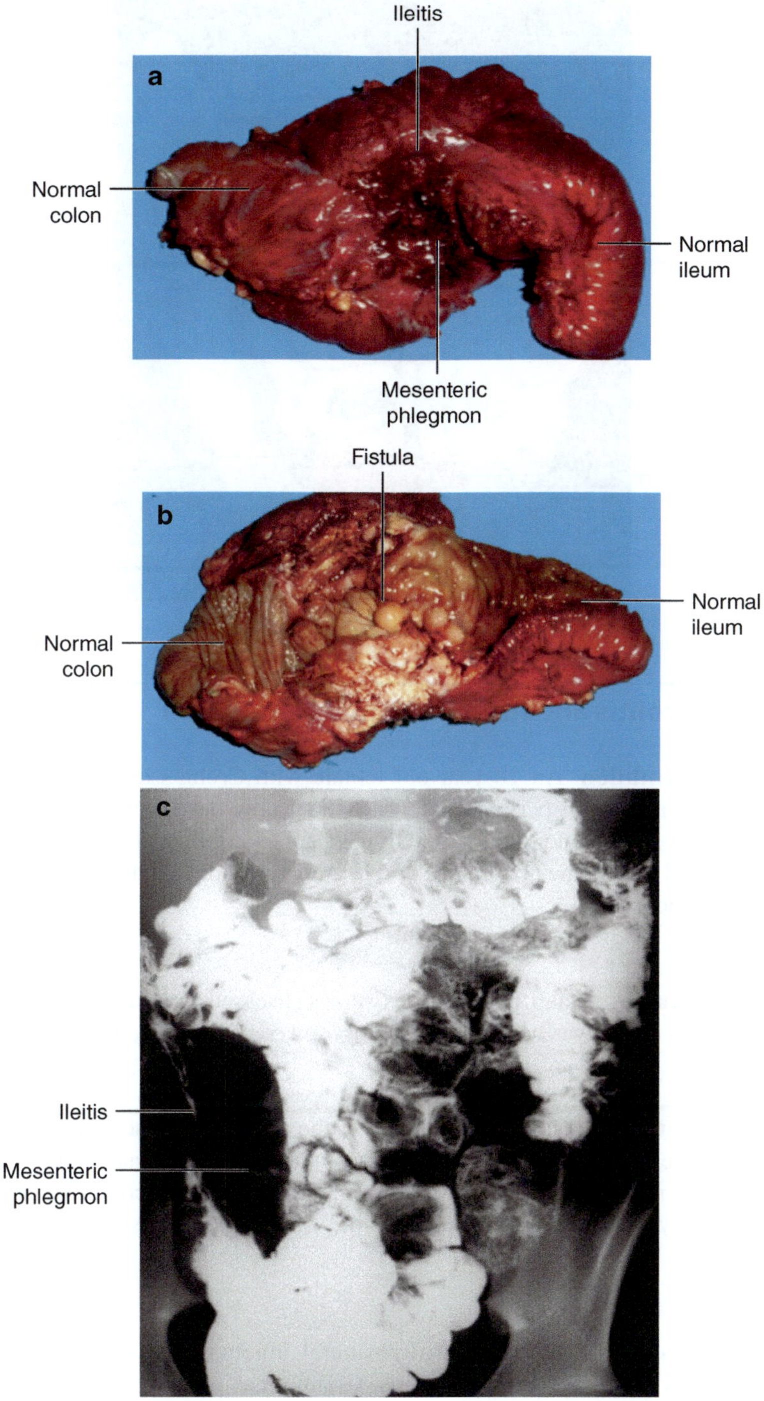

Fig. 4.1 (**a**–**d**) Ileocolitis with retroperitoneal fistula

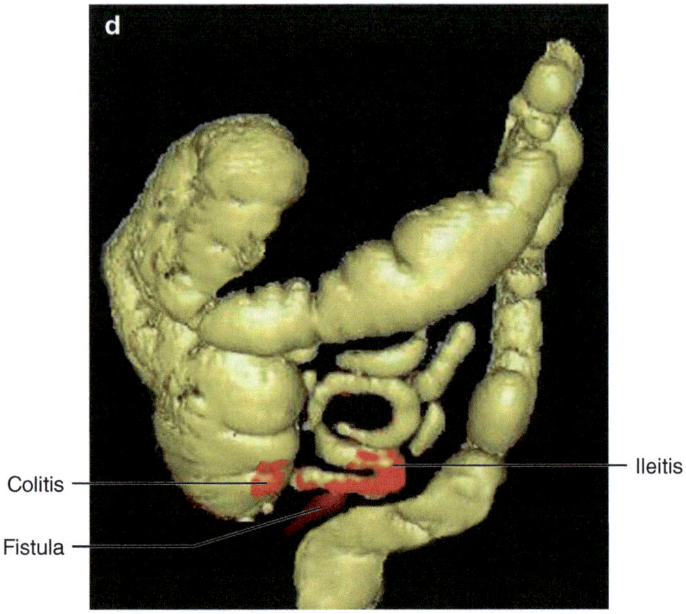

Fig. 4.1 (continued)

4.2 Ileocolitis and Retroperitoneal Phlegmon

Clinical Presentation An 18-year-old female with Crohn's disease for 11 years initially presenting with perianal fistulas. Patient now has fever, weight loss, and recurrent right-sided abdominal pain. On physical exam, the patient has features of chronic steroid intake, the abdomen is moderately distended, and there is significant right-sided tenderness.

Diagnostic Studies Small bowel series shows diseased terminal ileum and right colon. The left colon was normal on colonoscopy (see Fig. 4.2c, d, e).

Surgical Treatment A mass was found in the area of the ascending colon and hepatic flexure with severe stricture of the lumen. The terminal ileum was also inflamed. The mass was adherent to the stomach with a gastrocolic fistula. A right hemicolectomy was performed with closure of the gastric fistula site (see Fig. 4.2a, b).

Pathology Crohn's ileocolitis with transmural inflammation of the colon, with stricture, sinus tracts, and acute serositis. Granulomas are present, the margins of resection are normal, and the segment of gastric wall showed extrinsic inflammation.

Follow-Up This patient had an uneventful recovery and is doing well 4 years later.

Comment This patient has severe disease with multiple fistulas. The area surrounding the terminal ileum and ascending colon is encased in a chronic phlegmon, and there is a separate gastrocolic fistula. The presenting symptoms of abdominal pain and weight loss are similar to those seen in the previous patient. Fever is a common finding due to the presence of intestinal bacteria in the phlegmon. Resection of the diseased bowel, including the phlegmon and closure of the gastric fistula, is the treatment of choice. The stomach itself was free of Crohn's disease in this case (Fig. 4.2).

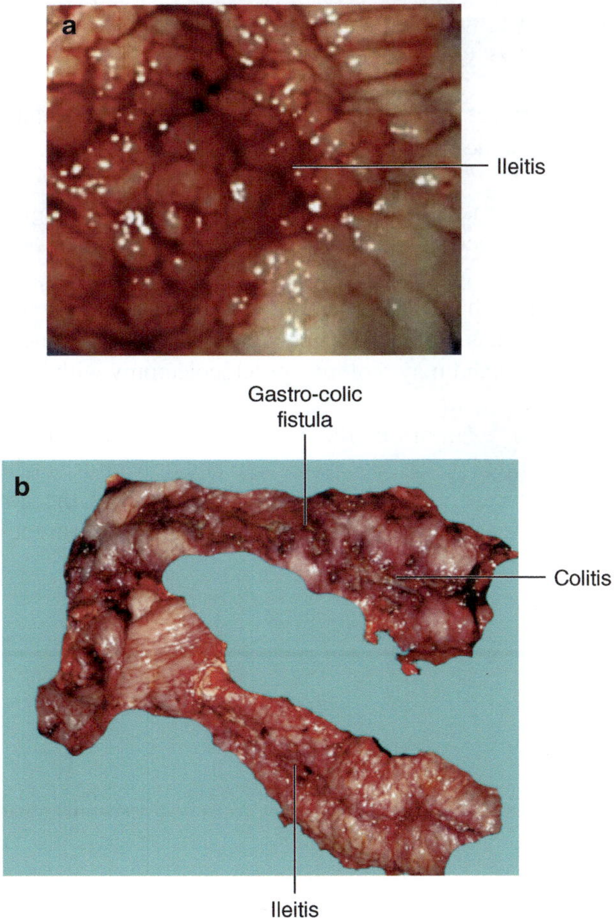

Fig. 4.2 (a–e) Ileocolitis and retroperitoneal phlegmon

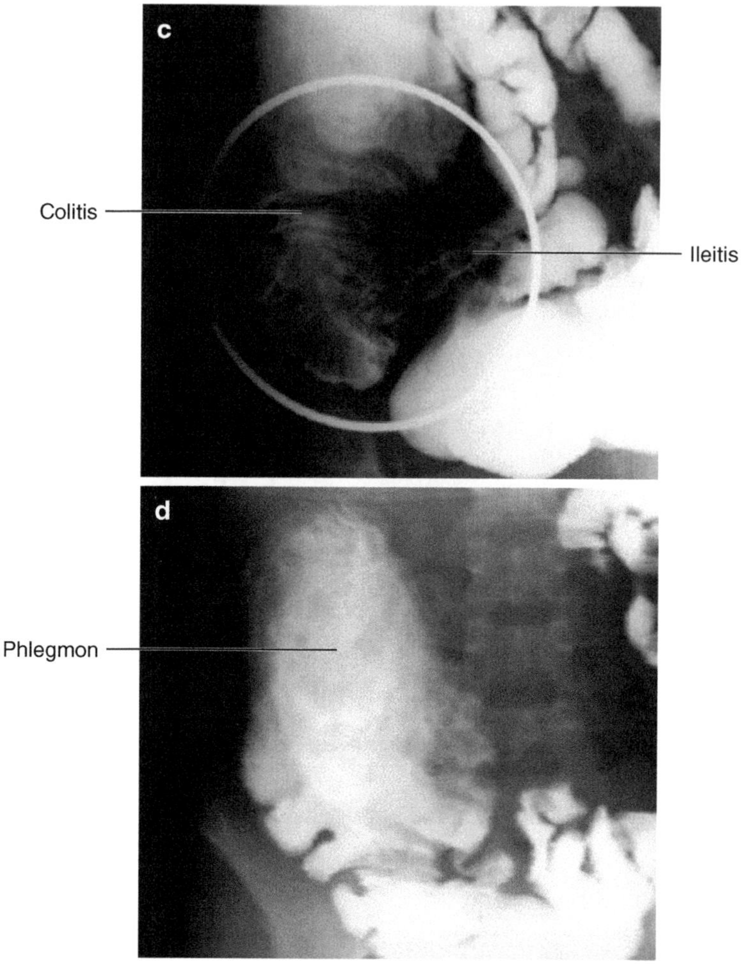

Fig. 4.2 (continued)

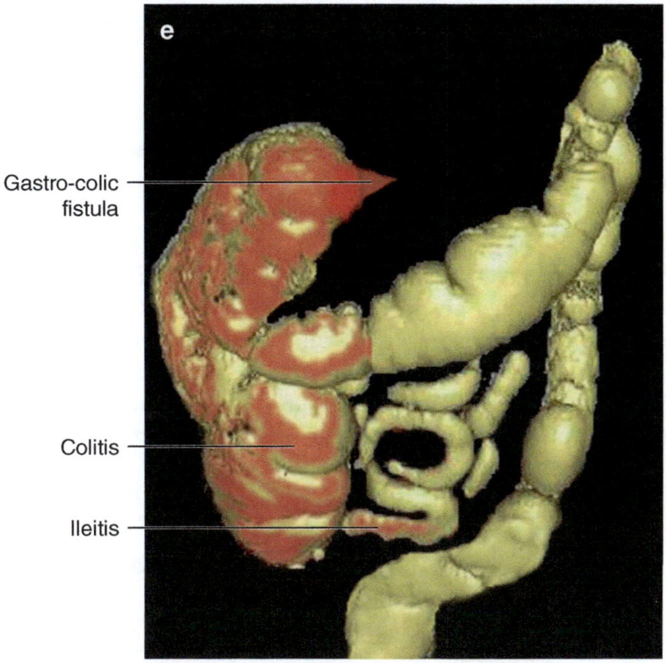

Fig. 4.2 (continued)

4.3 Ileocolitis with Pelvic Abscess

Clinical Presentation A 37-year-old male with Crohn's disease for 4 years. Now developed fever, weight loss, and colicky abdominal pain present for 5 weeks. On physical exam, the patient appears chronically ill, with significant weight loss, fullness, and tenderness in the right lower quadrant.

Diagnostic Studies CT scan of the abdomen showed a mass in the right lower quadrant with a dilated right ureter. Small bowel series showed a 15 cm segment of Crohn's disease in the terminal ileum, and colonoscopy revealed a normal colon except for mild inflammation in the cecum (see Fig. 4.3b, c).

Surgical Treatment This patient had disease of the terminal ileum with a 5 cm chronic abscess behind the cecum producing ureteral dilatation. An ileocolic resection with anastomosis was performed (see Fig. 4.3a).

Pathology Crohn's ileocolitis with severe activity, ulcerations, and deep fissures in the ileal segment and mild inflammation in the cecum. Epithelioid granulomas are present. The proximal margin is normal, but there is microscopic inflammation in the distal margin.

Follow-Up He had an uneventful postoperative recovery and is doing well 10 years later.

Comment In this patient, the small bowel fistula ends in a small chronic abscess. The location over the right ureter gives rise to hydronephrosis. Resection of the diseased bowel eliminates the source of the abscess allowing the ureteral dilatation to return to normal. The extent of the disease in this patient is limited to a short segment. Since this is his first operation at age 37, this patient is more likely to have a good prognosis than younger patients and those with more extensive disease (Fig. 4.3).

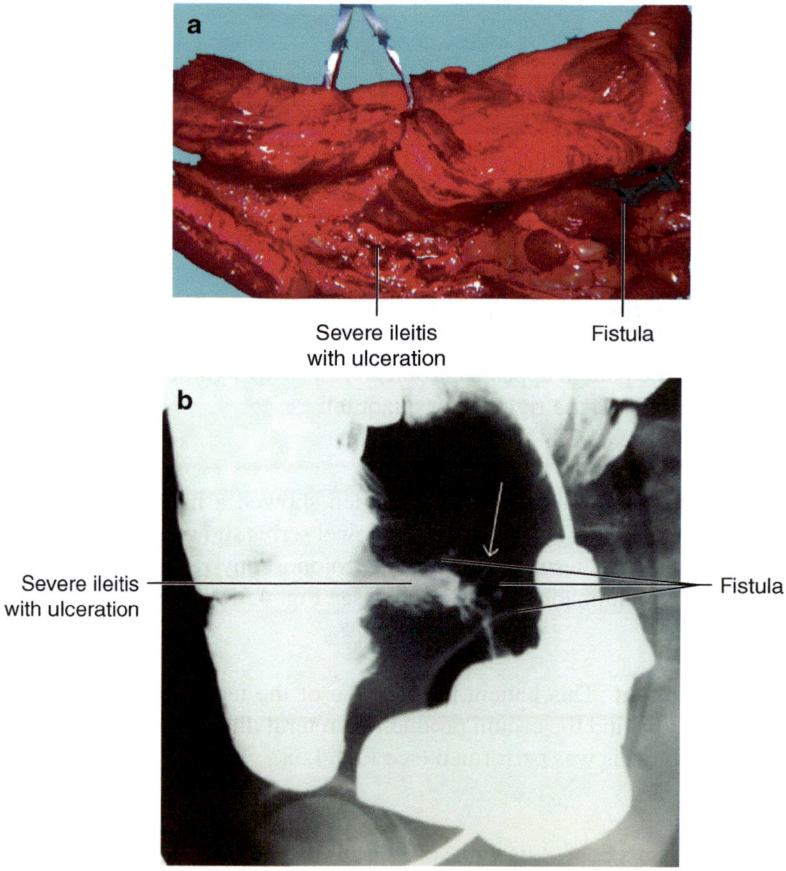

Fig. 4.3 (**a**–**c**) Ileocolitis with pelvic abscess

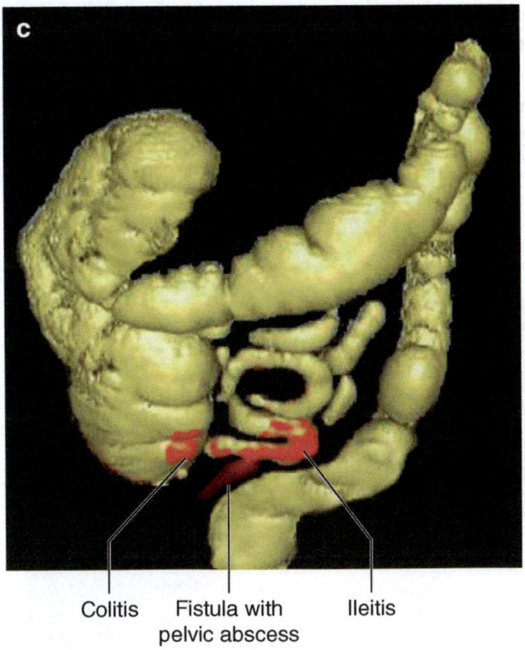

Fig. 4.3 (continued)

4.4 Ileocolitis with Pelvic Abscess

Clinical Presentation A 30-year-old woman with long-standing history of Crohn's disease. She had an extensive previous bowel resection with residual 4 ft of small intestine. Six months before this admission, she had percutaneous drainage of a pelvic abscess. She now comes in with severe left lower quadrant pain and fever.

Diagnostic Studies Abdominal films showed severe colonic dilatation with a stricture at the rectosigmoid junction. CT scan showed recurrent Crohn's disease at the rectosigmoid with marked stricture and possible pelvic collection (see Fig. 4.4d, e).

Surgical Treatment Patient had a sigmoid colostomy and drainage of a pelvic abscess followed by rectosigmoid resection with end sigmoid colostomy and Hartmann's closure of the rectum 6 weeks later (see Fig. 4.4a, b, c).

Pathology Rectosigmoid segment with pericolonic abscess, fistula tract, and chronic granulomatous inflammation. The findings are consistent with secondary involvement by Crohn's disease.

Follow-Up The patient did well following surgery. The rectal segment which is severely inflamed was left in place since there was extensive perirectal inflammation. Completion proctectomy was performed 6 months later.

Comment This patient has very aggressive Crohn's disease. At age 30, she has required multiple operations, and the length of bowel involvement is very extensive. It is interesting, however, that she is nutritionally stable with the remaining short segment of small bowel and colon. She has never required intravenous hyperalimentation. The rectum was recently removed and also showed severe inflammation with a very tight stricture. She is currently doing well with a sigmoid colostomy (Fig. 4.4).

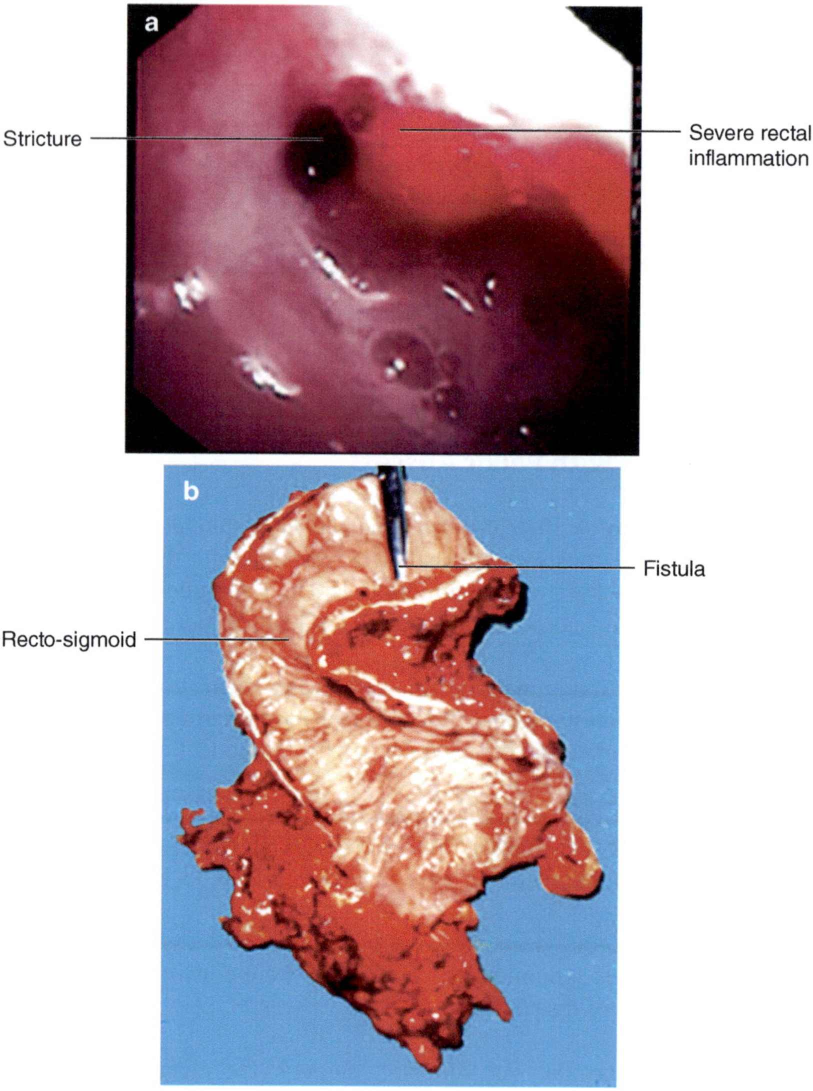

Fig. 4.4 (**a**–**e**) Ileocolitis with pelvic abscess

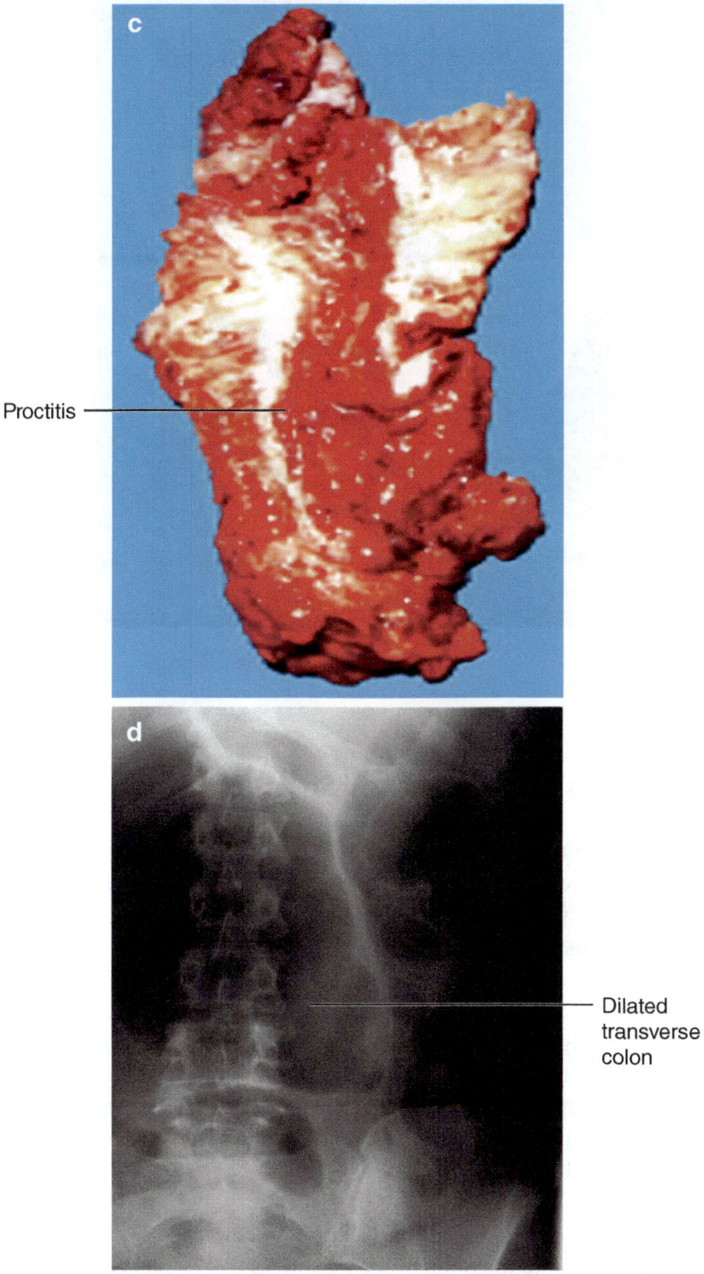

Fig. 4.4 (continued)

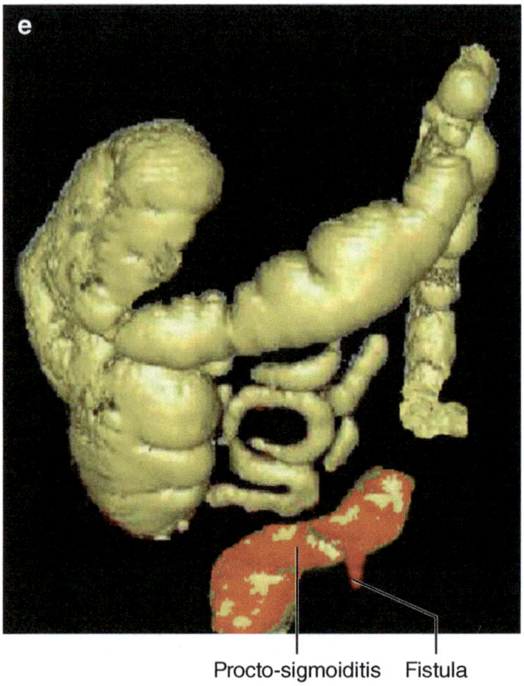

Fig. 4.4 (continued)

4.5 Ileocolitis with Fistula and Stricture

Clinical Presentation A 26-year-old patient with Crohn's ileocolitis who previously had an ileocolic resection and now presents with a retroperitoneal fistula and a narrow stricture in the distal sigmoid colon. He is admitted with abdominal pain and severe weight loss.

Diagnostic Studies CT scan of the abdomen showed chronic dilatation of the colon with thickening of the wall. A fistula is present in the right lower quadrant with a phlegmon. Colonoscopy showed mild proctitis, unable to pass pediatric endoscope past the sigmoid stricture. On physical exam, there is abdominal tenderness in the right lower quadrant, and a second stricture is present in the distal rectum on digital exam (see Fig. 4.5c, d).

Surgical Treatment He underwent a subtotal colectomy with Hartmann's closure of the rectum and Brooke ileostomy (see Fig. 4.5a, b).

Pathology Active Crohn's colitis with segmental transmural inflammation, stricture, ulcerations, and fissures. Multiple epithelioid granulomas are present. The ileum is unremarkable.

Follow-Up He is well with the ileostomy 3 years later.

Comment This 26-year-old patient is undergoing his second operation for Crohn's disease. He initially had a limited ileocolic resection and now requires a colectomy for colitis with a narrow stricture of the sigmoid colon. He underwent total colectomy with a Brooke ileostomy and is well. The residual rectum is diseased with a narrow distal stricture, and it is unlikely that he will be able to have an ileorectal anastomosis in the future. Eventually the patient should undergo an intersphincteric proctectomy since there is a significant risk of developing an anorectal cancer (Fig. 4.5).

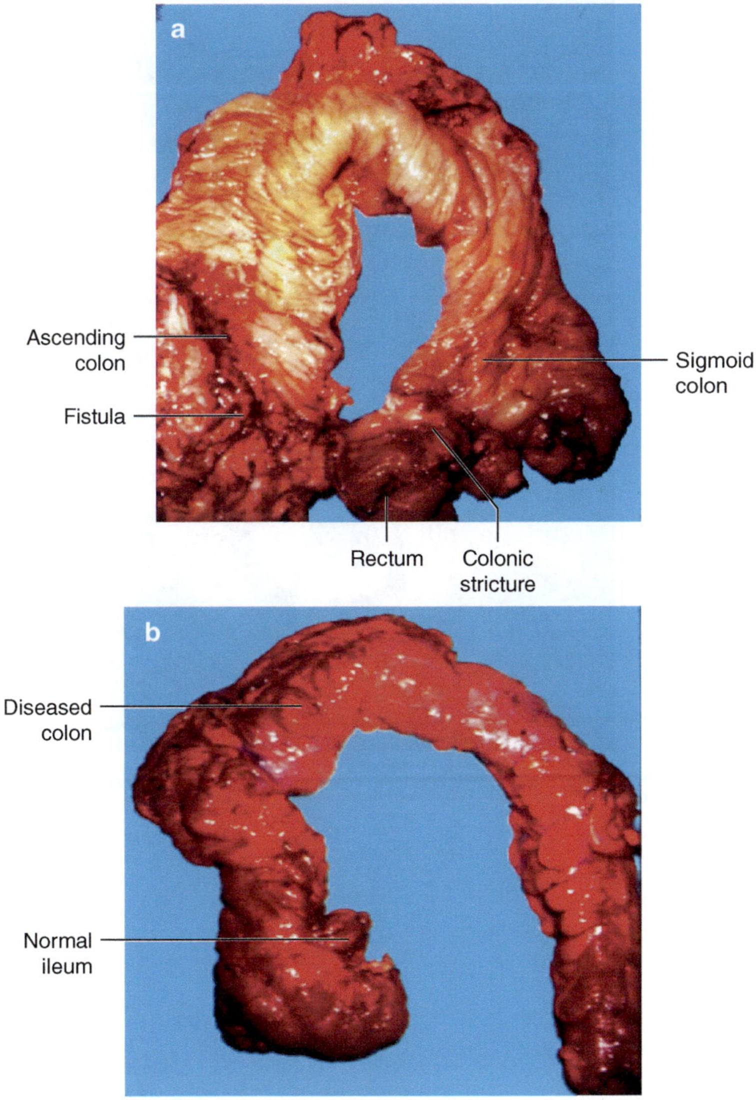

Fig. 4.5 (**a**–**d**) Ileocolitis with fistula and stricture

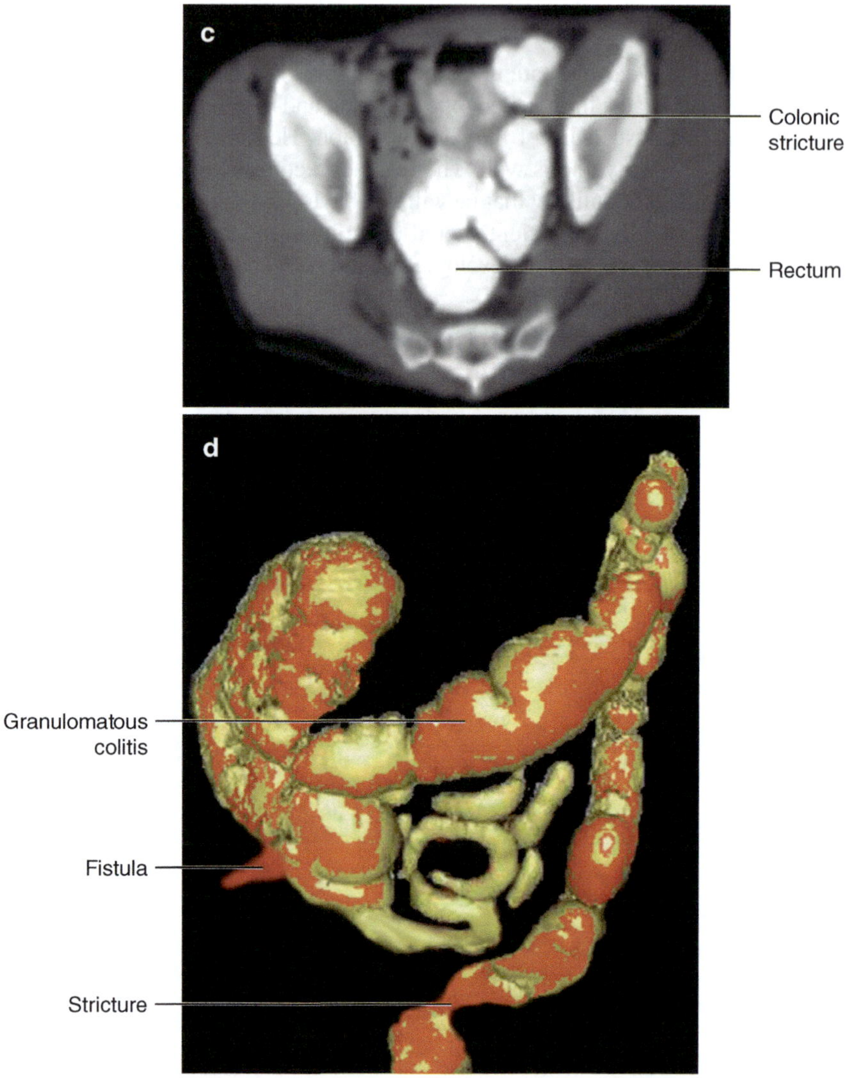

Fig. 4.5 (continued)

4.6 Ileocolitis with Recto-Vaginal Fistula

Clinical Presentation A 35-year-old woman with 12-year history of Crohn's disease. She had two previous intestinal resections prior to this admission. Patient now has recurrent disease in the terminal ileum and residual disease in the colon and rectum. There is a severe rectal stricture and a rectovaginal fistula associated with incontinence. She also has had severe weight loss and symptoms of partial obstruction.

Diagnostic Studies CT scan shows air in the vagina, rectal stricture, and disease in the terminal ileum (see Fig. 4.6c).

Surgical Treatment Recurrent disease in the neoterminal ileum and severe colitis with narrowing of the rectum and rectovaginal fistula originating at the dentate line. The patient underwent a proctocolectomy and Brooke ileostomy (see Fig. 4.6a, b).

Pathology Active Crohn's ileocolitis with ulcerations, transmural chronic inflammation, and epithelioid granulomas.

Follow-Up This patient had an uneventful recovery and is doing well 4 years later.

Comment This patient has recurrent disease in the neoterminal ileum and severe proctocolitis with a rectovaginal fistula. The rectum has a severe stricture, and repair of the rectovaginal fistula is not feasible in these cases. Proctocolectomy with resection of the disease in the ileum and a Brooke ileostomy is the appropriate treatment for these patients. The proctectomy is performed with an abdominal and a perineal team working simultaneously, thereby expediting the operation. The perineal wound is closed primarily after excising the rectovaginal fistula. Patients with a Brooke ileostomy have a lower recurrence potential than those with intestinal anastomosis (Fig. 4.6).

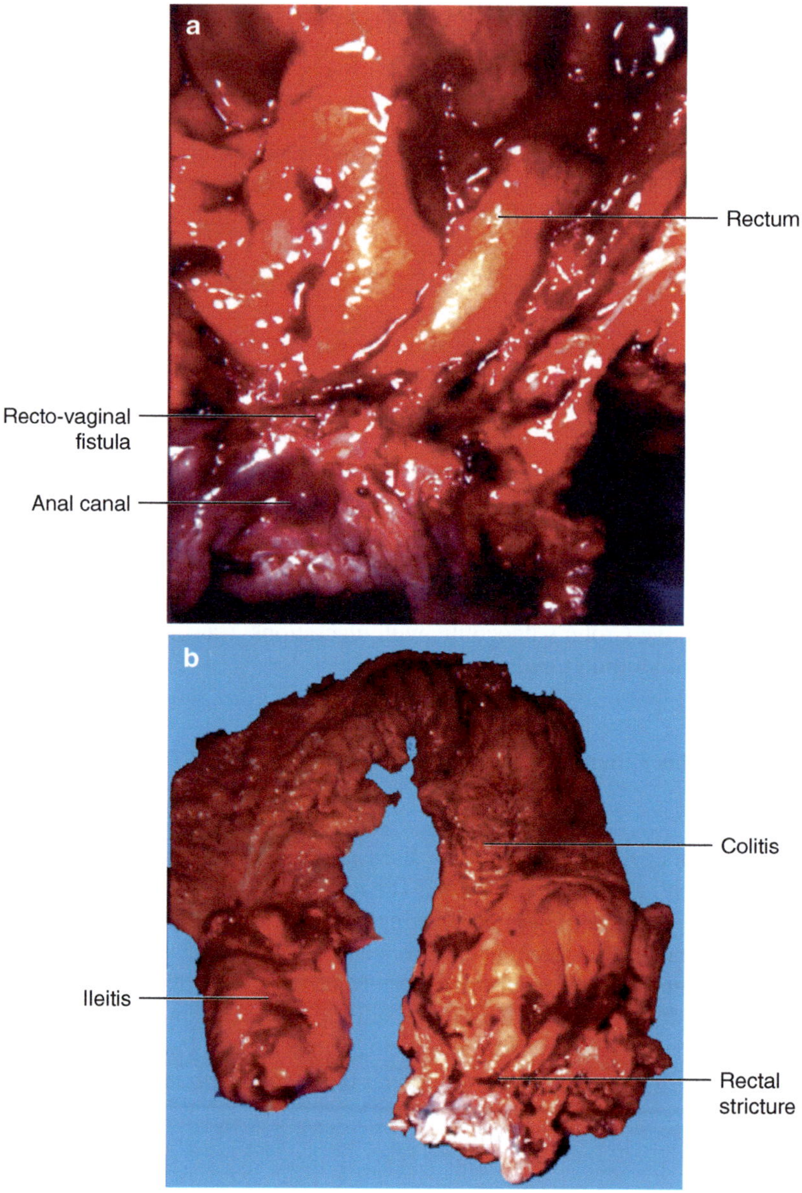

Fig. 4.6 (**a**–**c**) Ileocolitis with recto-vaginal fistula

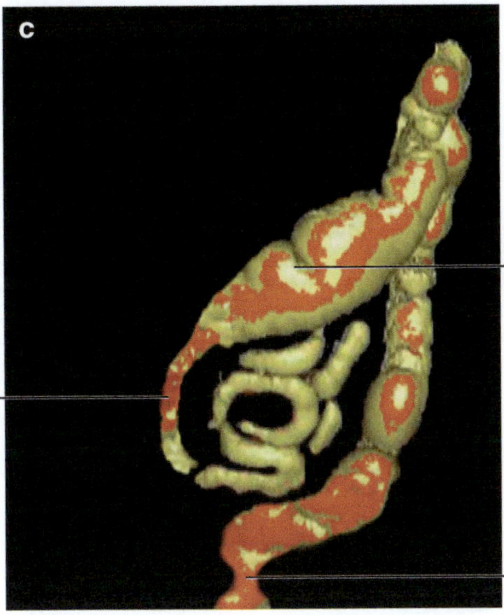

Fig. 4.6 (continued)

Further Reading

Greenstein AJ, Meyers S, Sher L, Heimann T, Aufses AH Jr. Surgery and its sequelae in Crohn's colitis and ileocolitis. Arch Surg. 1981;116:285–8.

Heimann TM, Bolnick K, Aufses AH Jr. Prognostic significance of severe preoperative lymphopenia in patients with Crohn's disease. Ann Surg. 1986;203:132–5.

Ileocolitis, Obstruction, and Perianal Disease

5

Tomas M. Heimann and Robert J. Kurtz

Patients with ileocolitis may also present with symptoms of obstruction from strictures in the small bowel or colon. Colonic strictures have the additional problem that if sufficiently narrow, surveillance of the colon by endoscopy may not be possible.

Perianal disease may also be the presenting feature of Crohn's disease. It may be manifested by the presence of a single perianal fistula with minimal symptoms. When severe, perianal disease may be extremely debilitating and refractory to treatment. In the worst cases, symptoms are only relieved when a stoma is performed. In patients requiring proctectomy, problems caused by delayed healing of the perineal wound are common in the presence of multiple fistulas. The last category in this section shows some of the diagnostic problems in patients initially thought to have ulcerative colitis who, after surgery, are found to have Crohn's ileocolitis. Fortunately, this group comprises only a small minority of patients.

5.1 Ileocolitis with Stricture

Clinical Presentation A 47-year-old woman with Crohn's for 15 years who now presents with increasing symptoms of intestinal obstruction characterized by cramps and bloating which have not improved with low residue diet and medical treatment.

Diagnostic Studies Small bowel series showed disease in the terminal ileum with moderate narrowing at the ileocecal valve. Colonoscopy was unremarkable except for mild inflammation in the cecum (see Fig. 5.1c, d).

T. M. Heimann (✉) · R. J. Kurtz
Department of Surgery, Icahn School of Medicine at Mount Sinai, New York, NY, USA
e-mail: Tomas.Heimann@mountsinai.org; Robert.Kurtz@mountsinai.org

T. M. Heimann (ed.), *Atlas of Surgical Treatment of Inflammatory Bowel Disease*, https://doi.org/10.1007/978-3-031-62431-5_5

Surgical Treatment She underwent an ileocolic resection with ileo ascending anastomosis (see Fig. 5.1a, b).

Pathology Enterocolitis with mild colonic ulcerations and transmural chronic inflammation of the terminal ileum. No granulomas are found.

Follow-Up She had an uneventful recovery and is well 2 years later.

Comment This patient had moderate symptoms of obstruction which did not respond to medical treatment. The symptoms were caused by a narrow stricture in the terminal ileum and could only be relieved with surgical resection. At the time of surgery, there was no dilatation of the proximal small bowel, but several pills were found in the ileum just proximal to the stricture. It is not infrequent to find vegetable fiber, pits, and even fecaliths at the site of obstruction. Proximal dilatation develops when the symptoms are chronic and surgical treatment is delayed (Fig. 5.1).

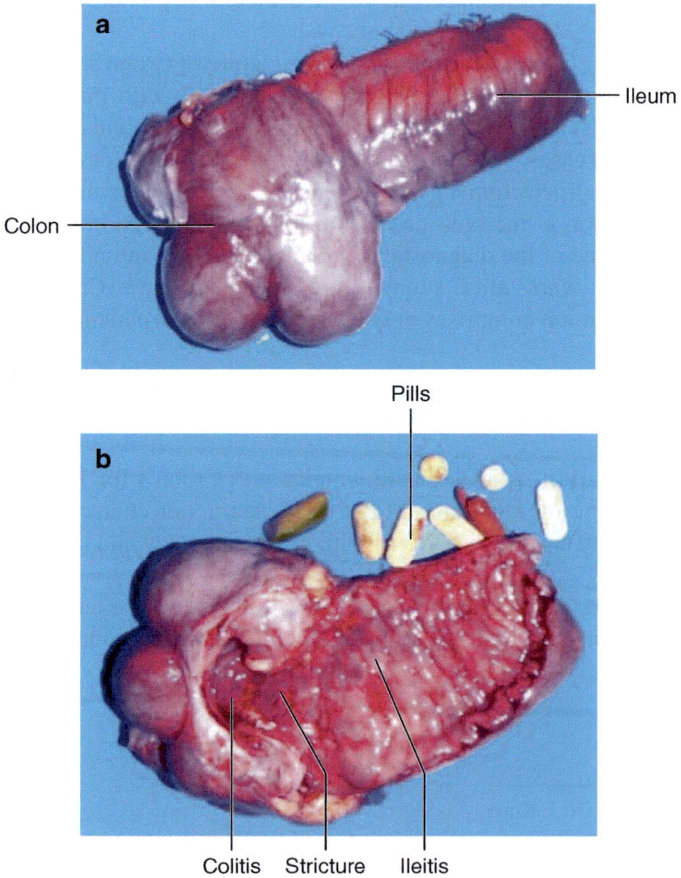

Fig. 5.1 (**a–d**) Ileocolitis with stricture

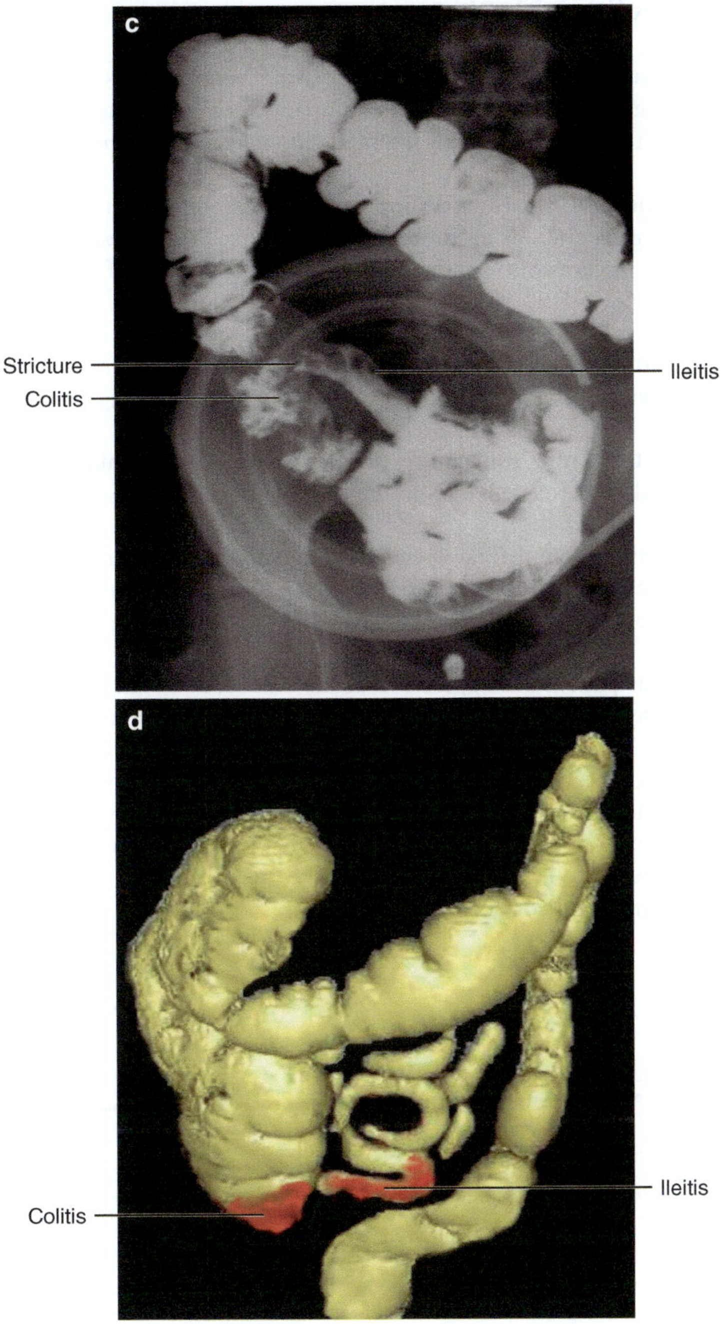

Fig. 5.1 (continued)

5.2 Ileocolitis with Obstruction

Clinical Presentation A 20-year-old man with Crohn's disease for 3 years presenting with right-sided abdominal pain, loose bowel movements, and weight loss. He is also severely anemic and has required a transfusion of 2 units of blood.

Diagnostic Studies Colonoscopy shows extensive Crohn's colitis in the right colon with deep linear ulcerations up to the hepatic flexure. Small bowel study confirms the presence of severe colitis and also shows a long segment of diseased terminal ileum (see Fig. 5.2c, d).

Surgical Treatment He underwent an extended ileocolic resection with right hemicolectomy and resection of 65 cm of diseased ileum (see Fig. 5.2a, b).

Pathology Active Crohn's ileocolitis with transmural chronic inflammation, linear ulcerations, and numerous epithelioid granulomas.

Follow-Up This patient had an uneventful recovery after surgery. In the next several months, he gained almost 10 lb. He has about 5–6 bowel movements per day and is doing well.

Comment This patient has aggressive Crohn's ileocolitis with a long segment of disease in the terminal ileum and severe disease in the right colon with long linear ulcerations, which account for his history of bleeding and anemia. In this case, the amount of blood loss was severe enough to require blood transfusions. An extended ileocolic resection was performed due to the extensive nature of his Crohn's disease. Although he has done well in the short term, this patient is at a very high risk for early recurrence since he has early onset and extensive disease requiring surgical treatment within 3 years of diagnosis (Fig. 5.2).

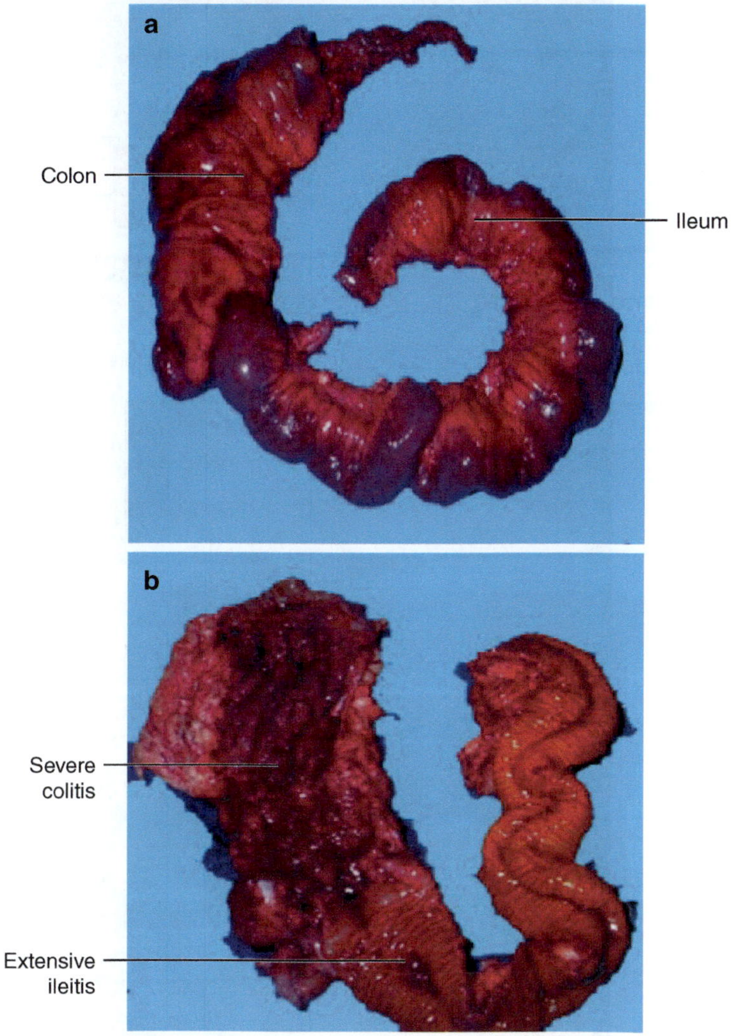

Fig. 5.2 (**a**–**d**) Ileocolitis with obstruction

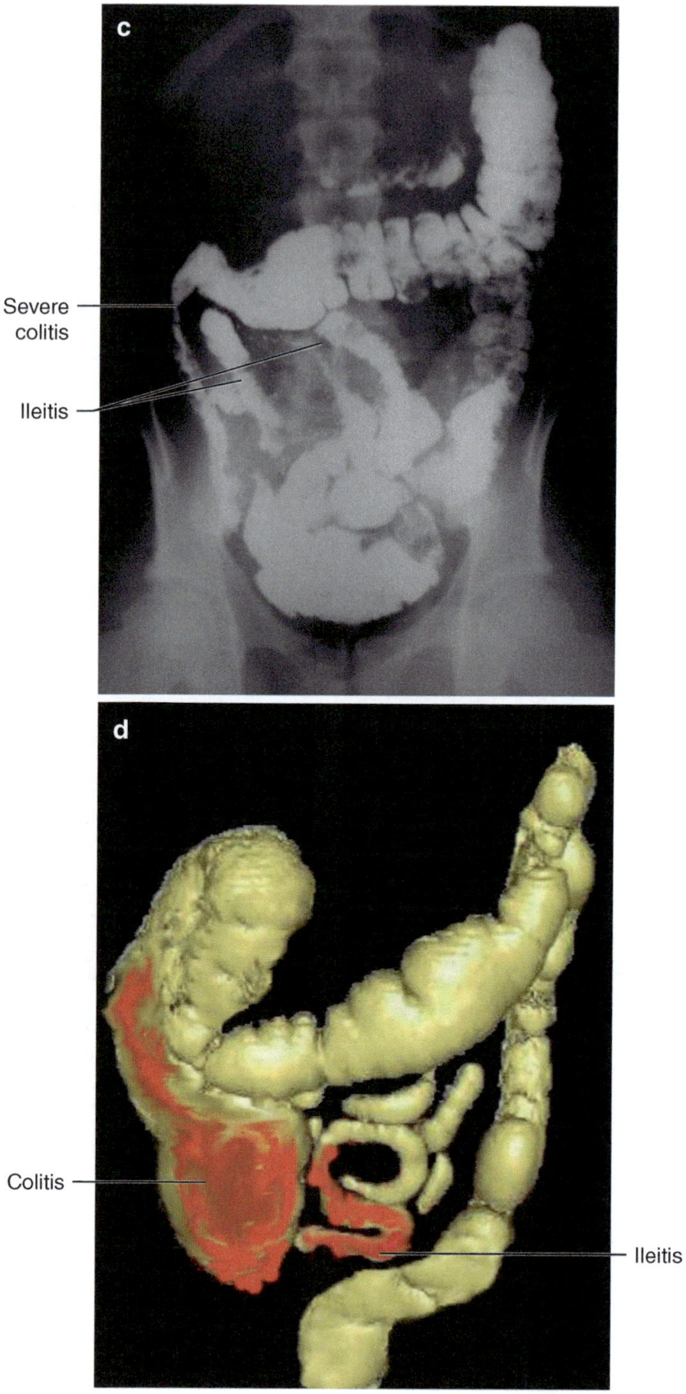

Fig. 5.2 (continued)

5.3 Ileocolitis with Chronic Stricture

Clinical Material A 39-year-old woman with Crohn's ileocolitis with a chronic stricture in the proximal transverse colon. Recently she has lost 10 lb due to difficulty eating with recurrent colicky abdominal pain and distention. On physical exam, there is moderate abdominal distention without palpable masses or tenderness.

Diagnostic Studies Colonoscopy showed diffuse colitis with rectal sparing and stricture of the proximal transverse colon. Small bowel series showed short segment of disease in the terminal ileum (see Fig. 5.3c, d).

Operative Treatment On exploration a 12 cm segment of disease in the terminal ileum and a mass in the proximal transverse colon was seen. The right, transverse, and descending colon showed Crohn's colitis. The patient was treated with a subtotal colectomy and ileorectal anastomosis (see Fig. 5.3a, b).

Pathology Crohn's ileocolitis with inflammatory stricture of the transverse colon, sinus tracts, and acute and chronic serositis. Margins of resection are unremarkable.

Follow-Up This patient did well following surgery and has been asymptomatic for 4 years.

Comment This patient had chronic ileocolitis with exacerbation of her symptoms caused by a narrow stricture in the transverse colon. Fortunately, she had rectal sparing and no perianal disease. A subtotal colectomy with limited ileal resection and ileorectal anastomosis was performed. This operation has a higher recurrence potential than colectomy with ileostomy, but it is worthwhile to attempt to delay the need for an ileostomy as long as possible. The use of adjuvant chemoprophylaxis has been shown to extend the disease-free interval (Fig. 5.3).

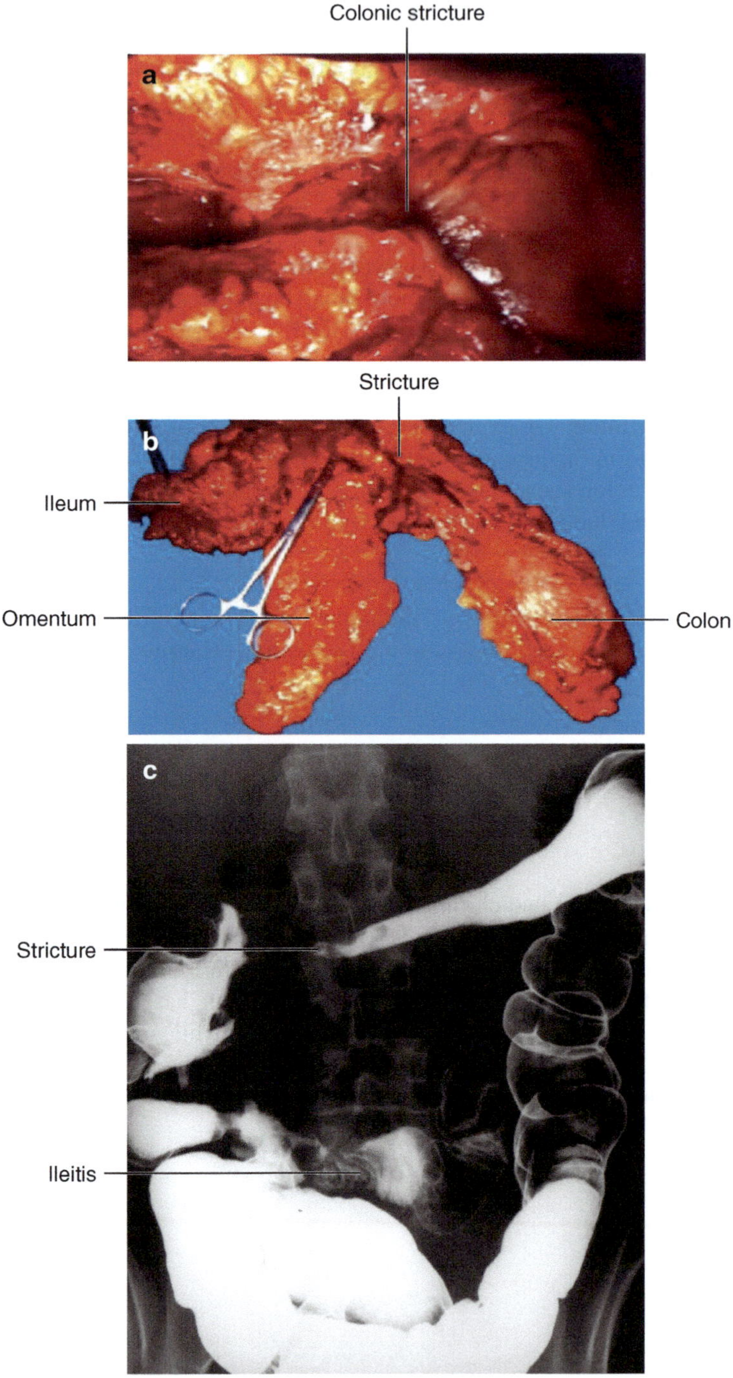

Fig. 5.3 (**a**–**d**) Ileocolitis with chronic stricture

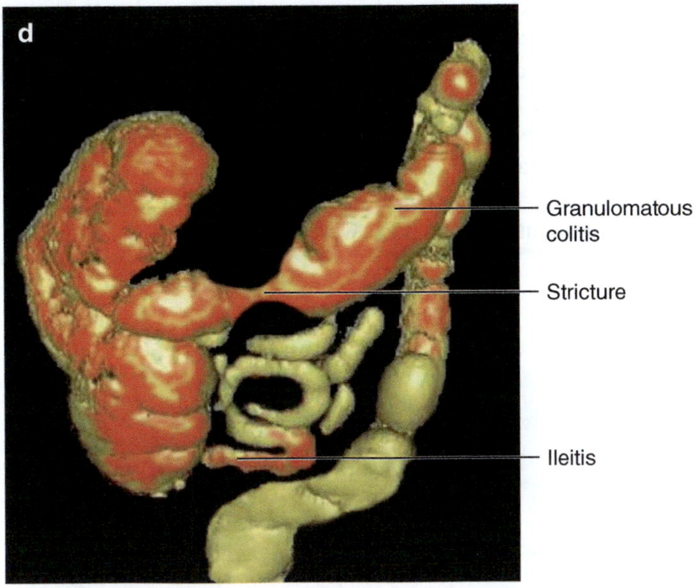

Fig. 5.3 (continued)

5.4 Ileocolitis with Obstruction and Fistula

Clinical Presentation A 57-year-old woman with Crohn's disease for 12 years presents with worsening symptoms of chronic obstruction and increasing inability to eat. Physical exam shows an emaciated woman with severe abdominal distention.

Diagnostic Studies Small bowel series showed disease in the terminal ileum with massive dilatation of the proximal small bowel. Colonoscopy showed a normal colon (see Fig. 5.4b, c).

Surgical Treatment After initial treatment with intravenous hyperalimentation, she underwent an extended ileocolic resection with ileotransverse anastomosis (see Fig. 5.4a).

Pathology Active Crohn's ileocolitis with stricture, ulcerations, and ileocecal fistulas. No granulomas are present. The resection margins are normal.

Follow-Up After a slow postoperative recovery, she did quite well. Within 6 weeks after surgery, she gained 20 lb, and the fluid retention caused by the low serum albumin was nearly resolved. She is well 2 years later.

Comment This is an extreme case of severe malnutrition due to chronic obstruction. The preoperative serum albumin was 1.1 g/dL, and she developed severe edema of the legs and secondary cellulitis. The fluid intake required by the intravenous hyperalimentation also aggravated this problem. Surgical correction of the obstruction by resecting the diseased segment restored her ability to eat allowing rapid tapering of the intravenous nutrition. Fortunately, the disease was localized to a single area, allowing for resection with one anastomosis, which healed well. Earlier surgical treatment would have lowered the risk considerably (Fig. 5.4).

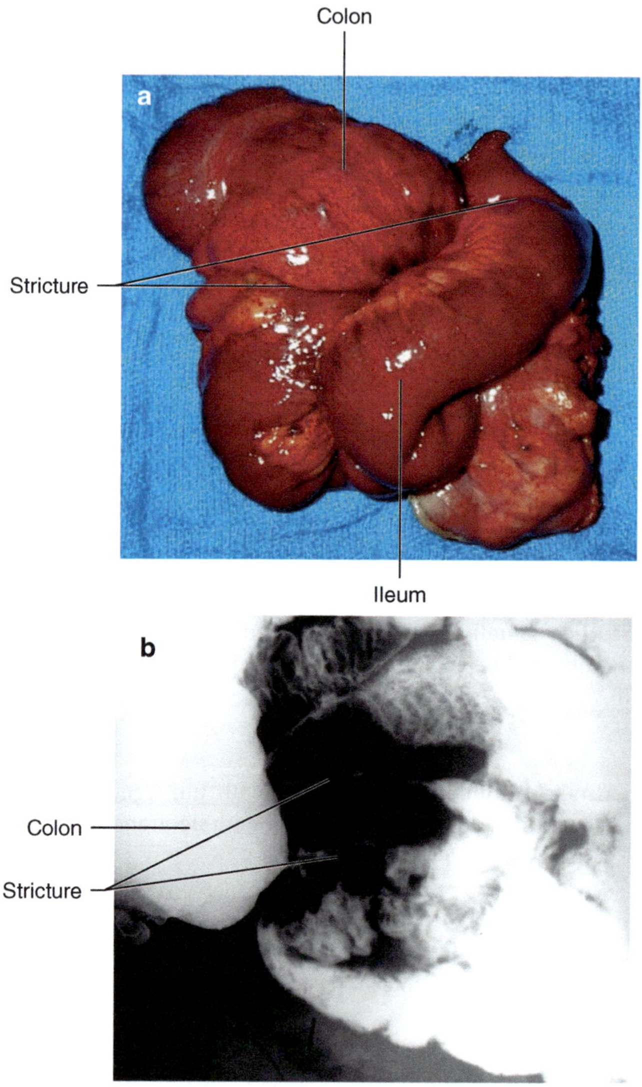

Fig. 5.4 (**a**–**c**) Ileocolitis with obstruction and fistula

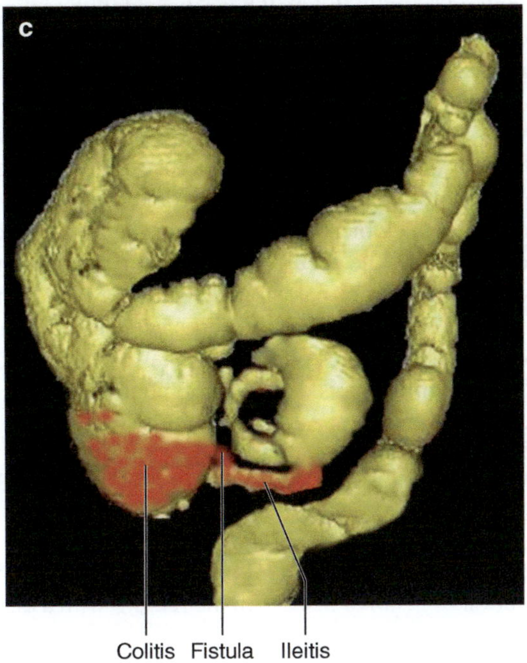

Fig. 5.4 (continued)

5.5 Ileocolitis with Severe Perianal Disease

Clinical Presentation A 31-year-old woman with 9-year history of Crohn's colitis with rectal sparing. In the past 3 years, she developed multiple perianal and rectovaginal fistulas. On physical exam, there are multiple perianal sinus tracts and rectovaginal fistulas. The sigmoid colon is palpable and tender (see Fig. 5.5c, d, e).

Diagnostic Studies Small bowel series showed normal small bowel, with inflammation of a short segment of terminal ileum. Colonoscopy demonstrated severe colonic inflammation with minimal disease in the rectum.

Surgical Treatment Examination under anesthesia revealed eight perianal fistulas and two rectovaginal fistulas. She underwent a total colectomy with Hartmann's closure of the rectum and Brooke ileostomy. Twelve centimeter of terminal ileum and the entire colon showed chronic inflammation (see Fig. 5.5a, b).

Pathology Terminal ileum and colon showing Crohn's ileocolitis with fissures, inflammatory polyps, and acute and chronic serositis. Epithelioid granulomas are present. Both margins showed microscopic inflammation.

Follow-Up This patient initially did well but returned with recurrent disease at the ileostomy 15 months later. Following a period of medical treatment, she required excision of the terminal ileum 4 years later for multiple fistulas.

Comment This patient has aggressive Crohn's disease with severe perianal fistulas. She underwent a subtotal colectomy with Brooke ileostomy. She also has disease of the terminal ileum, which recurred shortly after the ileocolectomy and required a second resection. The recurrent disease in the neoterminal ileum presented with a severe stricture and parastomal fistulas. Many patients with severe Crohn's proctitis find the decision to undergo proctectomy a difficult one. However, rectal preservation in patients, where ileorectal anastomosis is not feasible, is not wise, since there is a significant risk of development of cancer in the remaining rectum (Fig. 5.5).

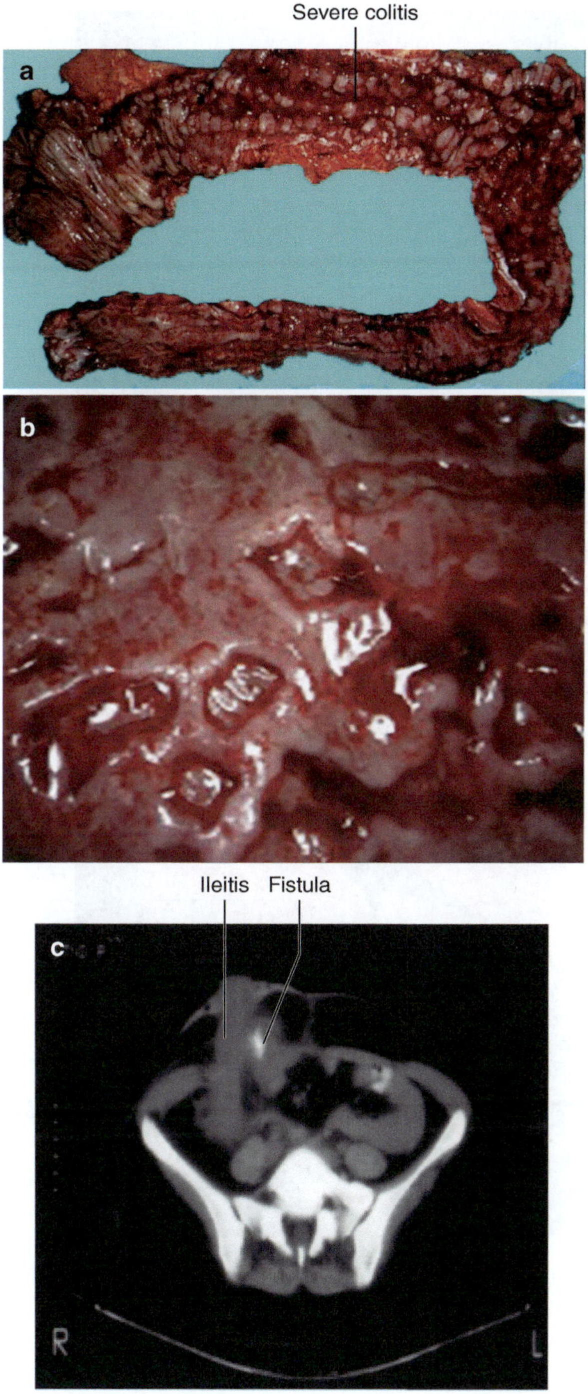

Fig. 5.5 (**a**–**e**) Ileocolitis with severe perianal disease

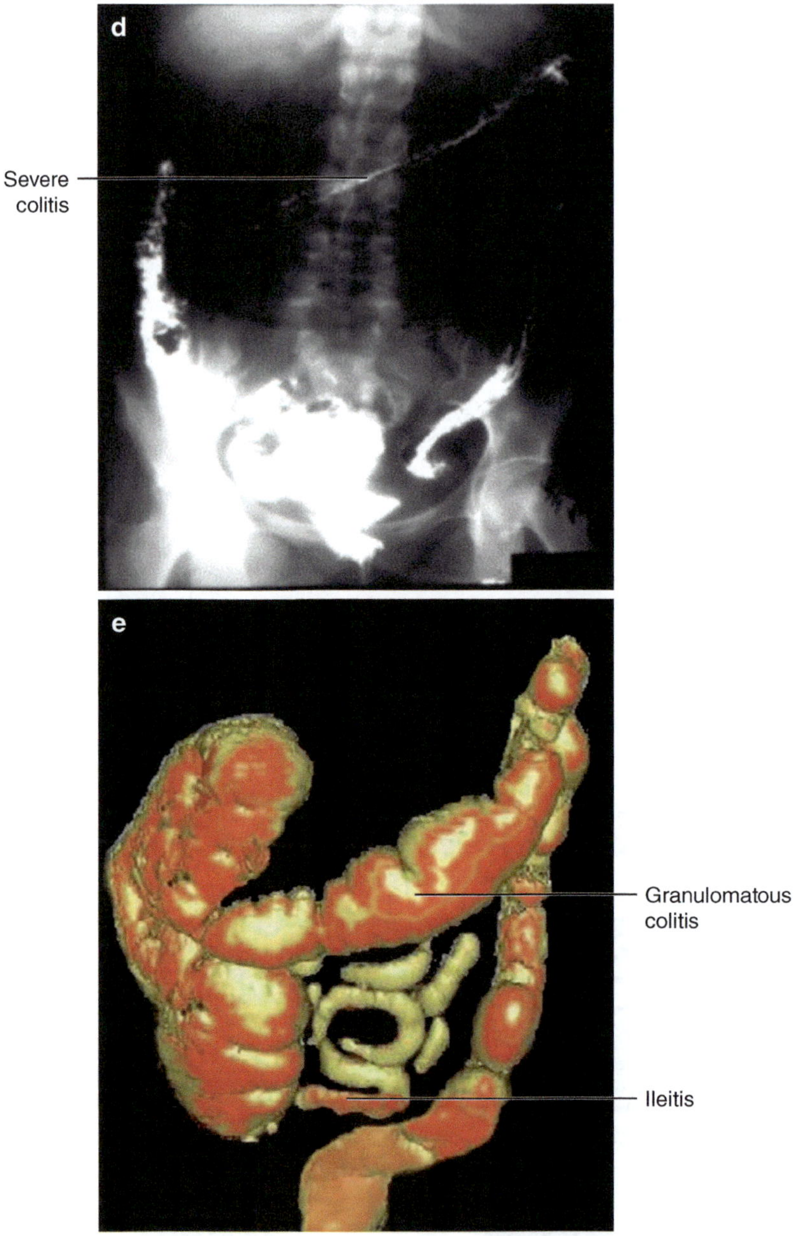

Fig. 5.5 (continued)

5.6 Ileocolitis with Severe Perianal Disease

Clinical Presentation A 40-year-old woman with a 13-year history of Crohn's disease manifested by multiple perianal and rectovaginal fistulas. Five years earlier, she underwent a loop transverse colostomy for rectal bleeding.

Diagnostic Studies Rectal inflammation with stricture at the rectosigmoid on endoscopy, severe perianal disease. CT scan showed severe left-sided colitis (see Fig. 5.6b, c).

Surgical Treatment At the time of surgery, she was found to have a severely inflamed rectum with perianal disease and benign stricture at the rectosigmoid. Less severe inflammatory changes in the distal ileum and proximal colon. She underwent a total colectomy, subtotal proctectomy, and Brooke ileostomy (see Fig. 5.6a).

Pathology Colon and rectum showed active Crohn's colitis with ulcerations, fissures, transmural chronic inflammation, and stenosis. Numerous epithelioid granulomas were present. The ileum showed slightly active Crohn's ileitis with patchy mural fibrosis and granulomas.

Follow-Up She did well following surgery and subsequently developed a peri-ileostomy fistula 3 months later, which did not require further surgical treatment. She underwent a perineal proctectomy 2 years later. The perineal wound required revision and took almost 1 year to finally heal.

Comment Bleeding is an uncommon manifestation of Crohn's disease and usually results from erosion of a vessel on the mesenteric side of an ulcerated segment of the bowel. In general, a patient with extensive ileocolitis, such as this one, should have an initial colectomy with an ileostomy unless the bleeding is from the rectum. Completion proctectomy should be performed within a year after the colectomy. Under elective conditions, it is possible to perform a resection of most of the rectum at the time of colectomy, leaving a short rectal segment that may be removed using a perineal approach at a later date, eliminating the need for a second laparotomy (Fig. 5.6).

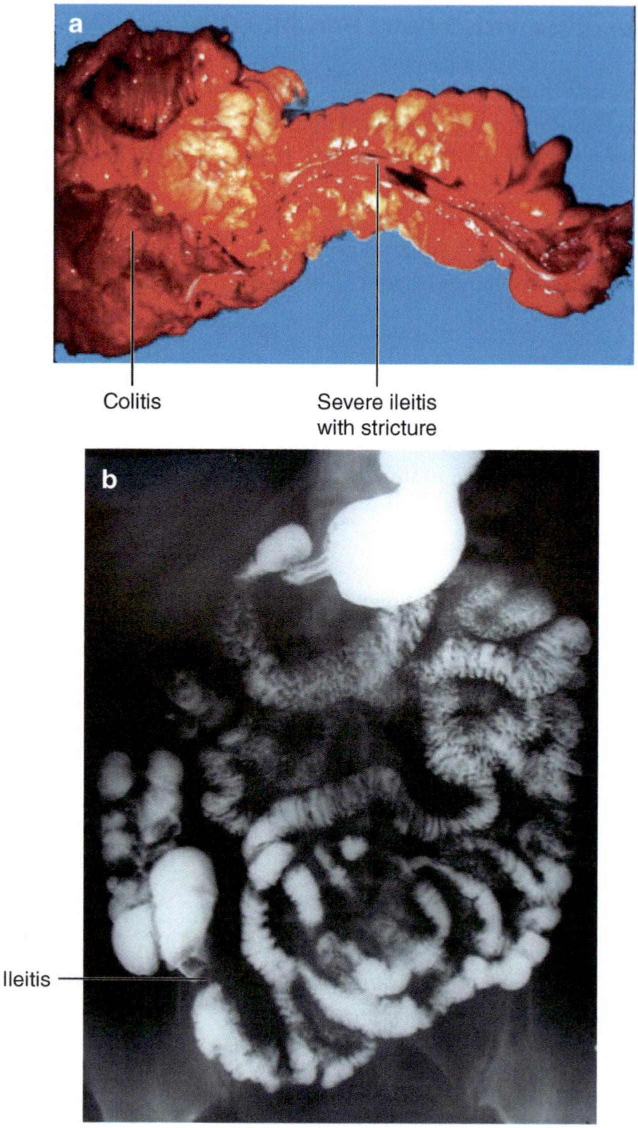

Fig. 5.6 (**a**–**c**) Ileocolitis with severe perianal disease

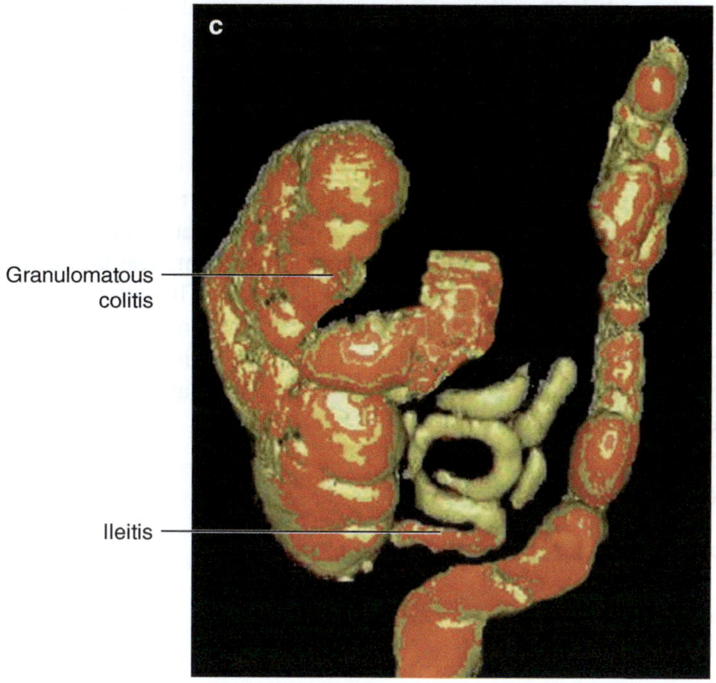

Fig. 5.6 (continued)

5.7 Ileocolitis, Fistula, and Perianal Disease

Clinical Presentation A 38-year-old man with a long-standing history of Crohn's disease who now presents with severe weight loss and anemia.

Diagnostic Studies CT scan and small bowel studies showed ileovesical and ileorectal fistulas. Colonoscopy showed severe perianal disease and cecal inflammation (see Fig. 5.7d).

Surgical Treatment He underwent an ileocolic resection, with ileostomy, and limited sigmoid resection, with Hartmann's closure of the rectum and mucous fistula (see Fig. 5.7a, b, c).

Pathology Severe Crohn's disease of the ileum and cecum with fistulas to the cecum and rectum. Except for the fistula, the rectum is unremarkable.

Follow-Up He had a good recovery following surgery with weight gain of over 30 lb within 6 months and improvement of the anemia. He could eventually have an ileocolic anastomosis since the remaining colon is normal. There is residual severe perianal disease, which will require him to convert the sigmoid mucous fistula to a functioning colostomy. He is well 3 years later and refuses any further surgery.

Comment This patient had severe Crohn's ileocolitis unresponsive to medical treatment. He presented with severe weight loss, caused mostly by the inability to eat due to the severity of the perianal disease. Multiple entero-enteric and entero-vesical fistulas further complicated the surgical treatment. The ileocolic resection with Brooke ileostomy removed the proximal disease. The pelvis was difficult to evaluate due to the severe inflammatory changes; therefore, the decision was made to perform a limited sigmoid resection without anastomosis, and the need for further surgical resection would be evaluated at a later date after the patient's health improved (Fig. 5.7).

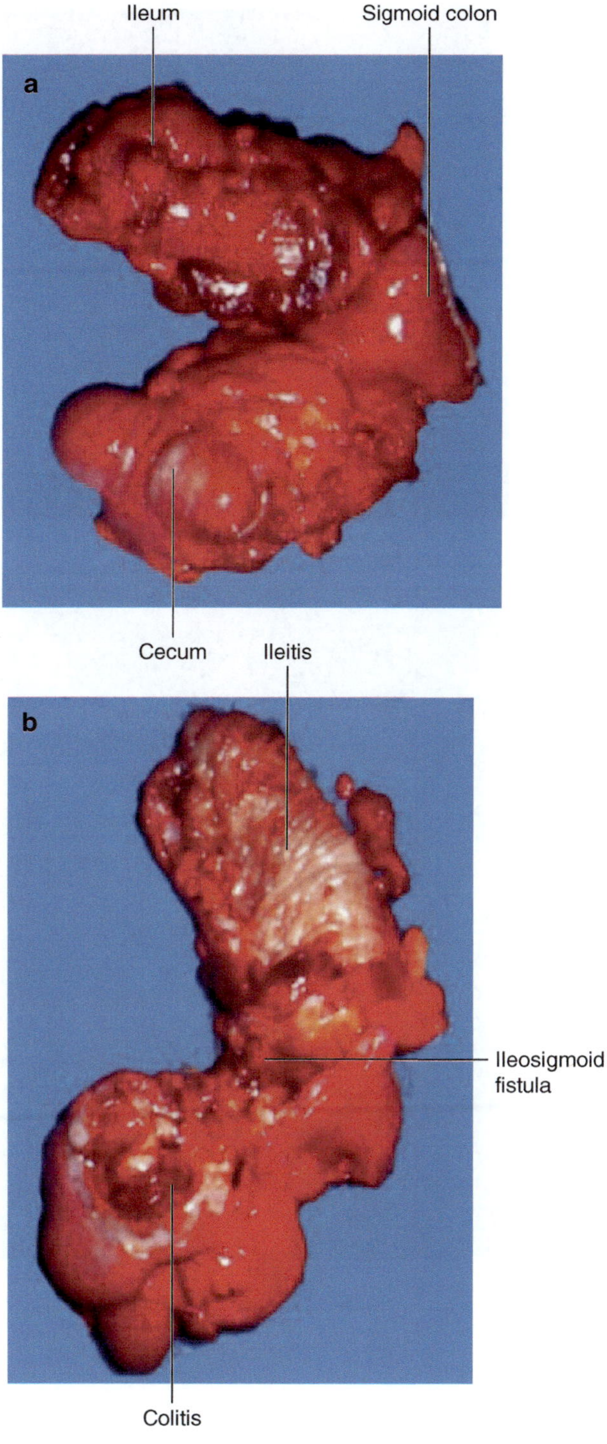

Fig. 5.7 (**a**–**d**) Ileocolitis, fistula and perianal disease

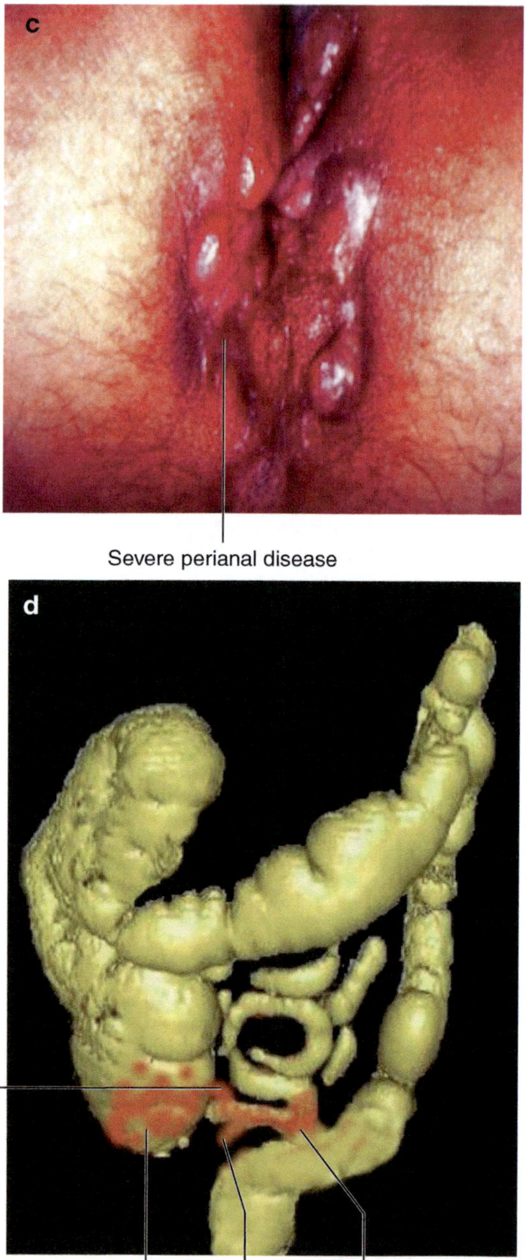

Fig. 5.7 (continued)

5.8 Ileocolitis Presenting as Ulcerative Colitis

Clinical Presentation A 35-year-old woman with a 16-year history of left-sided colitis, initially thought to be ulcerative colitis. At laparotomy for intractability, she was found to have colitis and inflammation in the terminal ileum consistent with Crohn's disease.

Diagnostic Studies Preoperative colonoscopy showed left-sided colitis (see Fig. 5.8c).

Surgical Treatment At laparotomy, the terminal ileum showed thickening of the bowel wall with creeping of the mesenteric fat consistent with Crohn's disease. Similar findings were seen in the left colon. She underwent an extended ileocolic resection with Brooke ileostomy (see Fig. 5.8a, b).

Pathology Segment of small intestine showing chronic ileitis and segment of colon with active nonspecific colitis.

Follow-Up This patient did well and had an ileorectal anastomosis 3 months later. She returned after 2 years with right upper quadrant pain, and ERCP showed multiple strictures of the right hepatic and common bile duct consistent with sclerosing cholangitis, which required a cholecysto-jejunostomy.

Comment Distinguishing ulcerative colitis from Crohn's colitis in some instances can be very difficult. Obtaining a small bowel study to rule out ileal disease is often helpful and may prevent surgical surprises, such as in this case. This patient was originally scheduled for an ileoanal pullthrough but underwent a subtotal colectomy with resection of the terminal ileum and ileostomy when she was found to have an inflamed terminal ileum consistent with Crohn's disease. The inflammation in the colon did not have specific features of Crohn's colitis even when the specimen was examined histologically. Since the rectum showed only mild disease, she was able to have an ileorectal anastomosis 3 months later (Fig. 5.8).

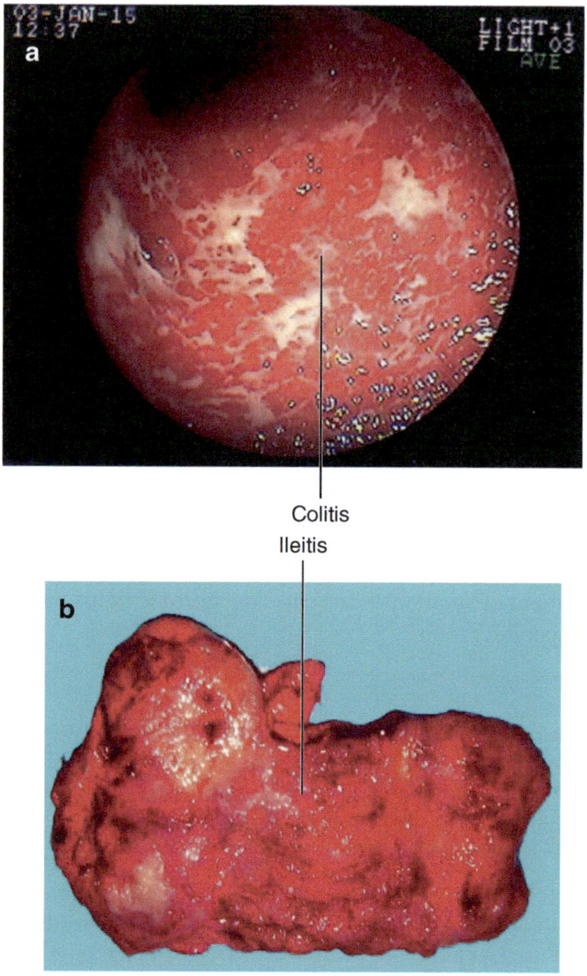

Fig. 5.8 (a–c) Ileocolitis presenting as ulcerative colitis

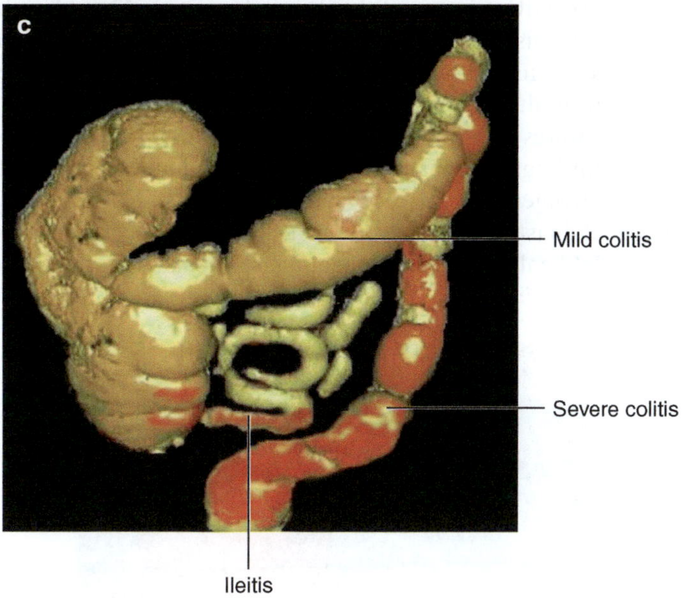

Fig. 5.8 (continued)

5.9 Ileocolitis Presenting as Ulcerative Colitis

Clinical Presentation A 43-year-old woman presenting with intractable ulcerative colitis. She underwent restorative proctocolectomy with mucosectomy and J-pouch anal anastomosis. Five years later, she developed a pelvic abscess and was found to have several fistulas at the ileoanal anastomosis including an anovaginal fistula.

Diagnostic Studies Pouch endoscopy showed edema, inflammation, and stricture at the ileoanal anastomosis with multiple perianal and anovaginal fistulas (see Fig. 5.9c).

Surgical Treatment Surgery confirmed the stricture at the ileoanal anastomosis with perianal and anovaginal fistulas. She underwent an abdominoperineal resection of the neorectum with Brooke ileostomy (see Fig. 5.9a, b).

Pathology Previous colectomy specimen showed universal ulcerative colitis with normal ileum. The pouch mucosa had chronic nonspecific inflammation, and the ileoanal anastomosis had multiple sinus tracts. No granulomas were seen.

Follow-Up The patient is doing well 4 years after abdominoperineal resection of the neorectum and Brooke ileostomy. The perineal wound healed well.

Comment This patient had typical ulcerative colitis and an ileoanal pullthrough operation was performed. She did well initially but 5 years later developed a large pelvic abscess with stricture of the ileoanal anastomosis and multiple perianal and rectovaginal fistulas. She initially required a loop ileostomy and eventually underwent excision of the pelvic pouch. Examination of the pouch showed inflammation with multiple sinus tracts at the ileoanal anastomosis. Although this patient has features of Crohn's disease, it is difficult to confirm the diagnosis based on the findings of nonspecific pouchitis and associated perianal fistulas, since these changes may also be seen in patients with ulcerative colitis, where the ileoanal anastomosis does not heal well. In this case, the late onset of fistulas after initial healing of the ileoanal anastomosis is more likely to represent Crohn's disease (Fig. 5.9).

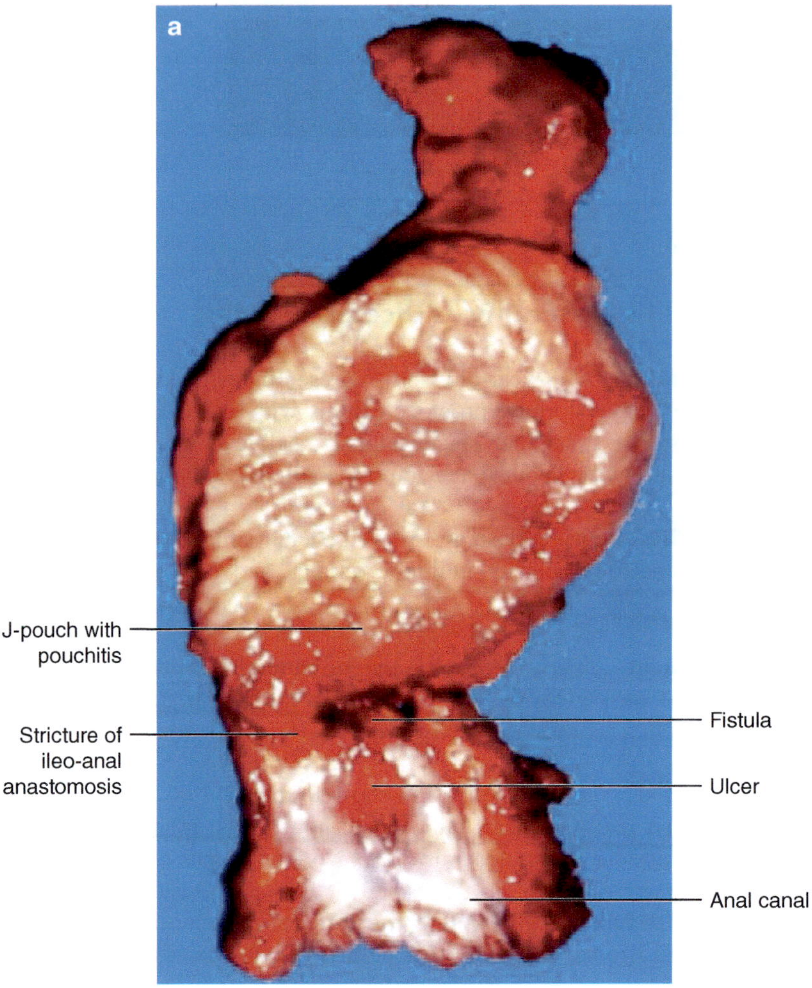

Fig. 5.9 (**a–c**) Ileocolitis presenting as ulcerative colitis

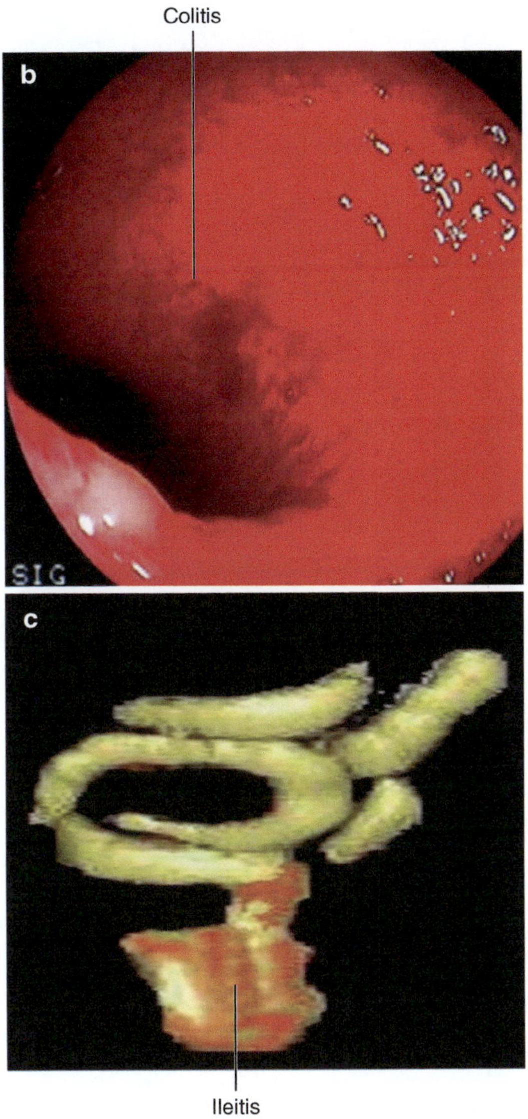

Fig. 5.9 (continued)

Further Reading

Greenstein AJ, Sachar DB, Tzakis A, Sher L, Heimann T, Aufses AH Jr. The course of enterovesical fistulae in Crohn's disease. Am J Surg. 1984;147:788–92.

Tartter PI, Heimann TM, Aufses AH Jr. Blood transfusion, skin test reactivity and lymphocytes in inflammatory bowel disease. Am J Surg. 1986;151:358–61.

6 Granulomatous Colitis

Tomas M. Heimann and Robert J. Kurtz

Granulomatous colitis may present as a limited segmental process or involve the entire colon and rectum. The features that lead to surgery are strictures with partial obstruction, intractability with diarrhea and bleeding, fistula with abscess formation, and perianal disease. Patients with segmental disease and those with rectal sparing are usually treated with resection and anastomosis.

Patients with severe rectal or perianal disease may require resection with ileostomy or colostomy. Distinguishing Crohn's colitis from ulcerative colitis may, on occasion, be quite difficult even after histologic examination of the resected colon. In general, patients with perianal disease should not undergo ileoanal pull-through operations even when examination of the colon reveals findings consistent with ulcerative colitis since the likelihood of failure is great. Patients in this category often behave like patients with perianal Crohn's disease and the possibility of serious complications resulting from exacerbation of the perianal disease is high. When possible, these patients should have a subtotal colectomy with ileorectal anastomosis. The final diagnosis of Crohn's disease may on occasion require several years to establish and may not become clear until there is recurrent disease in the small bowel or progression of perianal disease.

6.1 Segmental Granulomatous Colitis

Clinical Presentation A 56-year-old woman with Crohn's colitis for 10 years. She now has developed symptoms of left lower quadrant and pelvic pain associated with increasing constipation.

T. M. Heimann (✉) · R. J. Kurtz
Department of Surgery, Icahn School of Medicine at Mount Sinai, New York, NY, USA
e-mail: Tomas.Heimann@mountsinai.org; Robert.Kurtz@mountsinai.org

T. M. Heimann (ed.), *Atlas of Surgical Treatment of Inflammatory Bowel Disease*, https://doi.org/10.1007/978-3-031-62431-5_6

Diagnostic Studies Colonoscopy showed a stricture in the area of the distal sigmoid colon at 20 cm. CT scan showed a mass in the sigmoid colon with narrowing of the lumen. Small bowel series was normal (see Fig. 6.1b, c).

Surgical Treatment She underwent a segmental sigmoid resection with anastomosis (see Fig. 6.1a).

Pathology Sigmoid colon showing chronic inflammation and diverticulosis. The margins of resection are unremarkable.

Follow-Up This patient had an uneventful postoperative recovery. She is well 6 months later. She required repair of an incisional hernia, which developed in the lower portion of the incision. Several years later, she required an ileocolic resection for Crohn's ileocolitis.

Comment This type of segmental colitis presents with chronic pain and increasing obstructive symptoms. In older patients, it is often associated with the presence of sigmoid diverticula, and the diagnosis of Crohn's colitis may be difficult to differentiate from diverticulitis. Sigmoid resection with anastomosis is the treatment of choice. Observation of patients with Crohn's colitis and stricture carries some risk, since occasionally the narrowing may be due to the presence of a colonic adenocarcinoma. Progression of the disease to involve the small bowel and extension to the rest of the colon is not unusual, as seen in this case (Fig. 6.1).

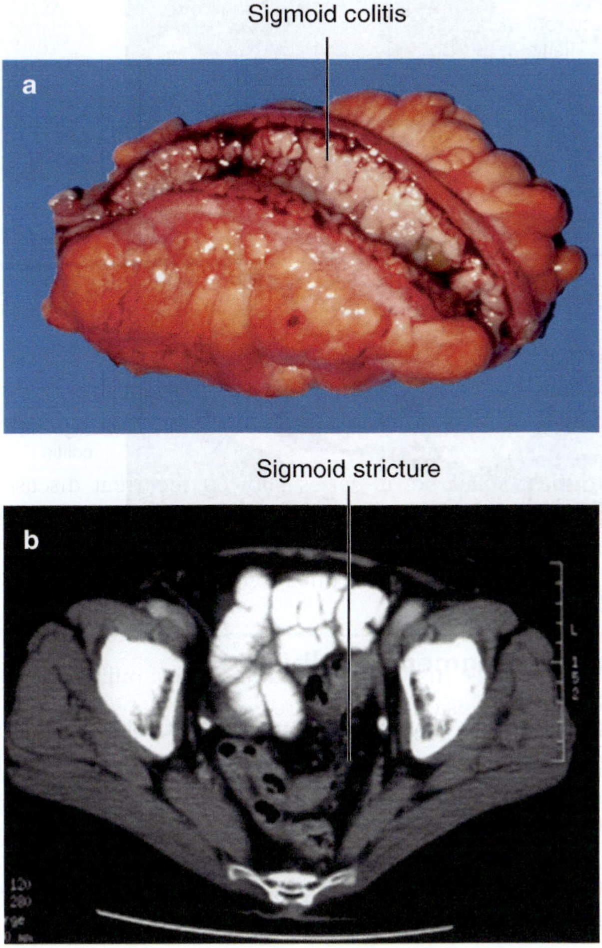

Fig. 6.1 Segmental Crohn's colitis

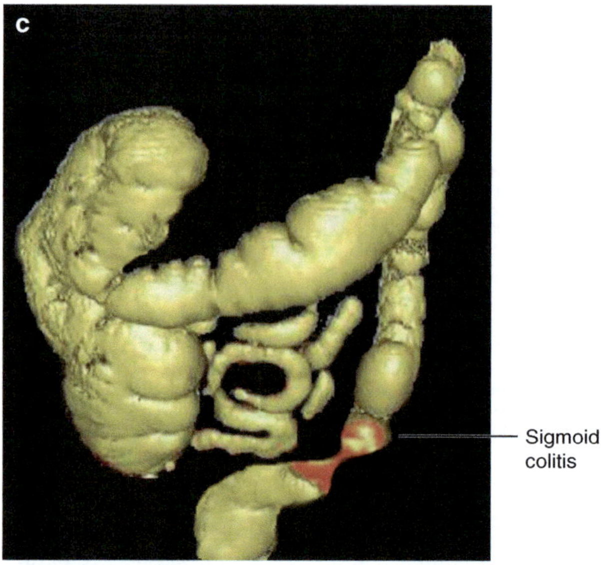

Fig. 6.1 (continued)

6.2 Recurrent Segmental Colitis

Clinical Presentation A 31-year-old woman with Crohn's colitis since age 16. She underwent a previous segmental sigmoid resection 5 years prior to this admission. She now comes in with recurrent disease manifested by a stricture at the site of the previous anastomosis.

Diagnostic Studies Colonoscopy showed a stricture at the descending colon with segmental colitis at this site (see Fig. 6.2b, c).

Surgical Treatment Secondary segmental resection of the descending colon with mobilization of the splenic flexure (see Fig. 6.2a).

Pathology, Active Crohn's colitis with inflammatory polyps. No granulomas were seen. The margins of resection are unremarkable.

Follow-Up This patient had an uneventful recovery after surgery and did well for several years. She now has progression of her colitis with involvement of nearly the entire colon and rectum and may require a proctocolectomy with ileostomy.

Comment This is an example of recurrent disease after segmental resection. This patient had a limited resection 5 years ago and now returns with a short segment of recurrent disease presenting as a stricture. Since the area of disease remained localized, she was able to have another segmental resection. Although the margins of resection are normal and there is no evidence of disease elsewhere in the intestinal tract, this young woman, with early onset of Crohn's disease and two intestinal resections, is at high risk of developing early recurrence. She now has extension of the disease involving most of the colon and rectum and after over 20 years of Crohn's disease may soon require a proctocolectomy and ileostomy (Fig. 6.2).

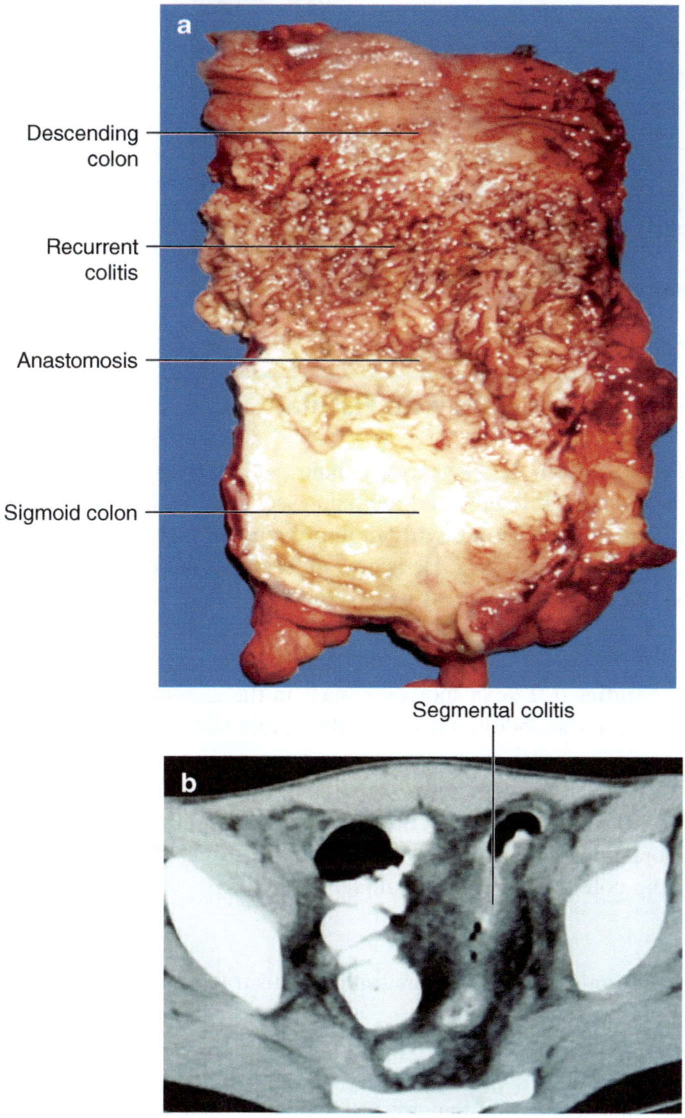

Fig. 6.2 Recurrent segmental colitis

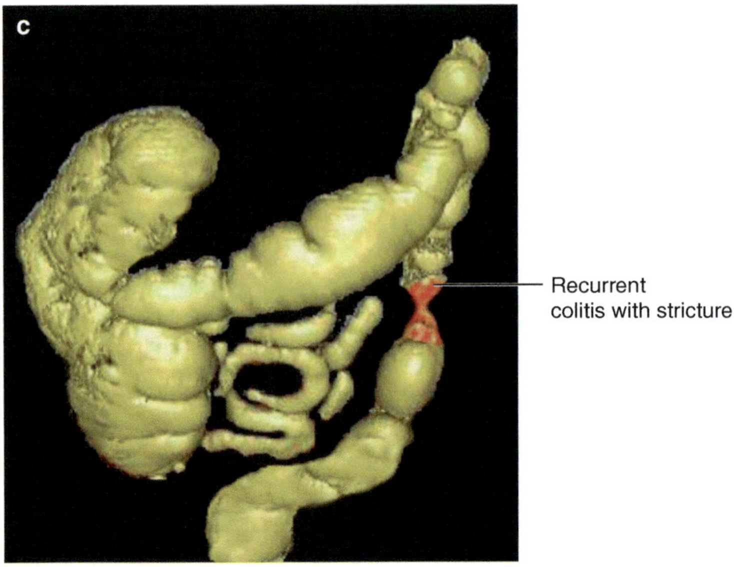

Fig. 6.2 (continued)

6.3 Segmental Colitis with Fistula

Clinical Presentation A 34-year-old male with Crohn's colitis for 12 years. Recently developed left lower quadrant pain associated with fever and night sweats. After treatment with antibiotics without improvement, he underwent drainage of an abscess in the left inguinal area. He is now afebrile but has enteric contents draining through the site where the abscess was opened.

Diagnostic Studies CT scan showed a mass in the area of the sigmoid colon with gas extending into the abdominal wall at the fistula site (see Fig. 6.3b, c).

Surgical Treatment This patient underwent a sigmoid resection with anastomosis and a temporary loop ileostomy. There was no residual abscess. The small bowel and remaining colon appeared normal (see Fig. 6.3a).

Pathology Crohn's colitis with penetrating sinus tracts and acute and chronic serositis. No granulomas are found.

Follow-Up This patient had an uneventful recovery. The loop ileostomy was closed 3 months later, and he is well 1 year after surgery.

Comment This patient presented with an abdominal wall abscess resulting from a sigmoid fistula. Once the abscess was incised, he improved but developed an enterocutaneous fistula. Treatment consisted of sigmoid resection with end-to-end anastomosis. In order to protect the anastomosis in this case, a temporary loop ileostomy was performed, which was closed 3 months later. We prefer to use loop ileostomies instead of loop colostomies for temporary diversion when the ileum is normal. These ileostomies are easier to care for than colostomies and closure is performed with a functional end to end stapled anastomosis using a small peristomal incision (Fig. 6.3).

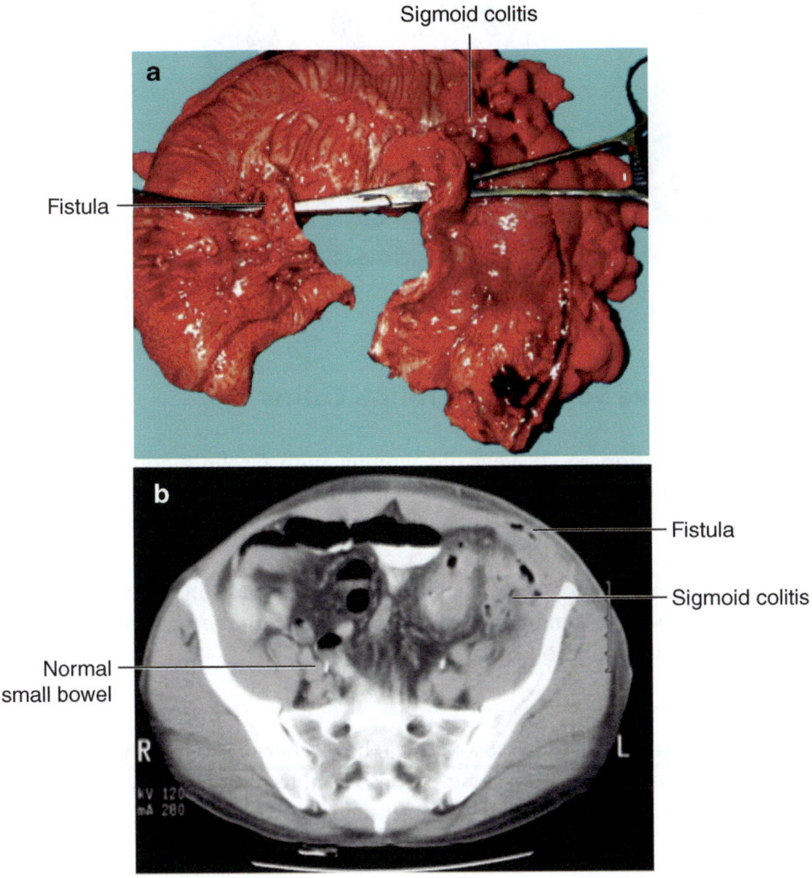

Fig. 6.3 Segmental colitis with fistula

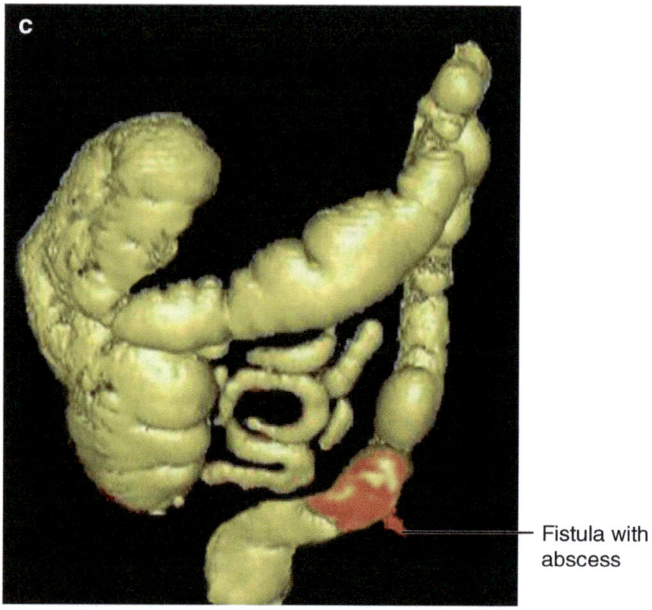

Fig. 6.3 (continued)

6.4 Extensive Segmental Crohn's Colitis

Clinical Presentation A 78-year-old woman with Crohn's colitis for 33 years. Recent increase in symptoms with weight loss and chronic anemia.

Diagnostic Studies Colonoscopy showed severe disease in the right colon with multiple pseudopolyps. Small bowel series showed a large paraesophageal hiatus hernia with normal small bowel (see Fig. 6.4c, d).

Surgical Treatment Large paraesophageal hiatus hernia, segmental colitis with an inflammatory mass in the transverse colon. A subtotal colectomy was performed with ileosigmoid anastomosis and repair of the hiatus hernia (see Fig. 6.4a, b).

Pathology Active Crohn's colitis with segmental inflammatory stenosis, fissuring, ulceration, and transmural chronic inflammation of the transverse colon. Occasional epithelioid granulomas are present. The remaining colon shows mild inflammation.

Follow-Up She had an uneventful recovery after surgery, her weight returned to normal, and the chronic anemia, which was previously unresponsive to iron, has improved significantly. She is doing well 5 years later.

Comment This patient has a long history of Crohn's disease and no previous operations. The indication for surgery is chronic anemia from blood loss from the inflamed colon. The area of most severe inflammation is the transverse colon. The left colon is unremarkable and the rectum is spared. She underwent a subtotal colectomy with ileosigmoid anastomosis and repair of a large paraesophageal hiatus hernia. Following surgery, her blood count rapidly returned to normal (Fig. 6.4).

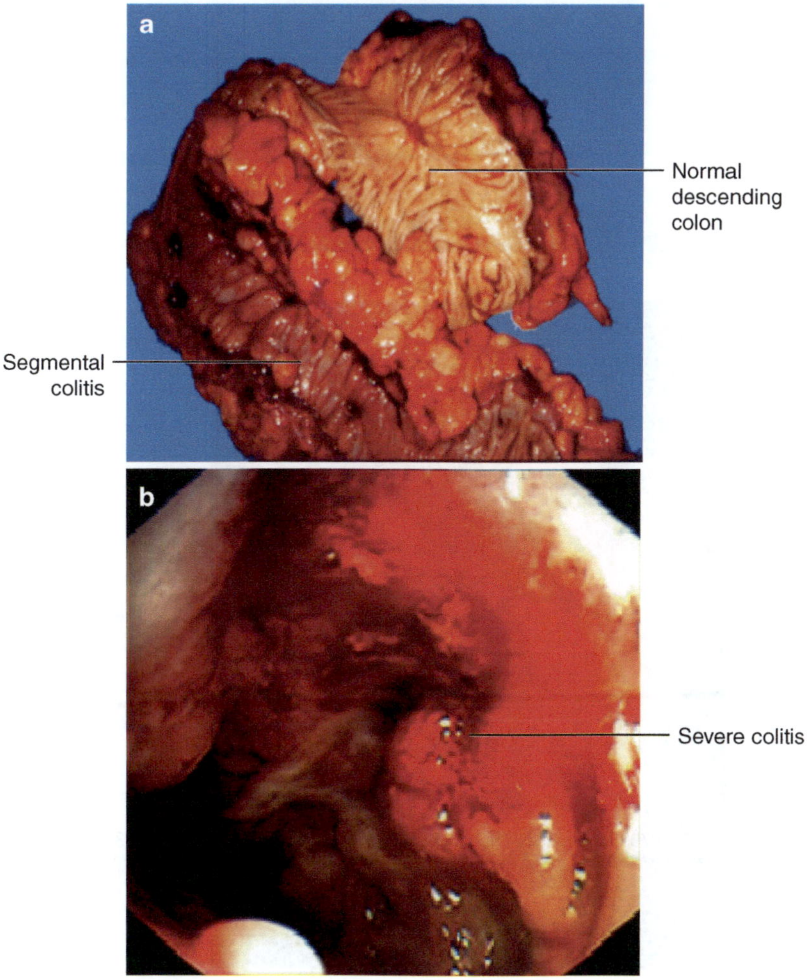

Fig. 6.4 Extensive segmental Crohn's colitis

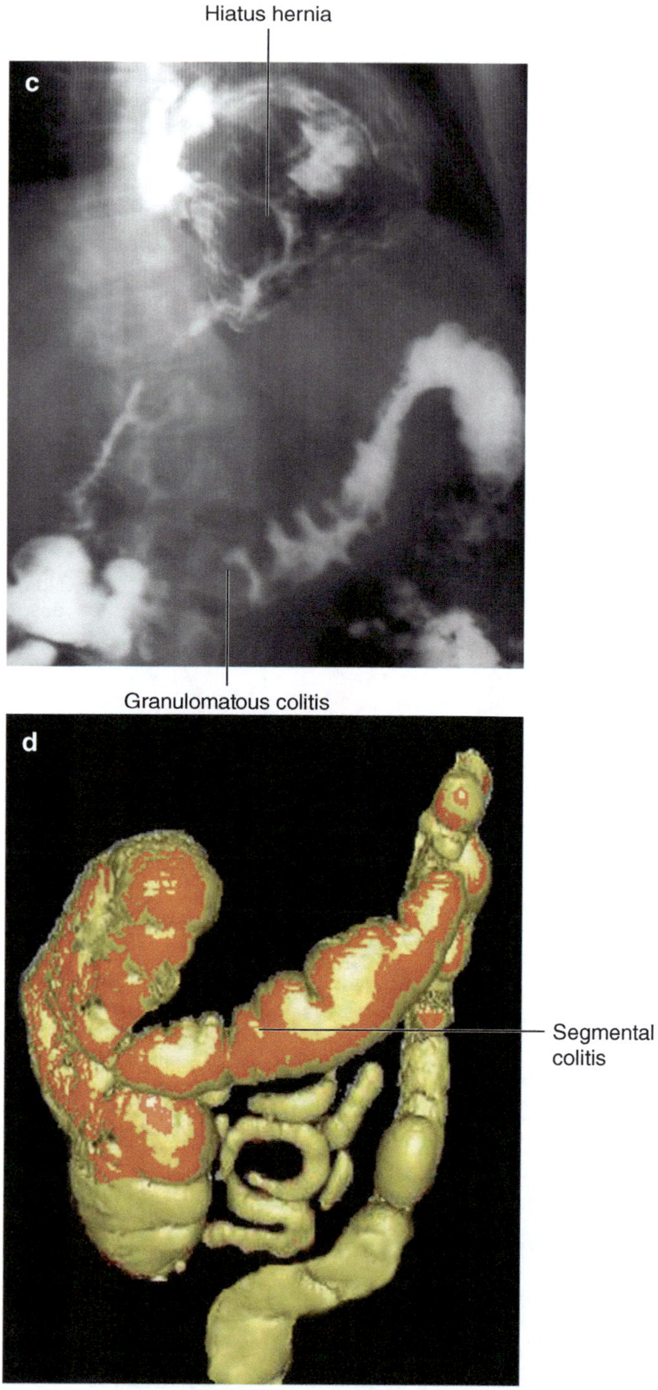

Fig. 6.4 (continued)

6.5 Granulomatous Colitis with Rectal Sparing

Clinical Presentation A 28-year-old woman with a 6-year history of colitis with rectal sparing. Her symptoms have increased recently and are manifested by abdominal pain and bloody diarrhea. She is chronically anemic but has not required any blood transfusions. The colon is palpable on abdominal exam, and she is tender in the left lower quadrant over the sigmoid colon.

Diagnostic Studies Colonoscopy showed mild rectal inflammation with severe colitis throughout the remaining colon with deep ulcerations and cobblestoning of the regenerating mucosa (see Fig. 6.5b).

Surgical Treatment This patient underwent a total colectomy with ileorectal anastomosis. The small bowel was normal (see Fig. 6.5a).

Pathology Severe granulomatous colitis with extensive ulceration, pseudopolyposis, and crypt abscesses.

Follow-Up She recovered well following surgery. Her anemia improved rapidly with oral iron supplements, and she is doing well several years later.

Comment This is a common presentation for patients with moderately severe granulomatous colitis. The rectum is often spared, and therefore, a subtotal colectomy with ileorectal anastomosis is feasible. These patients require continued medical treatment following surgery in order to prevent a recurrence in the neoterminal ileum and to avoid exacerbation in the residual rectum. Many of these patients eventually require further surgery and some may need resection of the rectum with a Brooke ileostomy. Most patients in this age group would rather have an anastomosis with a higher possibility of requiring further surgery than a permanent ileostomy and a lower recurrence potential (Fig. 6.5).

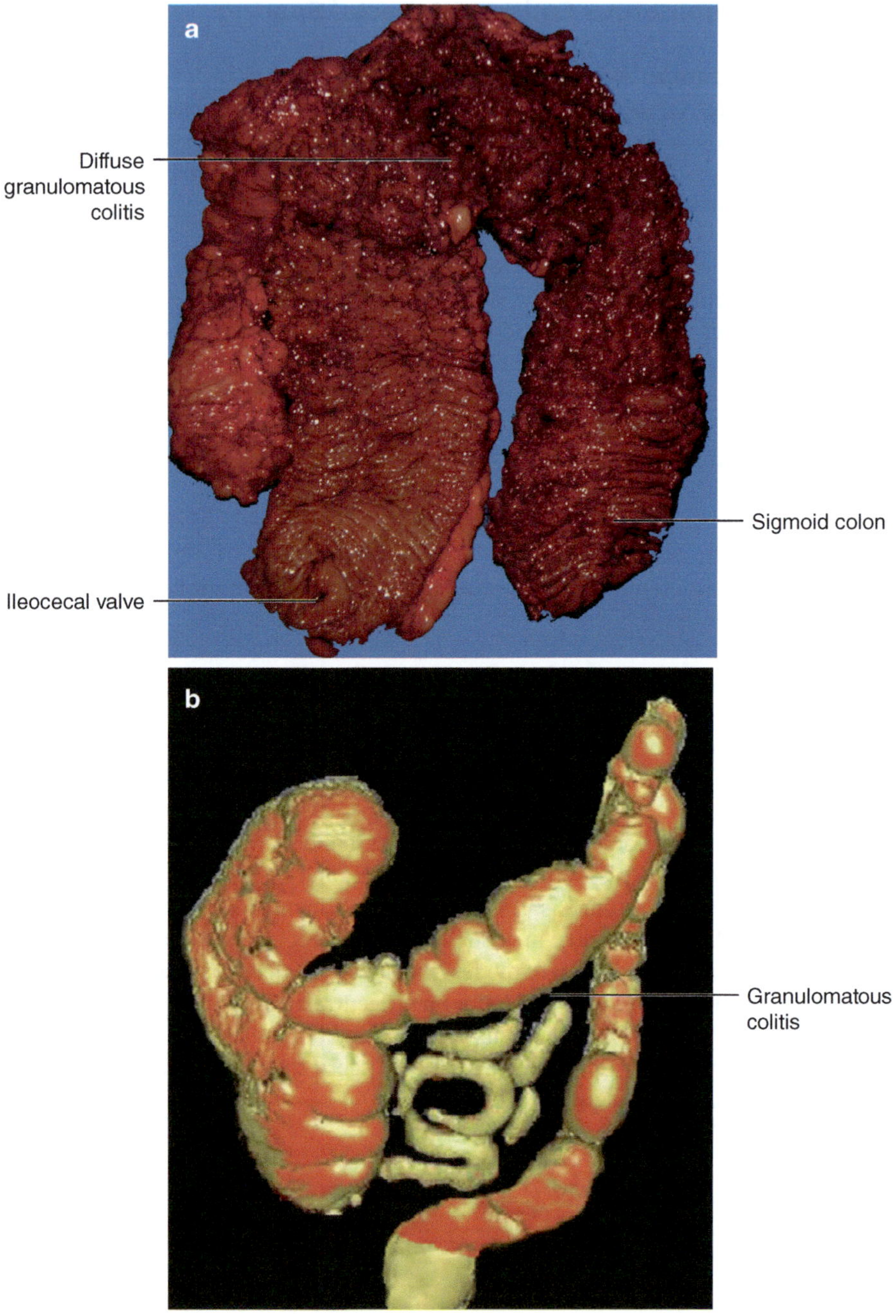

Fig. 6.5 Granulomatous colitis with rectal sparing

6.6 Granulomatous Proctitis with Stricture

Clinical Presentation A 37-year-old man with Crohn's disease for 20 years. He has severe granulomatous colitis with a perianal fistula and a stricture of the distal rectum, which precludes colonoscopic surveillance.

Diagnostic Studies Anorectal exam showed a healed fistulotomy scar. The distal rectum could be examined with difficulty using the smallest diameter pediatric sigmoidoscope and showed severe inflammation. Barium enema showed an 8 cm stricture of the distal rectum. Intraoperative endoscopy confirmed the presence of severe rectal disease and showed that the rest of the colon was unremarkable (see Fig. 6.6c).

Surgical Findings Normal small bowel and colon with severe anorectal disease. He underwent an abdominoperineal resection of the rectum with a sigmoid colostomy (see Fig. 6.6a, b).

Pathology Crohn's proctocolitis with transmural chronic inflammation and stricture. Multiple nonnecrotizing epithelioid cell granulomas are present.

Follow-Up He did well following surgery. The perineal wound healed well. He is currently asymptomatic and irrigates the colostomy every other day.

Comment This patient demonstrates the severity of rectal disease in granulomatous colitis. The perianal disease manifested by a perianal fistula was relatively mild and responded to surgical treatment. The severity of the rectal inflammation, however, produced a strictured ulcerated rectum, which eventually required surgical resection. Difficulty with surveillance colonoscopy as well as severity of symptoms unresponsive to medical treatment were the main indications for surgery. He has adapted well to the colostomy (Fig. 6.6).

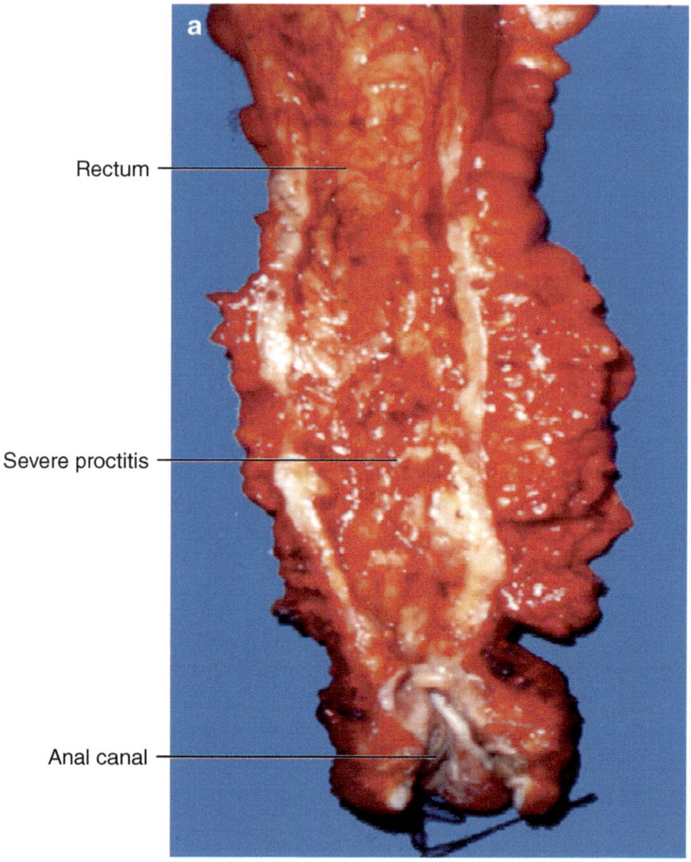

Fig. 6.6 Granulomatous proctitis with stricture

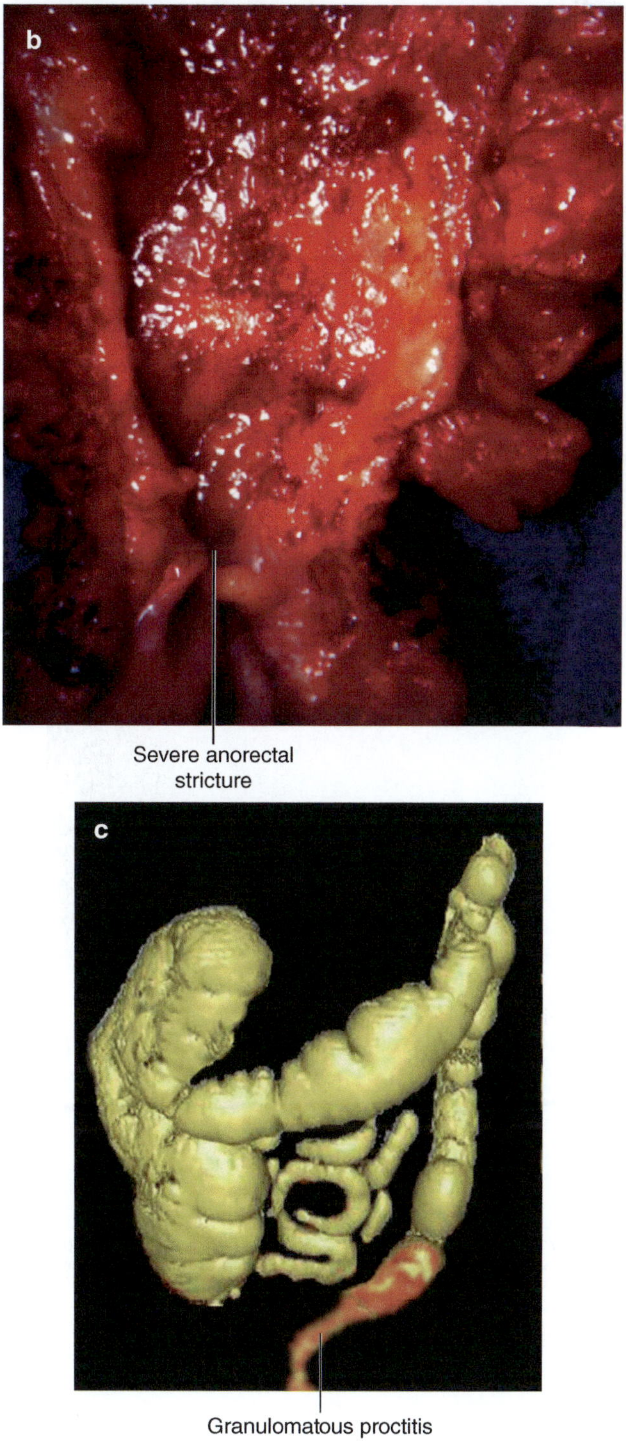

Fig. 6.6 (continued)

Further Reading

Greenstein AJ, Panveliwalla D, Katz LB, Heimann T, Donelly J, Pertsemlidis D, Geller S, Smith HS, Aufses AH Jr. Tissue carcinoembryonic antigen, dysplasia and disease duration in colonic inflammatory bowel disease. Am J Gastroenterol. 1982;77:212–5.

Heimann TM, Miller F, Martinelli G, Szporn A, Greenstein AJ, Aufses AH Jr. Correlation of presence of granulomas with clinical and immunologic parameters in Crohn's disease. Arch Surg. 1988;123:46–8.

Extensive Granulomatous Colitis

7

Tomas M. Heimann and Robert J. Kurtz

Extensive granulomatous colitis causes symptoms that mimic those seen in ulcerative colitis.

Granulomatous colitis differs, however, from ulcerative colitis in that it is more likely to form strictures and fistulas in adjacent organs that are common. In addition, the presence of perianal disease makes granulomatous colitis more difficult to treat. Patients with impassable strictures, which prevent surveillance of the colon, often require colectomy. In addition to intractability, colorectal cancer risk in granulomatous colitis seems to be increased and is probably similar to that seen in ulcerative colitis. The surgical treatment of granulomatous colitis, if the rectum is spared, is subtotal colectomy with ileorectal anastomosis.

When there is severe rectal or perianal disease, proctocolectomy may be necessary. Except in very unusual circumstances, patients with granulomatous colitis and colorectal cancer should undergo proctocolectomy and ileostomy.

7.1 Crohn's Presenting as Ulcerative Colitis

Clinical Presentation A 73-year-old man with the diagnosis of ulcerative colitis present for 30 years. Recent increase in symptoms with weight loss, diarrhea, and bleeding requiring hospitalization and blood transfusion. There was no improvement in his symptoms with a course of high-dose steroids.

Diagnostic Studies Severe colitis with multiple pseudopolyps seen on recent colonoscopy (see Fig. 7.1d).

T. M. Heimann (✉) · R. J. Kurtz
Department of Surgery, Icahn School of Medicine at Mount Sinai, New York, NY, USA
e-mail: Tomas.Heimann@mountsinai.org; Robert.Kurtz@mountsinai.org

T. M. Heimann (ed.), *Atlas of Surgical Treatment of Inflammatory Bowel Disease*, https://doi.org/10.1007/978-3-031-62431-5_7

Surgical Treatment A proctocolectomy and Brooke ileostomy were performed. The colon showed severe colitis without the typical stigmata of Crohn's disease, and the small bowel was normal (see Fig. 7.1a, b, c).

Pathology Severely active Crohn's proctocolitis with patchy ulcerations, inflammatory polyposis, and mucosal chronic inflammation. Lymphoid aggregates are present in the deep submucosa and subserosa with epithelioid cell granulomas seen in several sections.

Follow-Up The patient had an uneventful postoperative recovery. He developed a stricture of the ileostomy, which required a superficial revision 2 months later. He is doing well and returned to his normal weight. The perineal wound required several months to heal completely.

Comment This patient had recent exacerbation of his colitis manifested by severe diarrhea, weight loss, and bleeding. The endoscopic appearance of the colon was consistent with severe ulcerative colitis, and the small bowel was normal. The presence of epithelioid granulomas, however, was pathognomonic of granulomatous colitis. If this patient had been younger, he would have had an ileoanal pull-through procedure, since colonoscopic biopsies prior to surgery did not reveal the presence of granulomas and the appearance of the colon at the time of surgery was not typical of Crohn's disease. Although there was no perianal disease, the chance of failure after the ileoanal pull-through operation is significantly higher in patients with Crohn's colitis (Fig. 7.1).

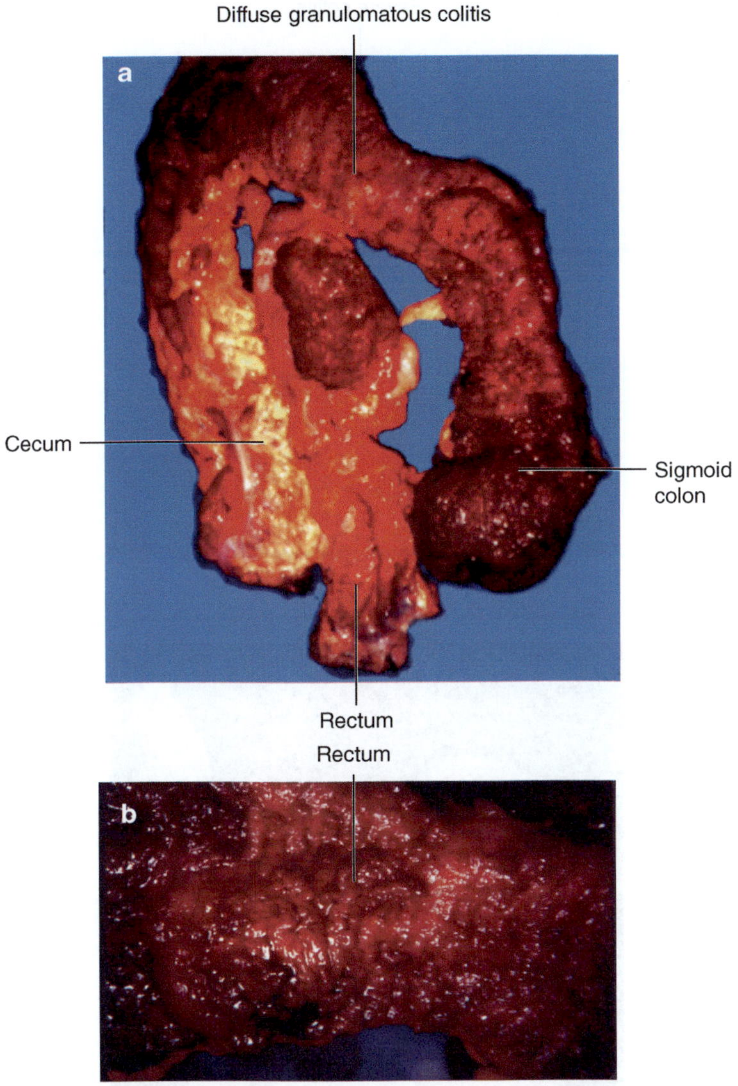

Fig. 7.1 (**a**–**d**) Crohn's presenting as ulcerative colitis

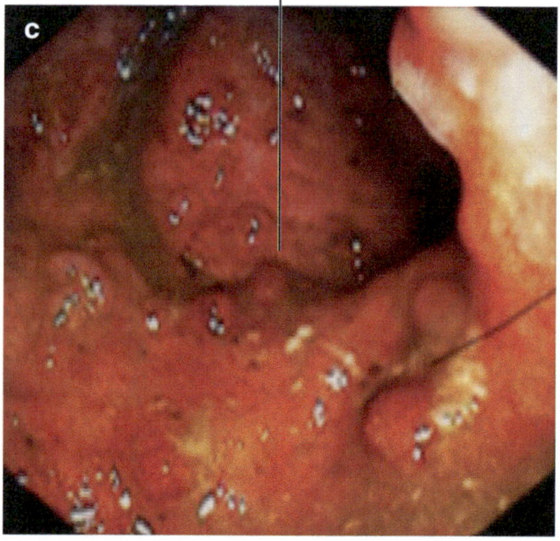

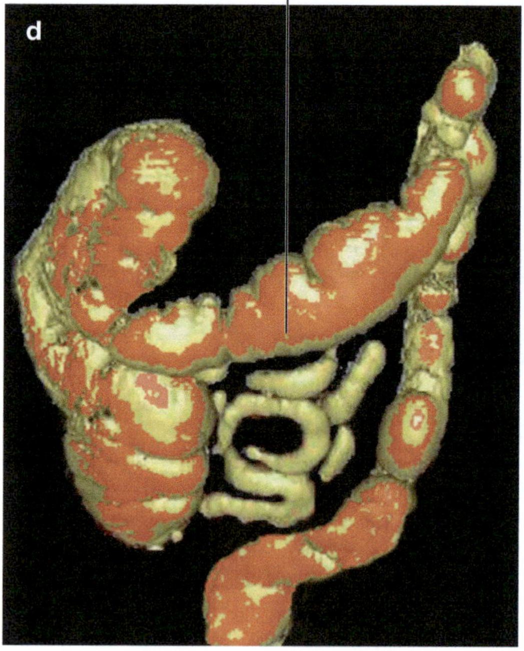

Fig. 7.1 (continued)

7.2 Crohn's Colitis with Gastrocolic Fistula

Clinical Presentation A 53-year-old man with a history of colitis for 33 years. This patient has a stricture in the transverse colon, which is causing increasing symptoms of obstruction. Physical exam showed mild abdominal distention. The patient also had a chronic perianal fistula.

Diagnostic Studies Barium enema showed a narrow stricture in the transverse colon. On colonoscopy, the colon and rectum showed inflammation up to the stricture site. The colonoscope could not be advanced past the stricture (see Fig. 7.2c, d).

Surgical Treatment He underwent a total proctocolectomy and Brooke ileostomy. At the time of surgery, a small cologastric fistula was found, which was treated with a limited wedge resection of the greater curve of the stomach. The perianal fistula was excised with the rectum (see Fig. 7.2a, b).

Pathology Crohn's colitis involving the entire colon and rectum with segmental inflammatory stenosis. No epithelioid were granulomas seen. The ileum was unremarkable.

Follow-Up He recovered well and is asymptomatic 3 years later. The perineal wound healed well.

Comment The gastrocolic fistula in this patient was asymptomatic and was not seen on the preoperative studies. His main symptom was partial obstruction from the colonic stricture. Since the entire colon and rectum were diseased and he also had perianal disease with a fistula, he required a proctocolectomy and Brooke ileostomy. The indications for surgery in this patient were obstructive symptoms with colonic distention and the inability to survey the colon since the stricture was too narrow to pass an endoscope. The perineal wound in patients with perianal disease often heals slowly and revisions may be necessary (Fig. 7.2).

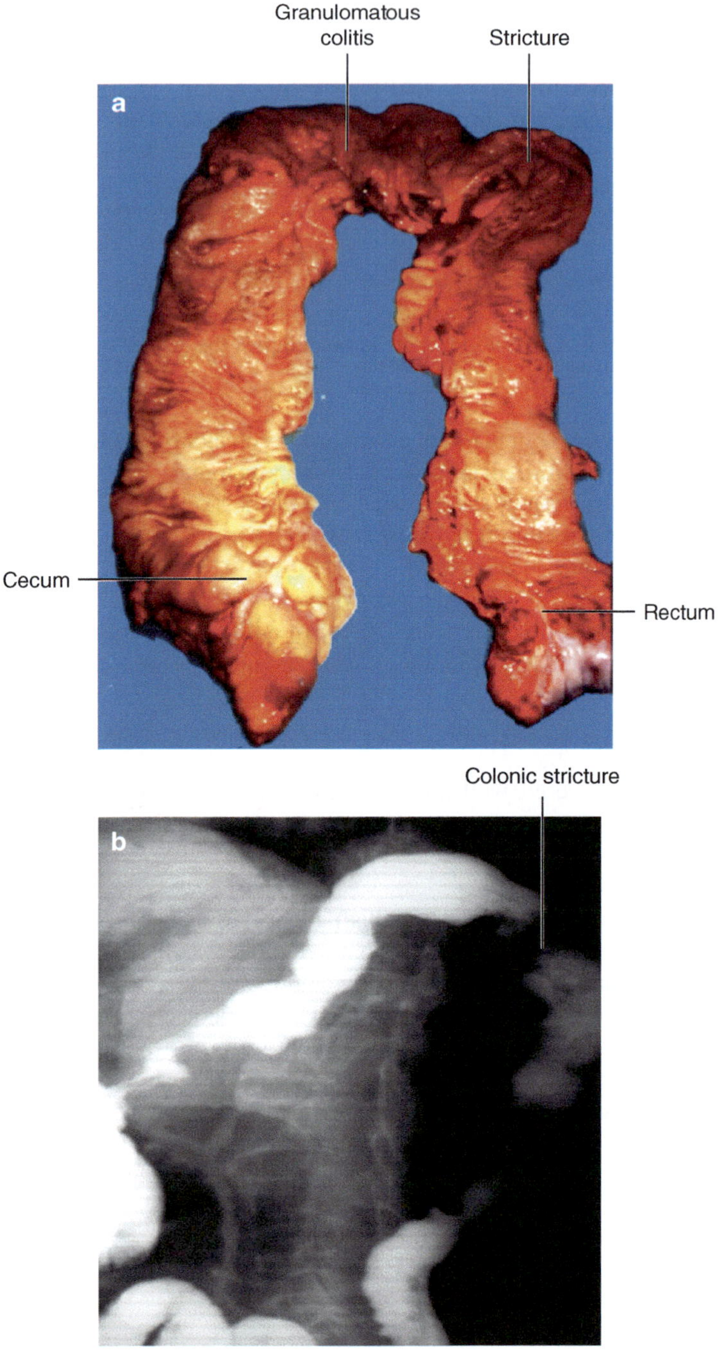

Fig. 7.2 (**a**–**d**) Crohn's colitis with gastrocolic fistula

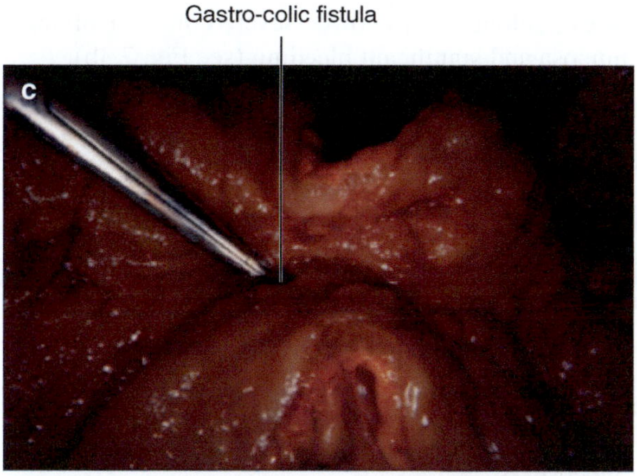

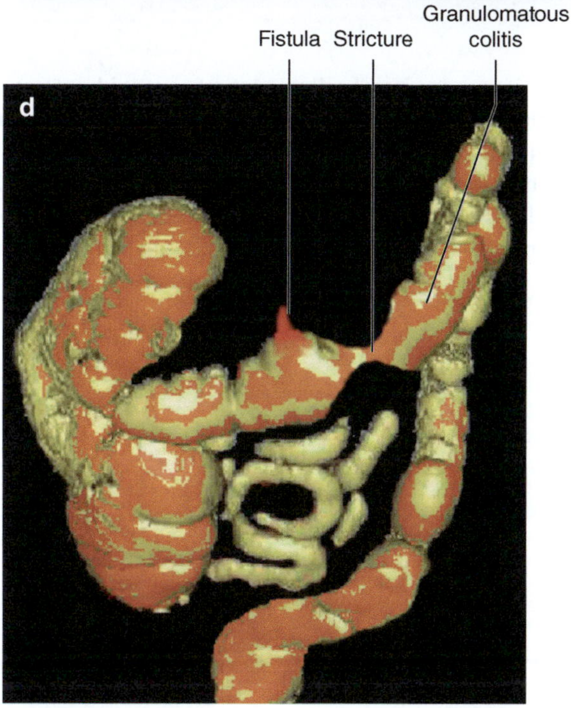

Fig. 7.2 (continued)

7.3 Crohn's Colitis with Bleeding

Clinical Presentation A 33-year-old Jehovah's Witness woman presenting with a recent onset of colitis manifested by rectal bleeding and severe diarrhea. She developed anemia, which did not improve with aggressive medical management of her Crohn's disease. As her hematocrit continued to decline and she would not accept blood products, surgical treatment became necessary.

Diagnostic Studies Colonoscopy showed severe colitis involving the entire colon with ulcerated mucosa and significant bleeding (see Fig. 7.3b).

Surgical Treatment Subtotal colectomy and ileostomy (see Fig. 7.3a).

Pathology Universal active Crohn's colitis with numerous aphthous ulcers and epithelioid granulomas. The ileal segment is unremarkable.

Follow-Up She has done well since surgery. The bleeding has stopped and her hemoglobin is stable. She had an ileorectal anastomosis performed 1 year later and remains well after 3 years.

Comment This patient was severely ill when first seen with intractable colitis. She was anemic and bleeding and did not respond to treatment with intravenous steroids. Following an urgent subtotal colectomy and ileostomy, she recovered rapidly and her hemoglobin returned to normal levels. She subsequently underwent ileorectal anastomosis and is doing well. In this patient, ileorectal anastomosis has a much lower risk of intraoperative blood loss than proctectomy, and she was very eager to have the ileostomy closed (Fig. 7.3).

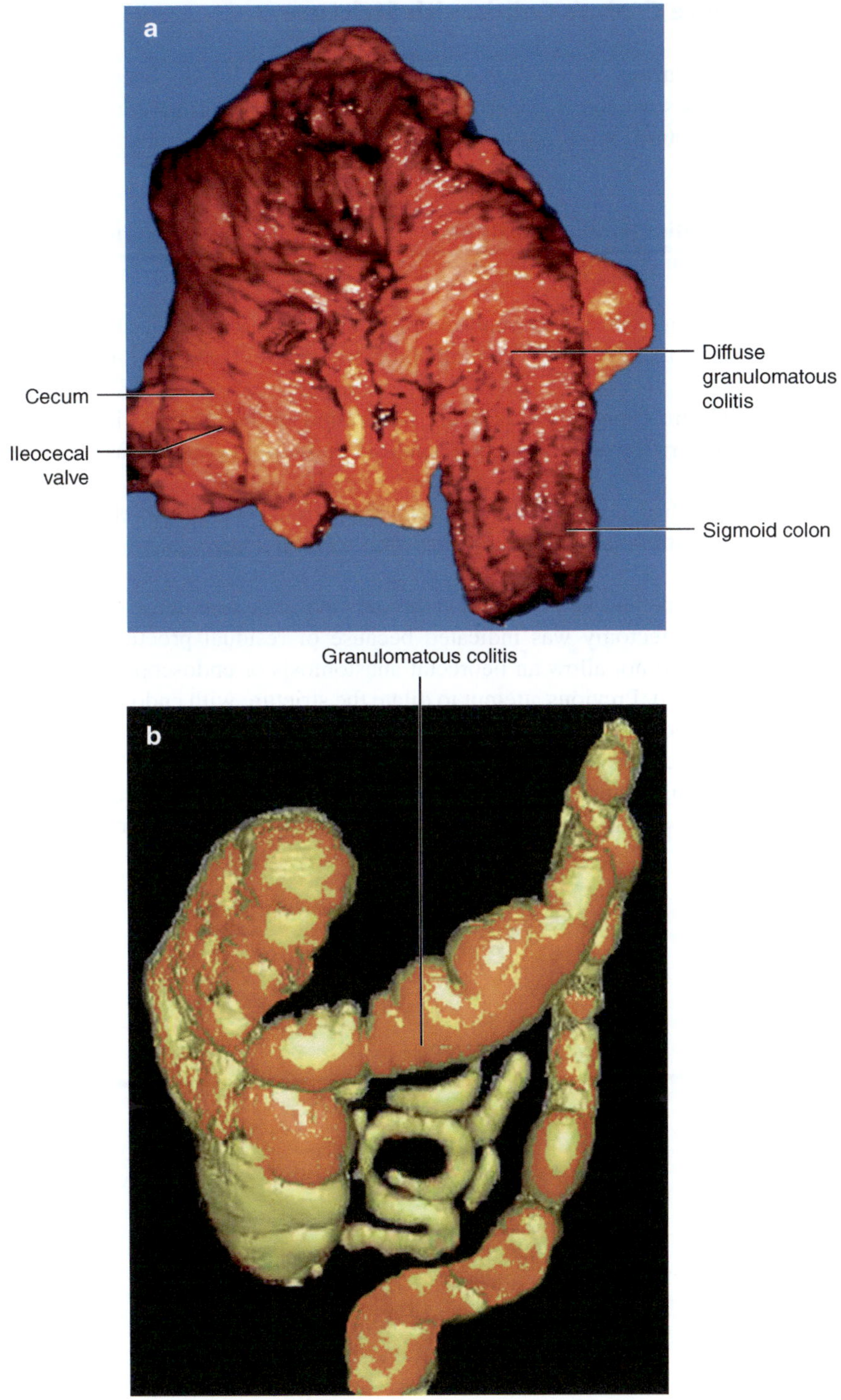

Fig. 7.3 (**a**, **b**) Crohn's colitis with bleeding

7.4 Severe Crohn's Colitis with Stricture

Clinical Presentation 24 year old woman with Crohn's disease since age 11. Has had 4 resections since age 17. Currently has an ileostomy and severe residual disease in the rectum with multiple strictures making endoscopic surveillance impossible.

Diagnostic Studies Normal small bowel series and ileoscopy. Severe stricture at anorectal junction (see Fig. 7.4b, c).

Surgical Findings She underwent completion proctectomy with abdominoperineal resection of the remaining sigmoid colon and rectum (see Fig. 7.4a).

Pathology Crohn's proctocolitis with transmural inflammation, inflammatory stricture and ulceration at the anorectal junction. Epithelioid granulomas are present.

Follow-Up She had an uneventful recovery, the perineal wound was closed primarily and healed without any problems. She is doing well 2 years later.

Comment This patient had minimal symptoms from the remaining disease in the rectum. The proctectomy was indicated because of residual proctitis and severe stricture which did not allow an ileorectal anastomosis or endoscopic surveillance of the rectosigmoid. Previous attempt to dilate the stricture with endoscopy resulted in a perforation of the rectum. In the absence of perianal sepsis, as in this patient, perineal wounds can be closed primarily with a good chance of rapid healing without infection. This patient has aggressive disease with early onset and has already had 5 operations. She is at high risk for further early recurrence of her Crohn's disease (Fig. 7.4).

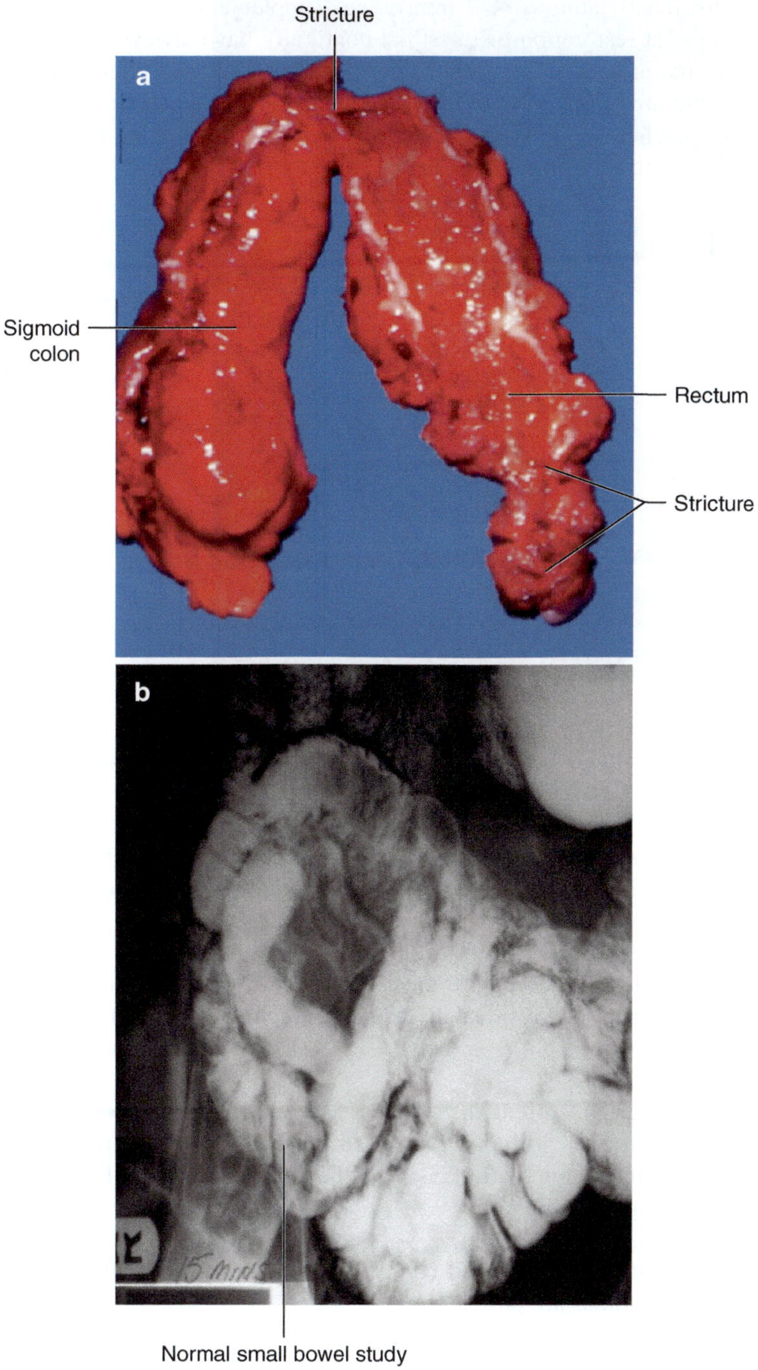

Fig. 7.4 (**a**–**c**) Severe Crohn's colitis with stricture

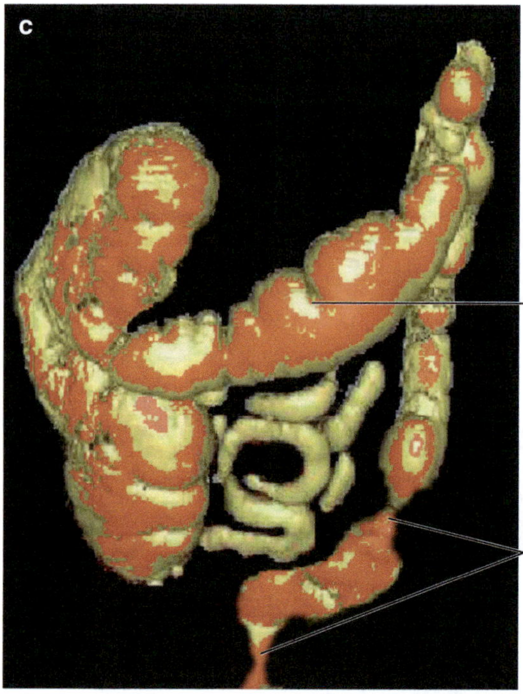

Fig. 7.4 (continued)

7.5 Severe Crohn's Colitis with Stricture

Clinical Presentation 27 year old woman with recurrent Crohn's disease 3 years following subtotal colectomy with ileorectal anastomosis. Her symptoms are severe diarrhea and weight loss.

Diagnostic Studies Endoscopy revealed recurrent disease at the ileorectal anastomosis and exacerbation of residual disease in the rectum with a distal rectal stricture (see Fig. 7.5c).

Surgical Findings Recurrent disease in 15 cm segment of neoterminal ileum. Severe residual proctitis with distal rectal stricture. She underwent abdominoperineal resection of the rectum with excision of the diseased terminal ileum and Brooke ileostomy (see Fig. 7.5a, b).

Pathology Segment of ileum and rectum with transmural chronic inflammation. Epithelioid granulomas are present.

Follow-Up She had an uneventful postoperative recovery. There is no evidence of recurrent disease 4 years later.

Comment This patient had granulomatous colitis with initial rectal sparing and underwent a subtotal colectomy with ileorectal anastomosis. Although there was some disease in the rectum, it was mild and the patient did not want an ileostomy. She returns 3 years later with severe exacerbation of the residual proctitis and recurrent disease in the neoterminal ileum. This time, proctocolectomy with Brooke ileostomy was the only treatment available. Proctocolectomy with ileostomy has a much lower recurrence potential than colectomy with ileorectal anastomosis, yet most of our younger patients opt for ileorectal anastomosis rather than ileostomy if the rectal disease is mild. These patients know that this may be a temporary solution but still want to delay the need for ileostomy as long as possible (Fig. 7.5).

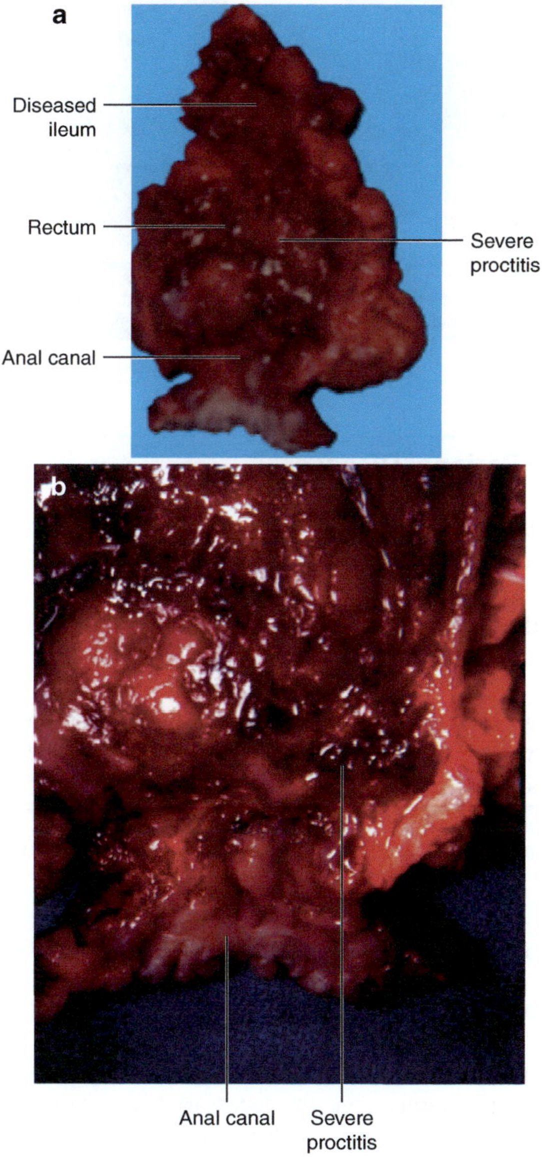

Fig. 7.5 (**a**–**c**) Severe Crohn's colitis with stricture

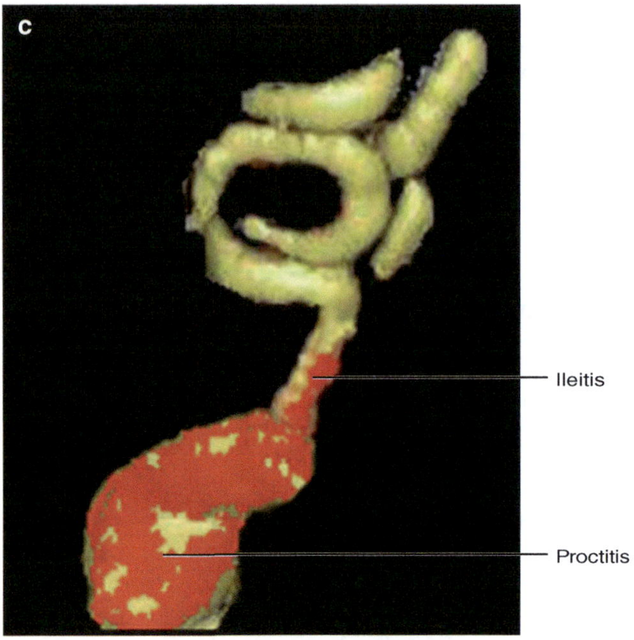

Fig. 7.5 (continued)

7.6 Severe Perianal Disease

Clinical Presentation A 38-year-old woman with Crohn's disease for 11 years presents with severe intractable perianal disease and multiple rectovaginal fistulas.

Diagnostic Studies Colonoscopy showed severe proctocolitis with multiple, extensive perianal and rectovaginal fistulas (see Fig. 7.6b).

Surgical Findings Severe proctocolitis with multiple perianal and rectovaginal fistulas. She underwent a total proctocolectomy with Brooke ileostomy. The small bowel was normal (see Fig. 7.6a).

Pathology Crohn's colitis with active transmural inflammation. No granulomas were found.

Follow-Up The perineal wound healed gradually following surgery, and 3 months later, a 3 × 2 cm area was still draining. This was treated conservatively with sitz baths and eventually healed several months later.

Comment This patient is an example of someone with granulomatous colitis and severe perianal disease. Surgery became necessary because of the increasing symptoms from the rectovaginal fistulas resulting in fecal incontinence. Healing of the perineal wound in the presence of multiple fistulas is always difficult. This patient eventually healed completely 6 months later. Occasionally a gracilis muscle flap may be necessary to fill the perineal space if the wound does not heal spontaneously. We usually wait at least 6 months before performing further surgery for the perineal wound (Fig. 7.6).

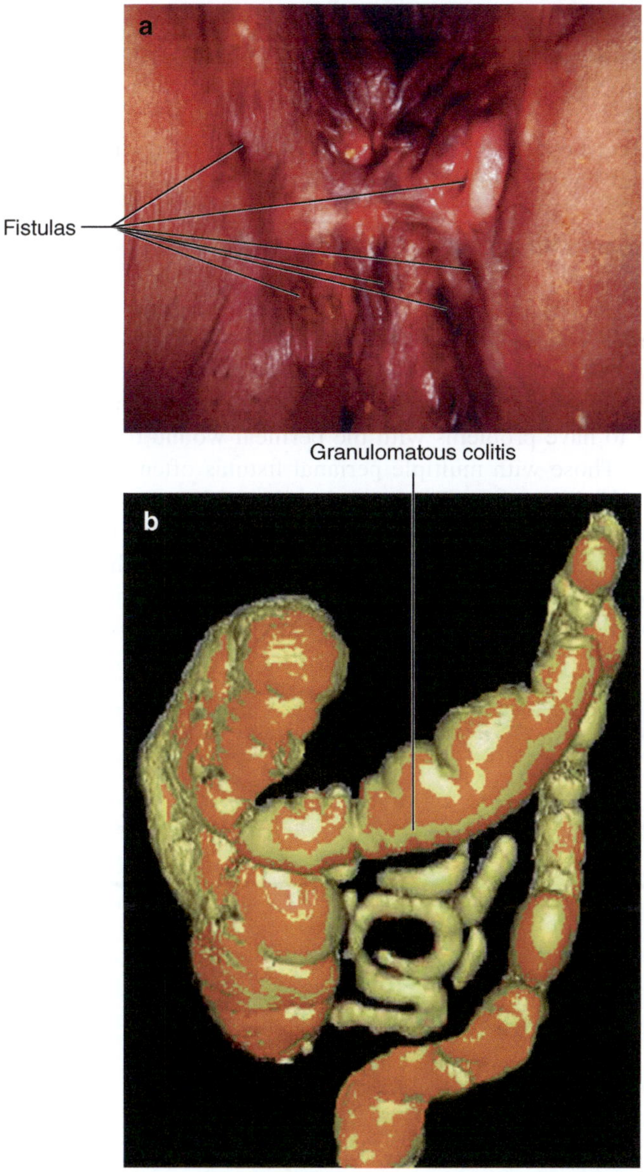

Fig. 7.6 (**a**, **b**) Severe perianal disease

7.7 Crohn's Colitis with Perianal Disease

Clinical Presentation A 52-year-old woman with Crohn's disease for 20 years. She had intractable colitis with perianal disease, which resulted in a total proctocolectomy and ileostomy. She had difficulty healing the perineal wound and required several surgical revisions. She is now being seen for severe perineal scarring and perineal pain. There are no residual fistulas, and the ileostomy is well healed.

Diagnostic Studies Small bowel series showed normal small bowel. CT scan and MRI of the pelvis showed no evidence of abscess or fistula (see Fig. 7.7c, d).

Surgical Treatment She underwent excision of the perineal scar with gracilis myocutaneous flap obtained from the right leg (see Fig. 7.7a, b).

Pathology Skin with hypertrophic scar.

Follow-Up The myocutaneous flap healed well, and she is markedly improved 3 years later.

Comment Patients with perianal Crohn's disease requiring proctectomy are more prone to have problems with the perineal wound than patients with ulcerative colitis. Those with multiple perianal fistulas often require wound revision such as seen in this patient. The result here was a hypertrophied scar with severe wound contracture. The use of gracilis myocutaneous flap in order to provide tissue to fill the perineum and skin to allow scar excision has provided excellent results. Most patients requiring these procedures have an unhealed perineal wound and usually require a gracilis muscle flap without the cutaneous component (Fig. 7.7).

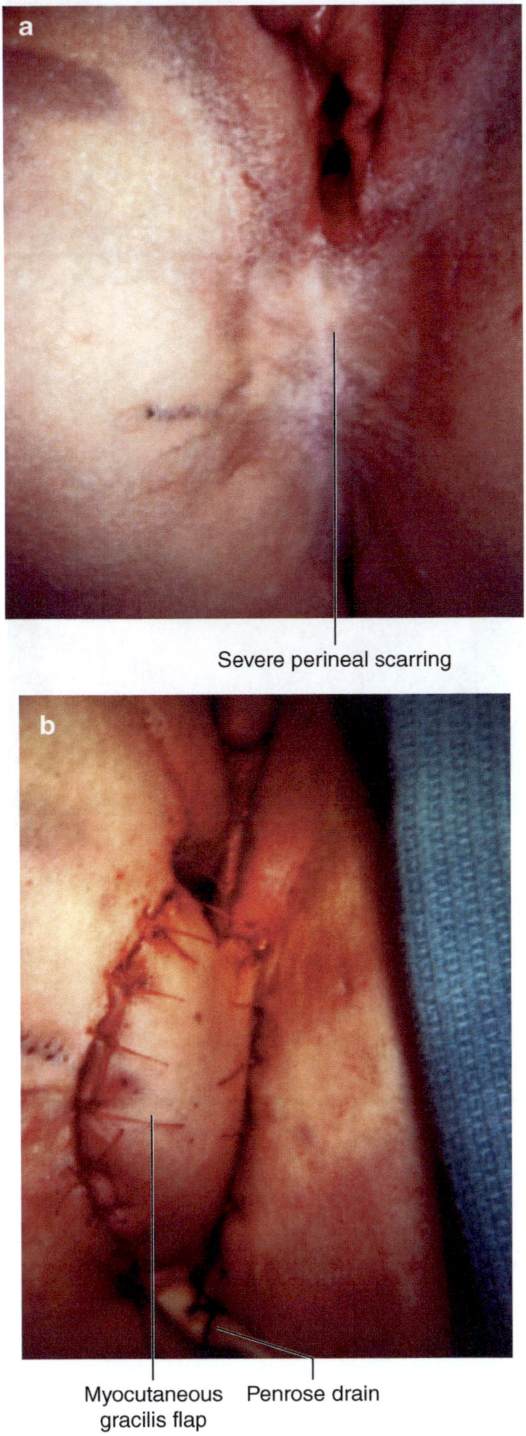

Fig. 7.7 (**a**–**d**) Crohn's colitis with perianal disease

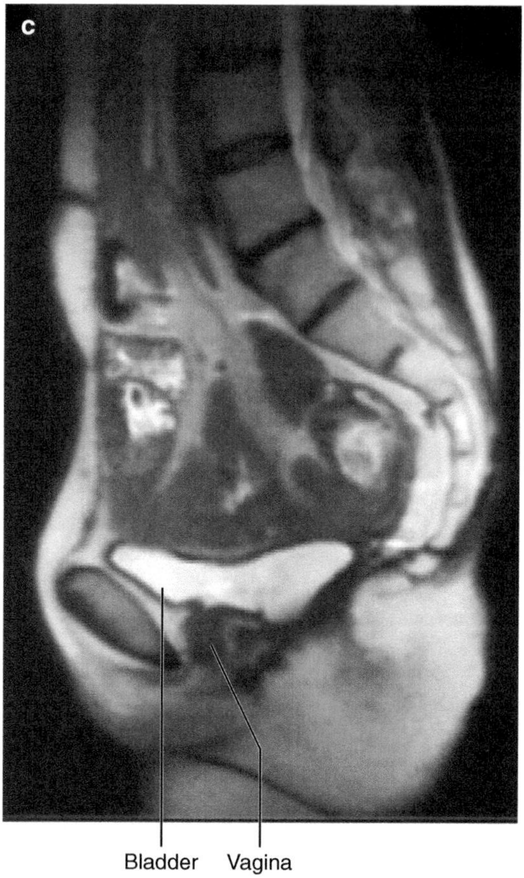

Fig. 7.7 (continued)

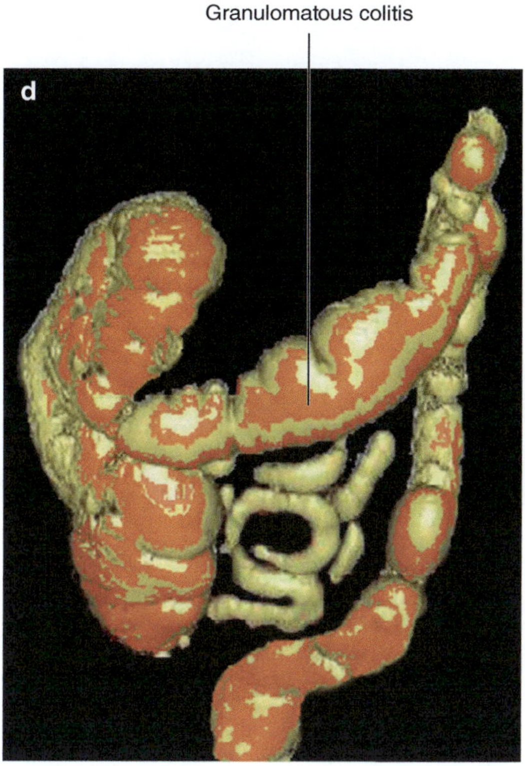

Fig. 7.7 (continued)

Further Reading

Greenstein A, Present DH, Sachar DB, Slater G, Heimann TM, Lachman P, Aufses AH Jr. Gastric fistulas in Crohn's disease: report of cases. Dis Col Rectum. 1989;32:888–92.

Heimann TM, Greenstein AJ, Mechanic L, Aufses AH Jr. Early complications following surgical treatment for Crohn's disease. Ann Surg. 1985;201:494–8.

Recurrent Ileitis with Obstruction and Stricture

8

Tomas M. Heimann and Robert J. Kurtz

The hallmark of Crohn's disease is the fact that it often recurs following surgical treatment. Recurrent disease has a predilection for anastomotic sites, and there is evidence that patients requiring multiple anastomosis are more likely to recur sooner than patients with ileostomy. Currently, postoperative chemoprophylaxis is indicated in patients with Crohn's disease after surgical resection in order to postpone the development of recurrence.

Patients with multiple previous operations who are at highest risk to develop recurrent disease should receive chemoprophylaxis after surgery even in the absence of any visible residual disease.

Recurrent ileitis often presents with symptoms of obstruction most often due to a stricture adjacent to the site of previous anastomosis. There is some evidence that end-end hand-sewn anastomosis are more likely to stricture sooner than side-to-side stapled anastomosis. Patients who originally presented with cicatrizing disease are prone to recur with strictures, while patients whose initial presentation was fistula and abscess tend to have fistulas and abscesses again when the disease recurs. In general, patients with cicatrizing disease tend to have longer symptom-free intervals between surgery than those presenting with recurrent abscess and fistula.

8.1 Recurrent Ileitis with Obstruction

Clinical Presentation A 29-year-old male with Crohn's disease since age 17 who returns 3 years after multiple strictureplasties and ileocolic resection with recurrent symptoms of obstruction. On physical examination, the patient appears thin from recent weight loss, and his abdomen is moderately distended.

T. M. Heimann (✉) · R. J. Kurtz
Department of Surgery, Icahn School of Medicine at Mount Sinai, New York, NY, USA
e-mail: Tomas.Heimann@mountsinai.org; Robert.Kurtz@mountsinai.org

T. M. Heimann (ed.), *Atlas of Surgical Treatment of Inflammatory Bowel Disease*, https://doi.org/10.1007/978-3-031-62431-5_8

Diagnostic Studies CT scan shows markedly dilated jejunum with a stricture in the mid small bowel. Small bowel series confirms these findings with a single stricture in the mid small bowel and collapsed distal ileum (see Fig. 8.1c, d).

Surgical Treatment The patient underwent a segmental resection of the small bowel at the site of the stricture with a stapled side-to-side anastomosis. The area of stricture was near the site of previous strictureplasty (see Fig. 8.1a, b).

Pathology Active Crohn's ileitis with transmural chronic inflammation and ulcerations. Non-necrotizing epithelioid cell granulomas are present. The resection margins are unremarkable.

Follow-Up Two months following surgery, the patient had gained 7 lb. His appetite had improved markedly, but he still had occasional cramps. He continues on medication for his residual Crohn's disease and for chronic arthritis.

Comment Marked dilatation of the small bowel is not uncommon in Crohn's disease. It results from chronic narrowing of the intestinal lumen to just a pinpoint opening. Initially, the patient may be able to compensate by adjusting his diet, but eventually, surgery becomes necessary to correct the problem. This patient had extensive small bowel disease. The site of previous strictureplasties was still open, but this stricture developed in an area of inflammation in the adjacent bowel (Fig. 8.1).

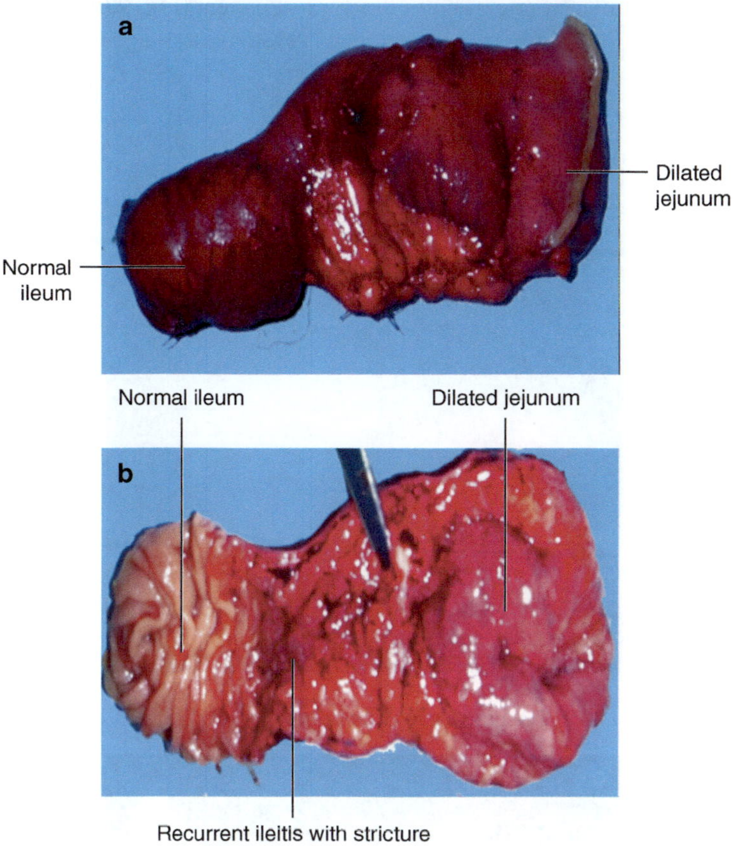

Fig. 8.1 Recurrent ileitis with obstruction

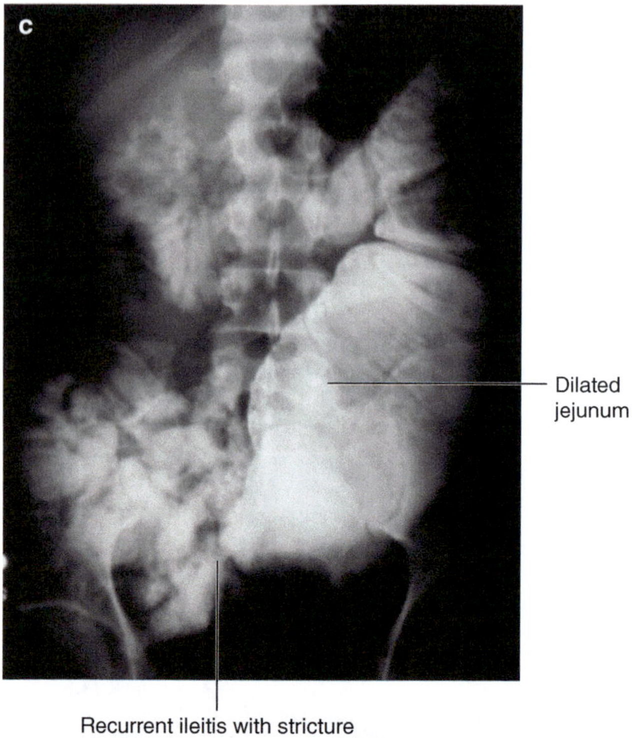

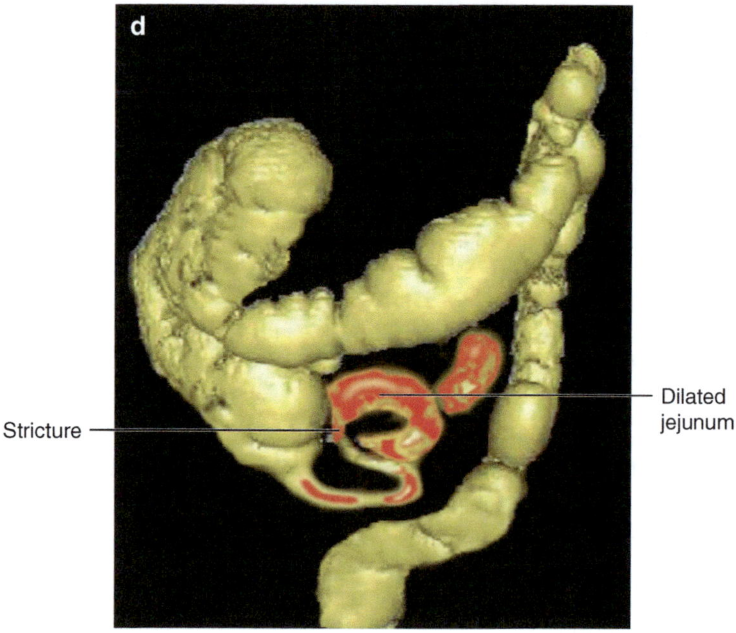

Fig. 8.1 (continued)

8.2 Recurrent Ileitis with Stricture

Clinical Presentation A 31-year-old male with nearly 20-year history of Crohn's disease. He had extensive small bowel resection about 10 years ago, followed by ileocolic resection and multiple strictureplasty 4 years ago for obstructive symptoms. He now returns with recent onset of increasing abdominal distention, cramps, and weight loss.

Diagnostic Studies Small bowel study showed short segment of remaining small bowel with dilated mid small bowel and multiple strictures. Colonoscopy showed a normal colon (see Fig. 8.2d, e, f).

Surgical Treatment The narrowed segment was limited to the mid small bowel with multiple strictures. The patient underwent a limited small bowel resection and three new strictureplasties (see Fig. 8.2a, b, c).

Pathology Severely active Crohn's enteritis with deep mucosal ulcerations, transmural inflammation, and inflammatory strictures. Nonnecrotizing epithelioid cell granulomas are present. Both margins show evidence of chronic inflammation.

Follow-Up His postoperative course was uneventful; he was able to regain the previously lost weight after surgery and has done well for 18 months.

Comment This patient has Crohn's disease since age 11 and has already required three operations. He has very aggressive disease of the small bowel with strong tendency to form strictures. Currently, the remaining 5 ft of small bowel is sufficient to maintain a normal nutritional status. The asymptomatic interval between operations seems to be decreasing, and this patient cannot afford to lose any more small bowel. He has so far required strictureplasties in six areas of the small intestine, and it is likely that further strictureplasties will be necessary in the future (Fig. 8.2).

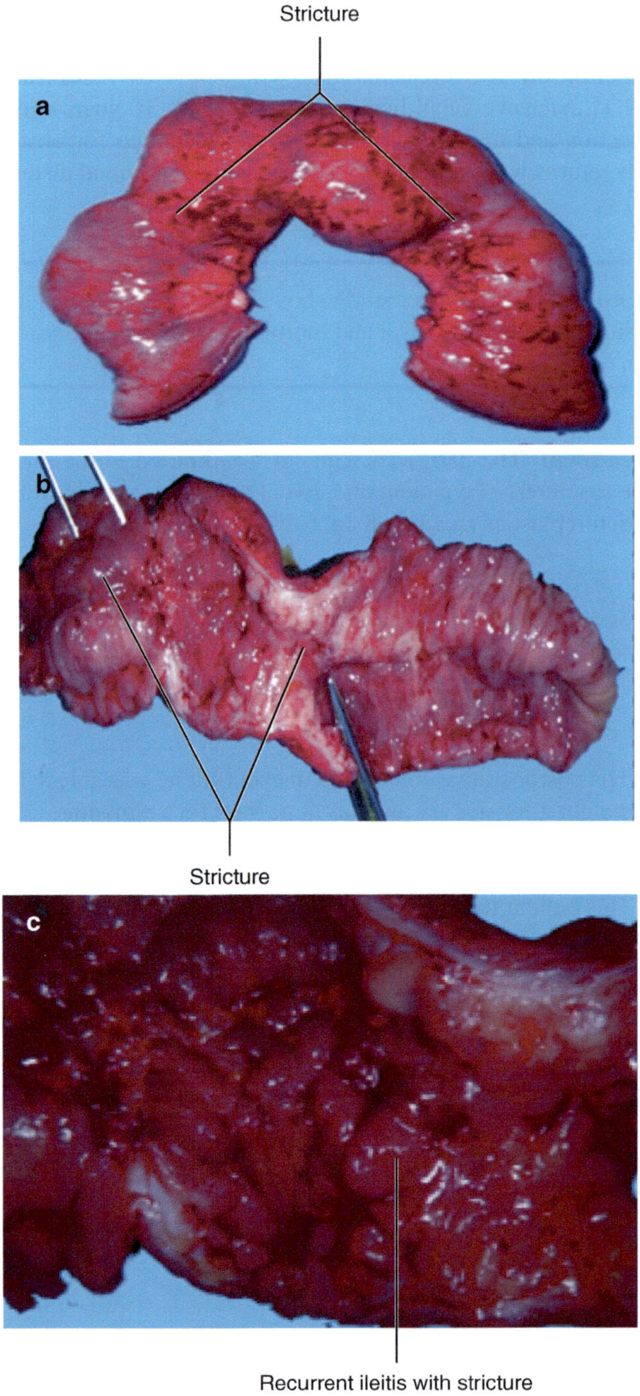

Fig. 8.2 Recurrent ileitis with stricture

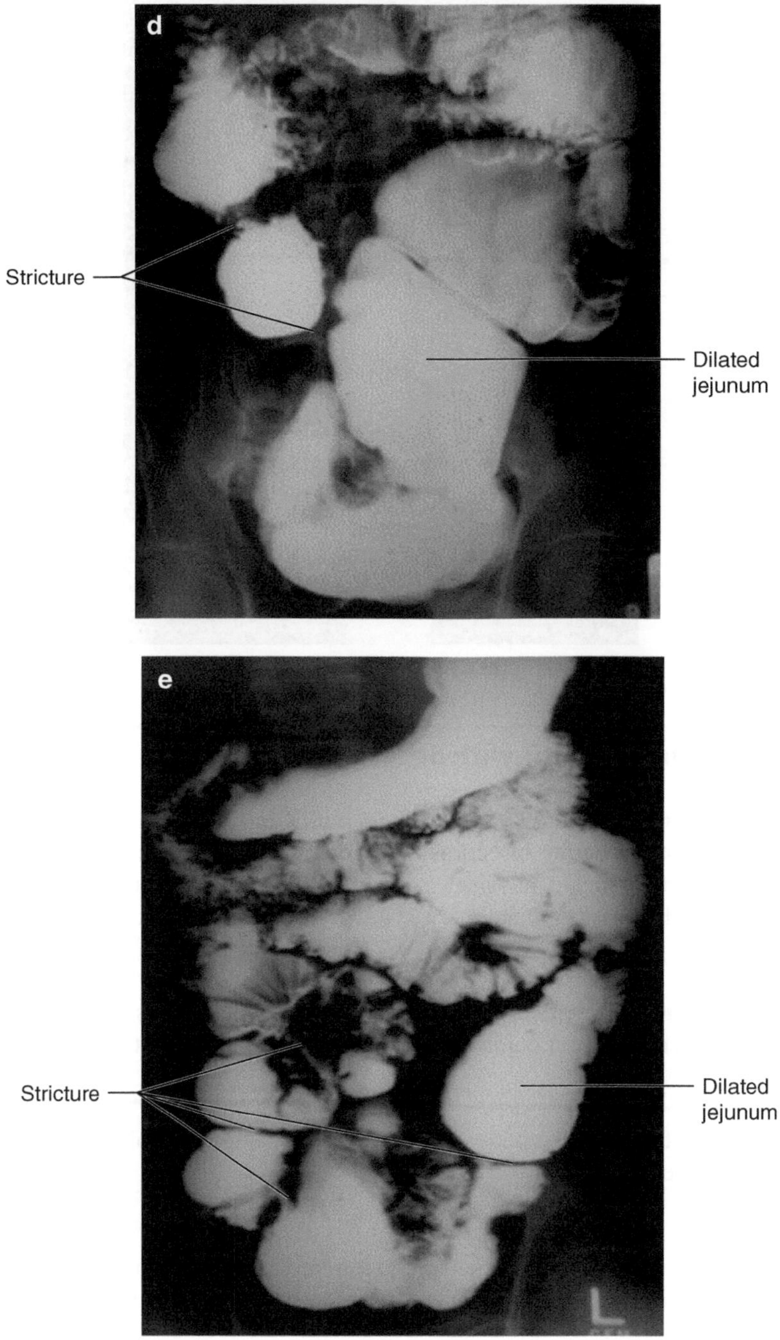

Fig. 8.2 (continued)

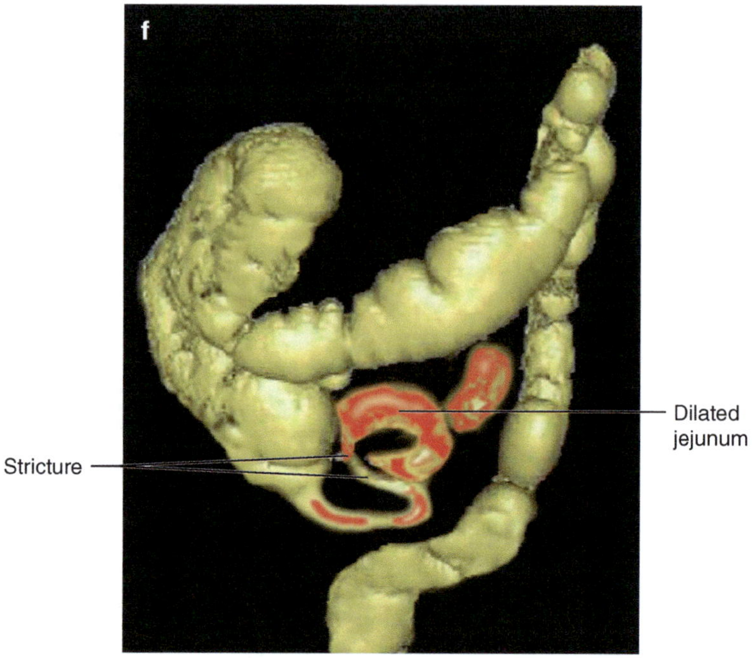

Fig. 8.2 (continued)

8.3 Recurrent Ileitis with Stricture

Clinical Presentation A 49-year-old male with Crohn's disease for 29 years. He had two previous ileocolic resections and now returns with recurrent episodes of intestinal obstruction. On physical exam, his abdomen is moderately distended without palpable masses or tenderness. Patient also has a chronic perianal fistula.

Diagnostic Studies Small bowel series shows recurrent Crohn's disease in the distal 20 cm of ileum. Recent colonoscopy showed a normal colon (see Fig. 8.3b, c).

Surgical Treatment This patient underwent a tertiary ileocolic resection with anastomosis (see Fig. 8.3a).

Pathology Crohn's ileitis with transmural inflammation, ulcerations, inflammatory stricture, and occasional granulomas. The colon is uninvolved. Resection margins are normal.

Follow-Up This patient had an uneventful recovery following surgery. He is well 1 year later.

Comment This patient has had two previous ileocolic resections and now returns with recurrent disease in the neoterminal ileum. The colon is normal although he has a chronic perianal fistula. The small bowel series shows that there is disease in the distal ileum only. This patient had a limited tertiary ileocolic resection with a wide side-to-side ileocolic anastomosis and is well 3 years later. Since this is his third operation, the risk of early recurrence is high, and he should remain on chemoprophylaxis indefinitely (Fig. 8.3).

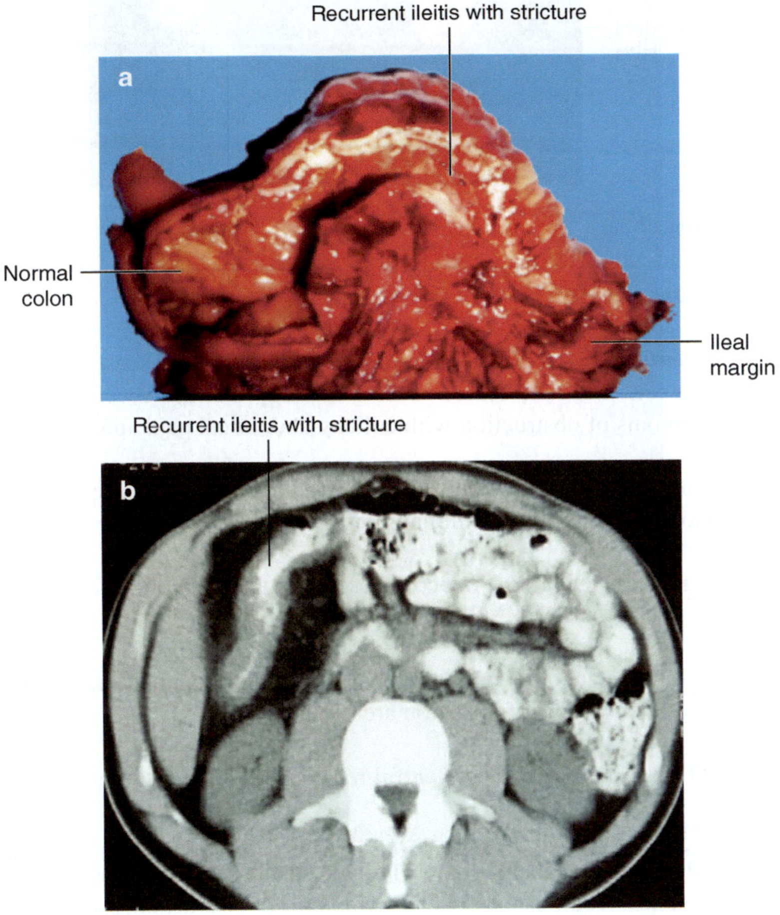

Fig. 8.3 Recurrent ileitis with stricture

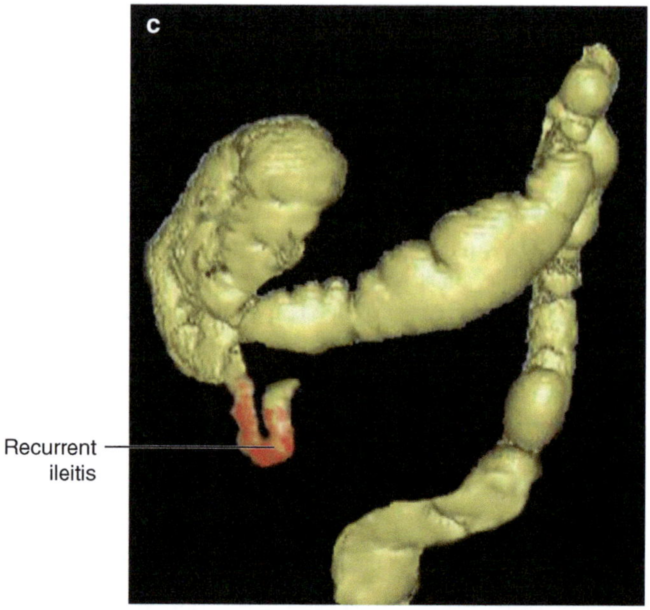

Fig. 8.3 (continued)

8.4 Recurrent Ileitis with Stricture

Clinical Presentation A 35-year-old woman with Crohn's disease for 20 years. She had a previous ileocolic resection 15 years ago and has recently developed increased symptoms of obstruction with colicky abdominal pain and weight loss.

Diagnostic Studies Small bowel series showed recurrent disease at the distal ileum. Colonoscopy showed rectal inflammation with stricture (see Fig. 8.4b, c).

Surgical Treatment Secondary ileocolic resection with ileocolic anastomosis (see Fig. 8.4a).

Pathology Crohn's ileocolitis with transmural chronic inflammation, granulomas, and ulceration. The margins of resection are normal.

Follow-Up This patient had an uneventful recovery following surgery. She is well 3 years later.

Comment Although this patient had only a single previous ileocolic resection and now presents with an ileal recurrence producing symptoms of obstruction, she is at a higher risk to develop problems because of the presence of disease in the rectum with a stricture at the anorectal junction. She underwent an uneventful secondary ileocolic resection and remains well 3 years later. Her prognosis depends on the severity of the rectal disease, and she may eventually require a proctectomy and ileostomy if the anorectal inflammation becomes impossible to control with medical treatment (Fig. 8.4).

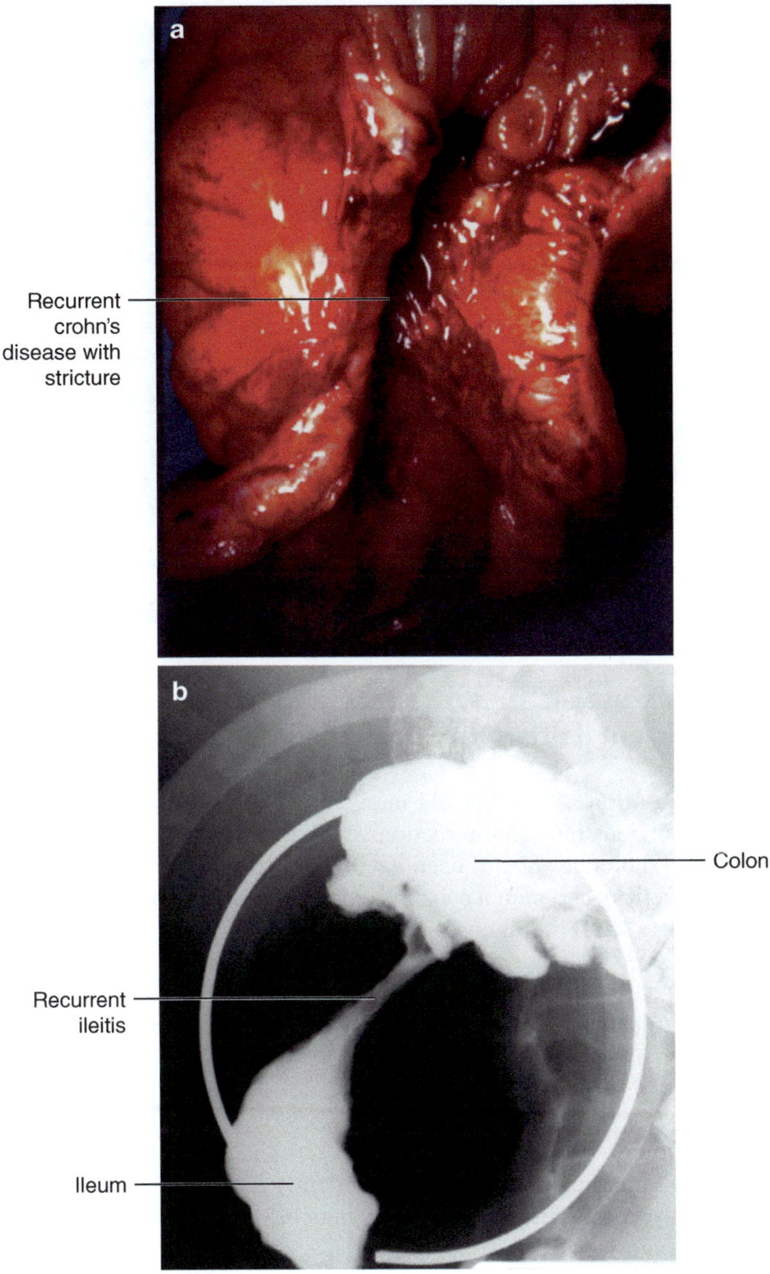

Fig. 8.4 Recurrent ileitis with stricture

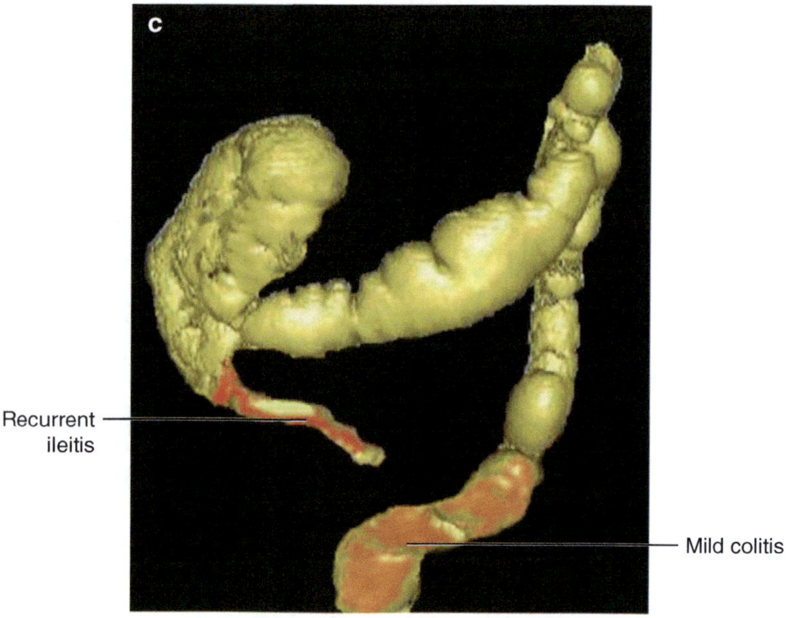

Fig. 8.4 (continued)

8.5 Recurrent Ileitis with Stricture

Clinical Presentation A 77-year-old man with Crohn's disease for 50 years. He has had four previous intestinal resections, with the last operation being 40 years ago. In the past 6 months, he has been having increasing symptoms of obstruction manifested by colicky abdominal pain, distention, and weight loss. He is now admitted with complete small bowel obstruction.

Diagnostic Studies Small bowel series showed recurrent disease with stricture at neoterminal ileum (see Fig. 8.5c, d).

Surgical Treatment Recurrent disease at neoterminal ileum with severe narrowing and marked proximal dilatation. The patient had about 6 ft of normal small bowel proximal to 1 ft of diseased ileum. He underwent a secondary ileocolic resection with anastomosis (see Fig. 8.5a, b).

Pathology Active Crohn's ileitis with inflammatory stricture, transmural chronic inflammation, and inflammatory polyps. The resection margins are normal. Granulomas are not present.

Follow-Up The patient had an uneventful recovery and is well on chemoprophylaxis.

Comment This patient has been well for nearly 40 years since the last operation. He now has a short stricture in the neoterminal ileum with increasing symptoms of obstruction. He underwent a limited ileocolic resection with relief of his symptoms. He has only 6 ft of normal small bowel remaining with most of the colon intact. He is able to maintain his weight and does not require any intravenous fluids. The fact that most of the colon is preserved and normal is probably responsible for his lack of excessive fluid loss from the intestinal tract (Fig. 8.5).

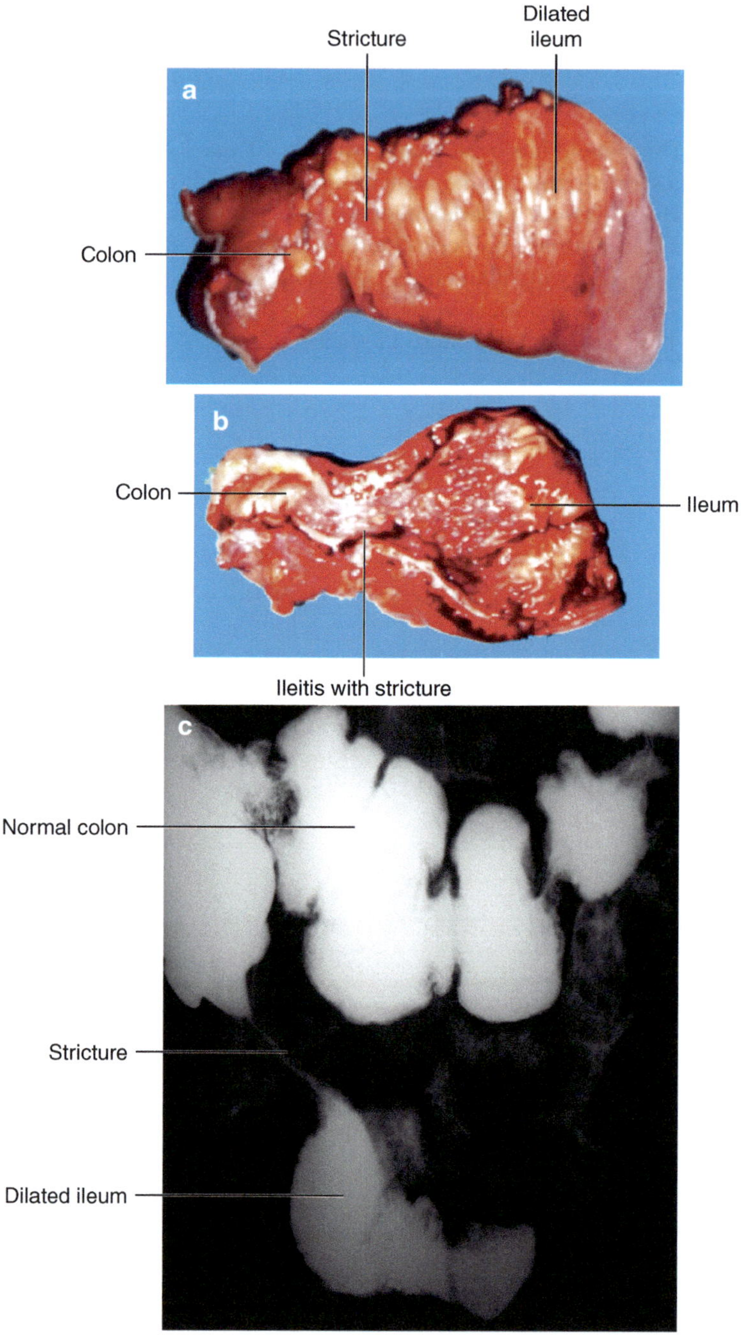

Fig. 8.5 Recurrent ileitis with stricture

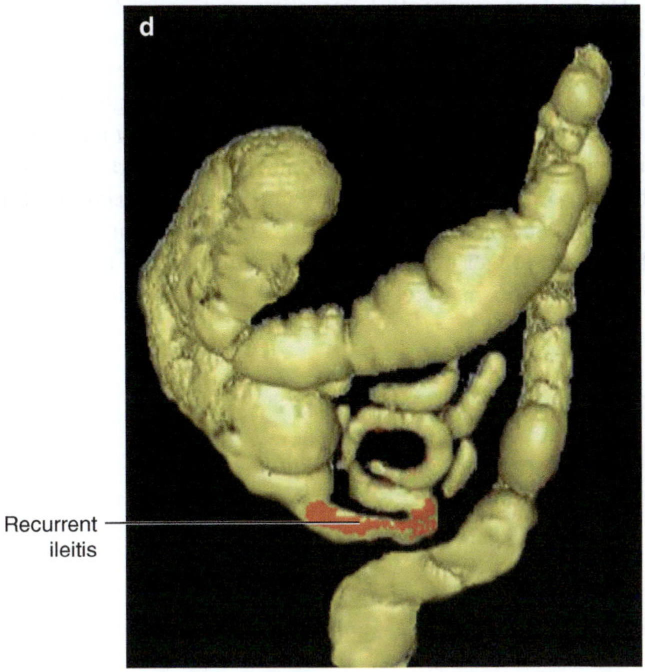

Fig. 8.5 (continued)

8.6 Recurrent Ileitis with Stricture

Clinical Presentation A 71-year-old man with a 30-year history of Crohn's disease and has three previous resections, the last one 13 years ago. Now comes in with recurrent colicky abdominal pain and weight loss.

Diagnostic Studies Colonoscopy showed narrowing of the neoterminal ileum. The colon is unremarkable. Small bowel series showed recurrent disease in the neoterminal ileum with a significant stricture and proximal dilatation (see Fig. 8.6c, d).

Surgical Treatment Secondary ileocolic resection with ileotransverse anastomosis (see Fig. 8.6a, b).

Pathology Active Crohn's ileitis with ulcerations and transmural chronic inflammation. No granulomas are seen. The proximal margin and colonic segments are unremarkable.

Follow-Up He had an uneventful recovery and is well 6 months later on chemoprophylaxis.

Comment This patient had a short segment of recurrence at the neoterminal ileum with a severe stricture. The previous anastomosis was an end-end anastomosis, and the lumen has narrowed to a very small diameter. We currently perform side-side anastomosis with a much larger lumen, which should prevent the occurrence of this type of problem for a longer period of time. Since this is the fourth resection in this patient, chemoprophylaxis is necessary to slow the progression of recurrent disease (Fig. 8.6).

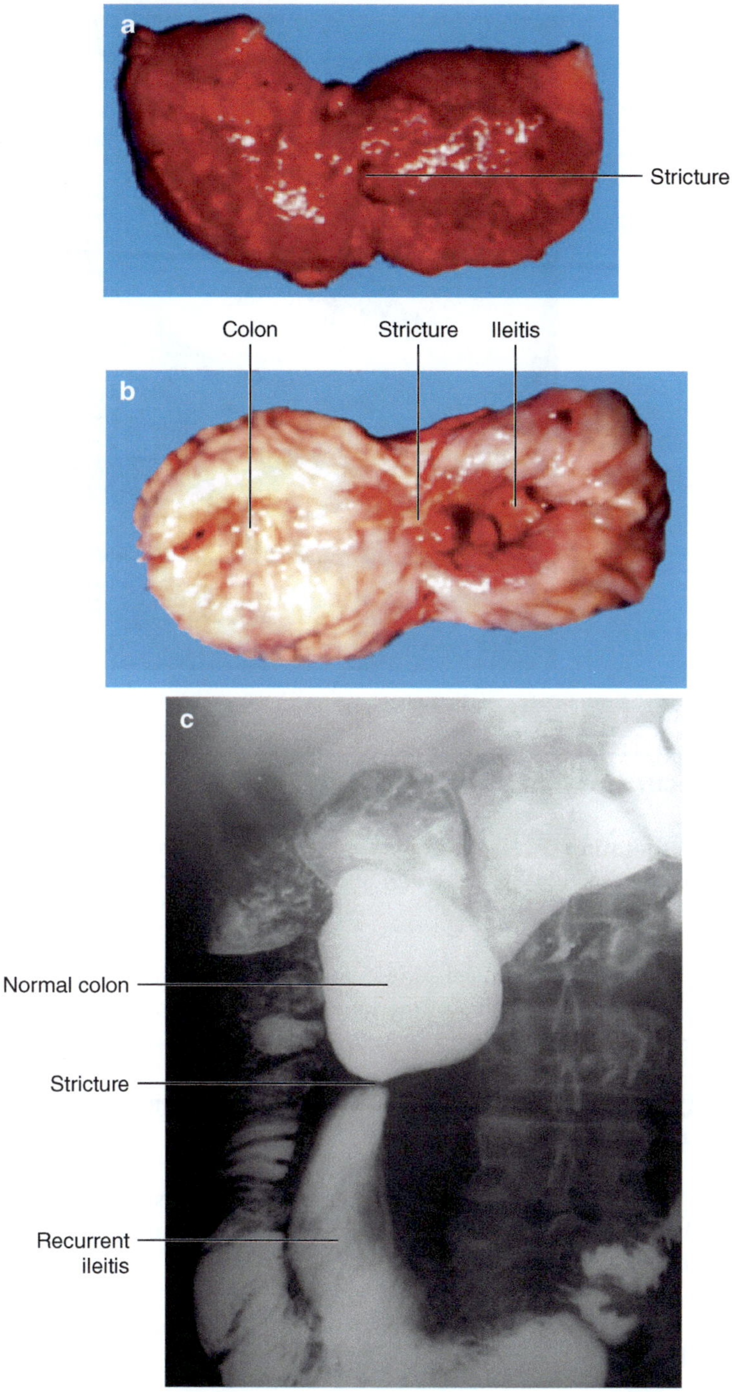

Fig. 8.6 Recurrent ileitis with stricture

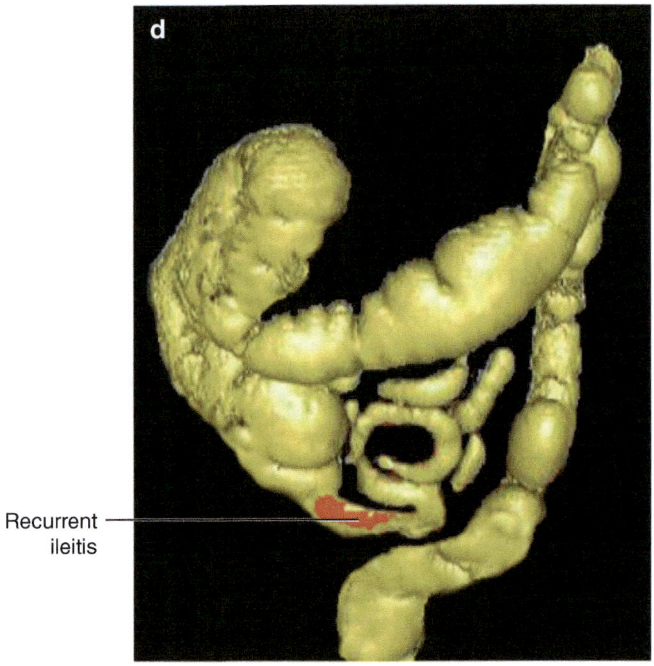

Fig. 8.6 (continued)

8.7 Recurrent Ileitis with Stricture

Clinical Presentation A 50-year-old woman with Crohn's disease since age 21. Had a previous resection 23 years ago and now has recurrent colicky abdominal pain and weight loss.

Diagnostic Studies Small bowel series showed recurrent disease in the neoterminal ileum with severe narrowing of the lumen. The colon appears normal on colonoscopy (see Fig. 8.7b, c).

Surgical Treatment She underwent a secondary ileocolic resection with ileo ascending anastomosis (see Fig. 8.7a).

Pathology Active Crohn's ileitis with ulcerations and transmural chronic inflammation and stricture. No granulomas are seen. The ileal margin and colonic segments are unremarkable.

Follow-Up She recovered well and is asymptomatic 1 year later on chemoprophylaxis.

Comment This patient had a limited recurrence with narrowing of the terminal ileum and obstructive symptoms. A secondary ileocolic resection was performed with a wide side-side anastomosis. Although she is likely to eventually develop recurrent disease again, the fact that 23 years have passed between operations makes her a low risk for early recurrence (Fig. 8.7).

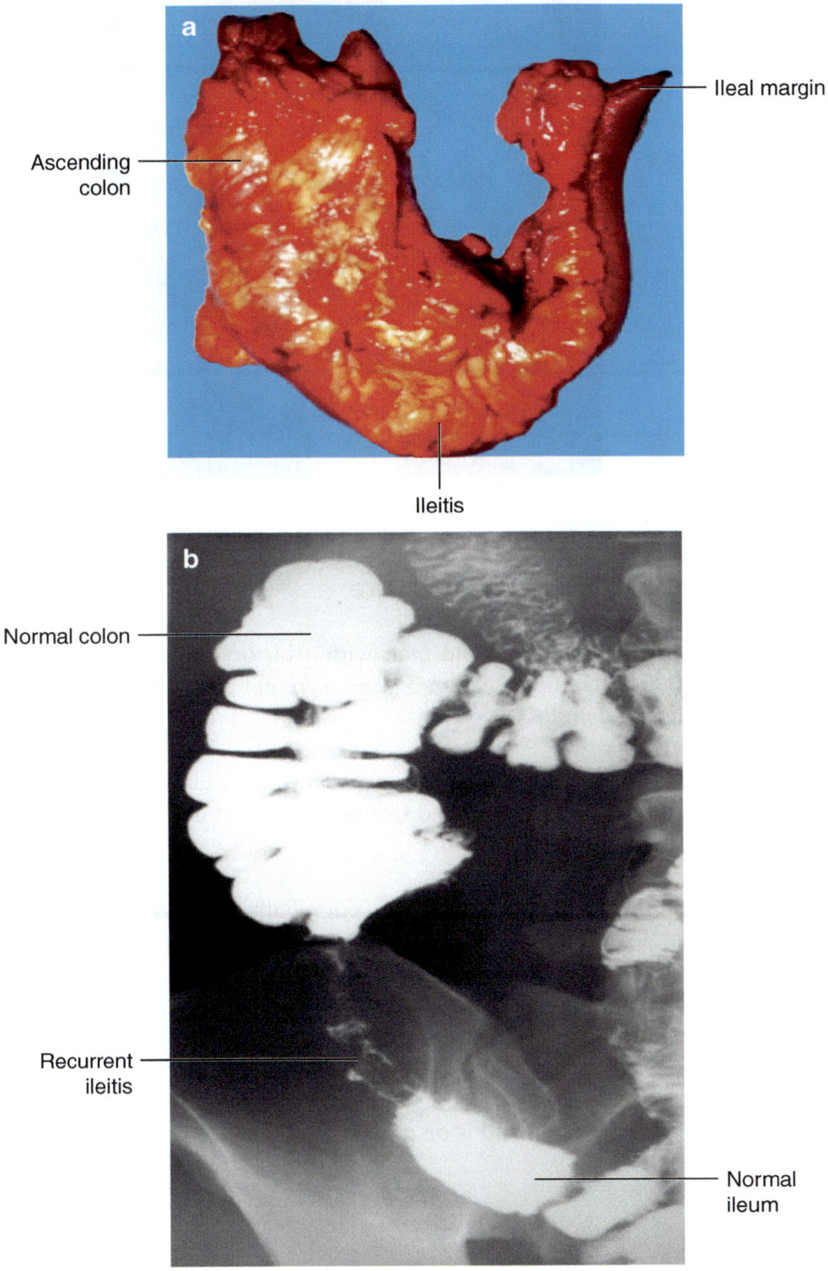

Fig. 8.7 Recurrent ileitis with stricture

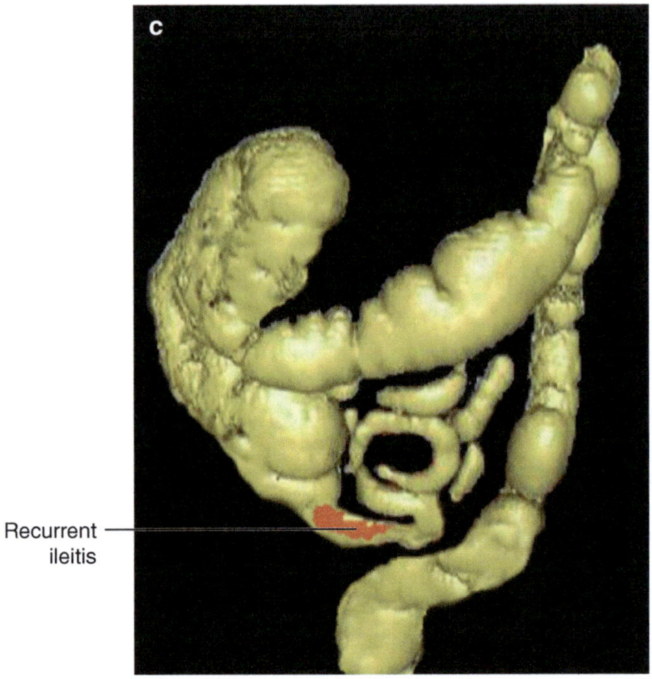

Fig. 8.7 (continued)

8.8 Recurrent Ileitis with Stricture

Clinical Presentation A 28-year-old man with a history of Crohn's disease for 10 years. He had an ileocolic resection 3 years ago and now returns with colicky abdominal pain and weight loss.

Diagnostic Studies Small bowel series shows recurrent disease at the neoterminal ileum with significant stricture. A second stricture is present in a skip area proximal to the neoterminal ileum (see Fig. 8.8b, c).

Surgical Treatment Secondary ileocolic resection with strictureplasty of the proximal stricture (see Fig. 8.8a).

Pathology Active Crohn's ileitis with ulcerations, transmural chronic inflammation, and stricture. Multiple epithelioid granulomas are present. The proximal margin and colonic segment are unremarkable.

Follow-Up He recovered well and is on chemoprophylaxis 1 year later.

Comment This patient has rapidly progressive disease. He has a severe stricture at the recent ileocolic anastomosis and a second skip area proximal to the recurrent disease in the neoterminal ileum. His symptoms have progressed in spite of prophylaxis with 6-MP. A secondary ileocolic resection was performed and a strictureplasty of the more proximal stricture. One year later, his symptoms are again increasing in severity (Fig. 8.8).

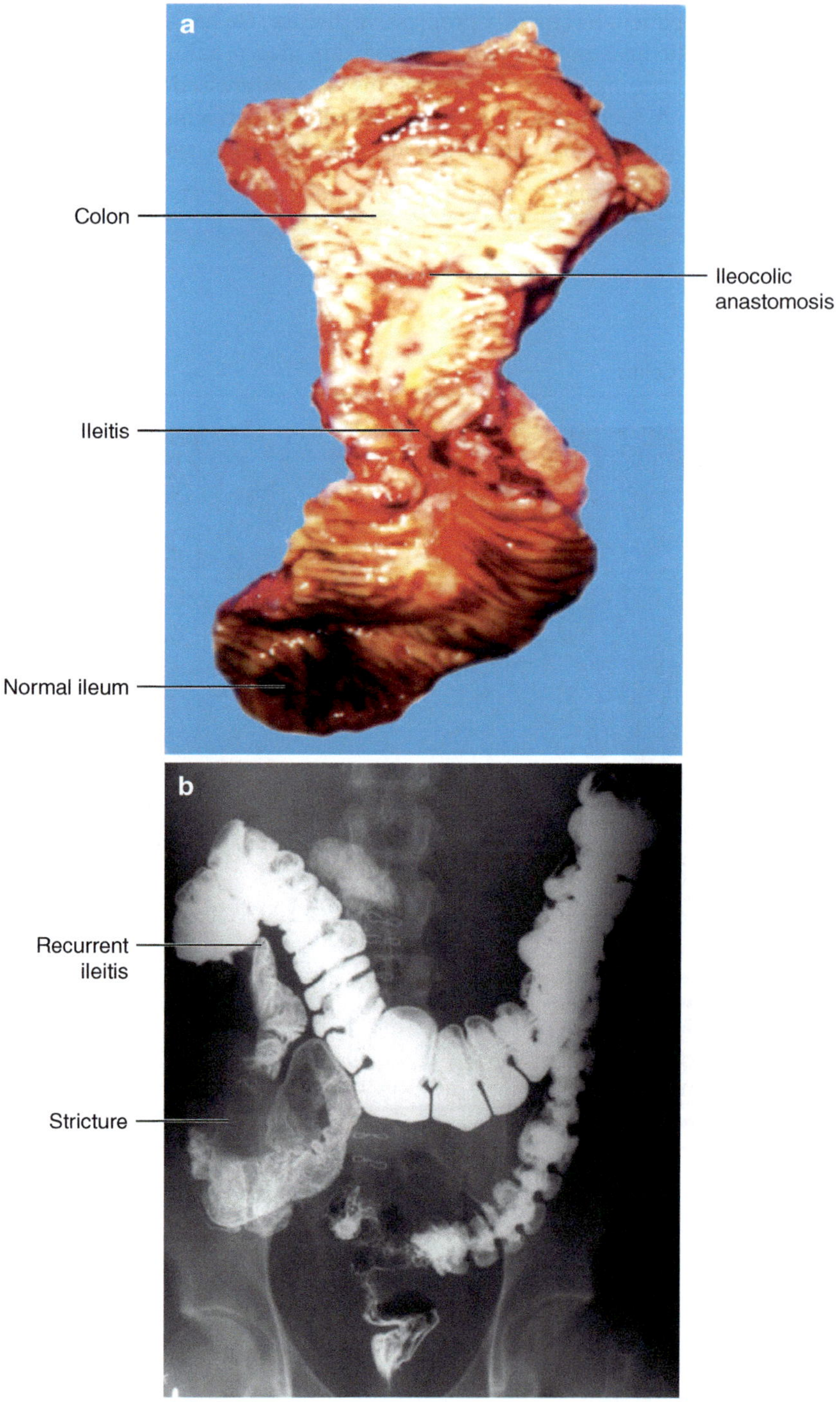

Fig. 8.8 Recurrent ileitis with stricture

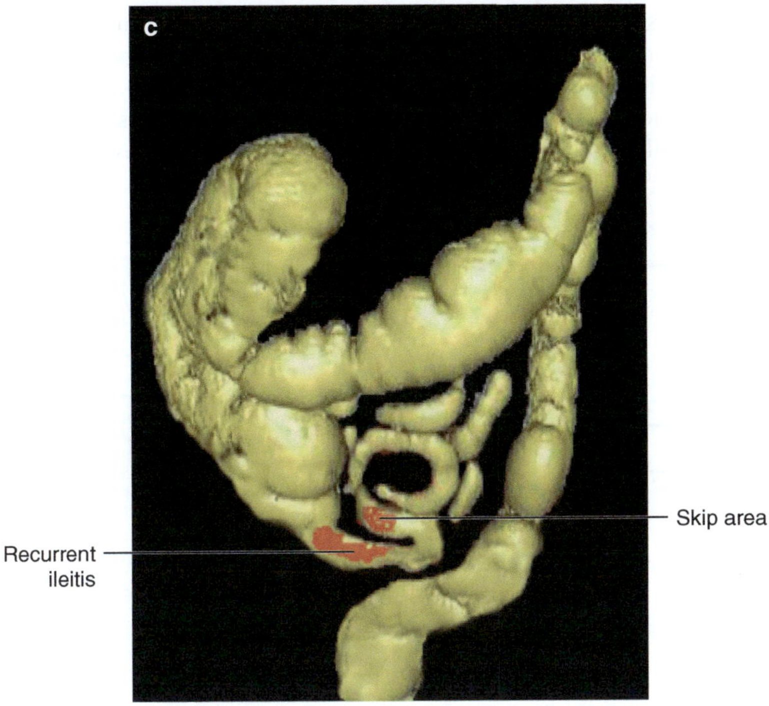

Fig. 8.8 (continued)

8.9 Recurrent Ileitis with Stricture

Clinical Presentation A 46-year-old man with Crohn's disease for 20 years. Has two previous intestinal resections, the last one 4 years ago. He now comes in with recurrent abdominal pain and severe diarrhea.

Diagnostic Studies Obstructive series and small bowel study show narrowing of the ileocolic anastomosis with significant proximal dilatation (see Fig. 8.9c, d).

Surgical Treatment Secondary ileocolic resection with excision of severely dilated ileum and ileotransverse anastomosis (see Fig. 8.9a, b).

Pathology Focal active chronic nonspecific inflammation. Severe ileal dilatation.

Follow-Up He is well 1 year later on chemoprophylaxis.

Comment This patient had severe ileal dilatation proximal to an ileocolic anastomosis with recurrent Crohn's disease. The degree of dilatation was extensive especially when taking into account that only 4 years have passed since the previous operation. A stricture is present at the anastomosis, which is best seen in the barium study. Tertiary ileocolic resection with wide side-side anastomosis eliminated the problem (Fig. 8.9).

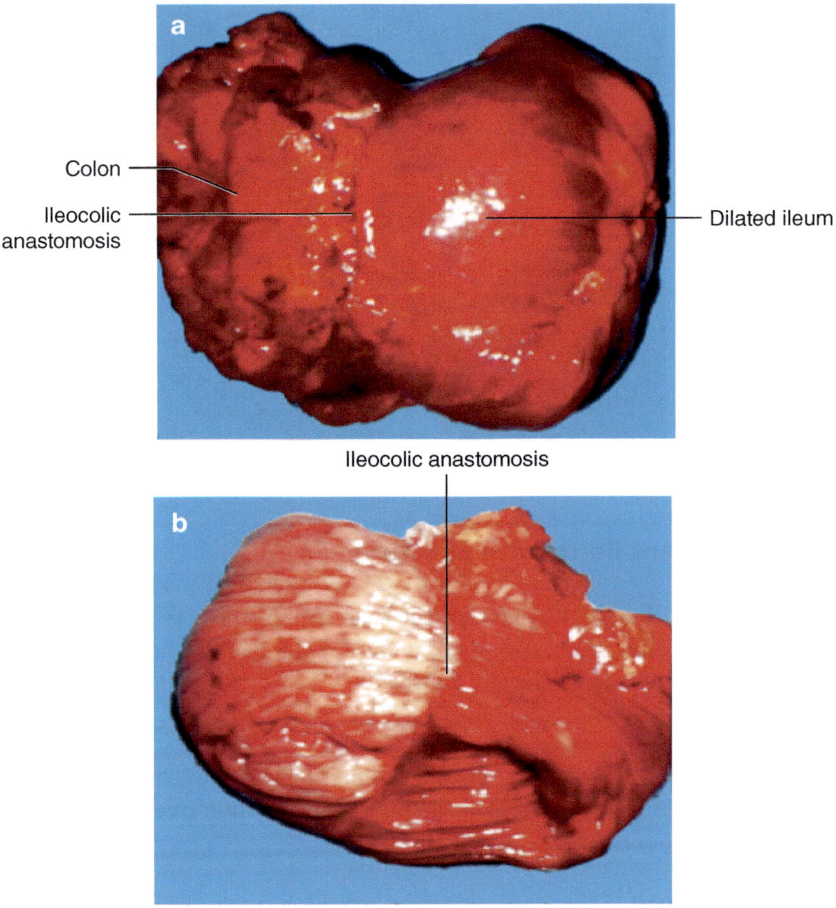

Fig. 8.9 Recurrent ileitis with stricture

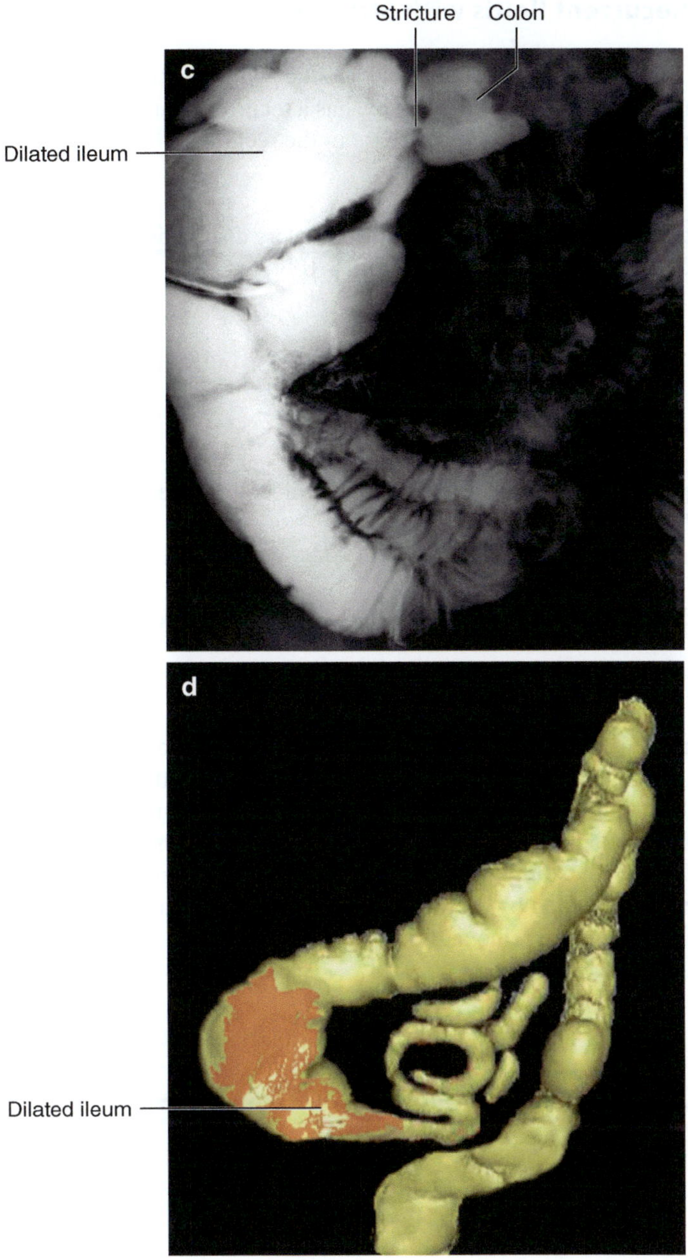

Fig. 8.9 (continued)

8.10 Recurrent Ileitis with Stricture

Clinical Presentation A 50-year-old woman with multiple previous abdominal operations for Crohn's disease. She now has a recurrence at the ileorectal anastomosis with exacerbation of residual disease in the rectum.

Diagnostic Studies Colonoscopy showed severe disease in the rectum with a stricture at the ileoanal anastomosis (see Fig. 8.10b).

Surgical Treatment Abdominoperineal resection of the rectum with Brooke ileostomy (see Fig. 8.10a).

Pathology Crohn's ileoproctitis with rectal ulceration, perianal fissures, and granulomas. The proximal margin is normal.

Follow-Up This patient had an uneventful recovery and is well 6 months following surgery.

Comment This patient had a subtotal colectomy with ileorectal anastomosis in the past. The residual disease in the rectum has progressed to the point that the mucosal layer of the distal rectum is severely ulcerated. The inflammation extends into the anal canal and the patient has severe pain. Abdominoperineal resection of the rectum and Brooke ileostomy resulted in marked improvement. Although this problem may have been avoided by recommending an ileostomy at the previous operation, these patients are often reluctant to have a stoma when an ileorectal anastomosis is still possible (Fig. 8.10).

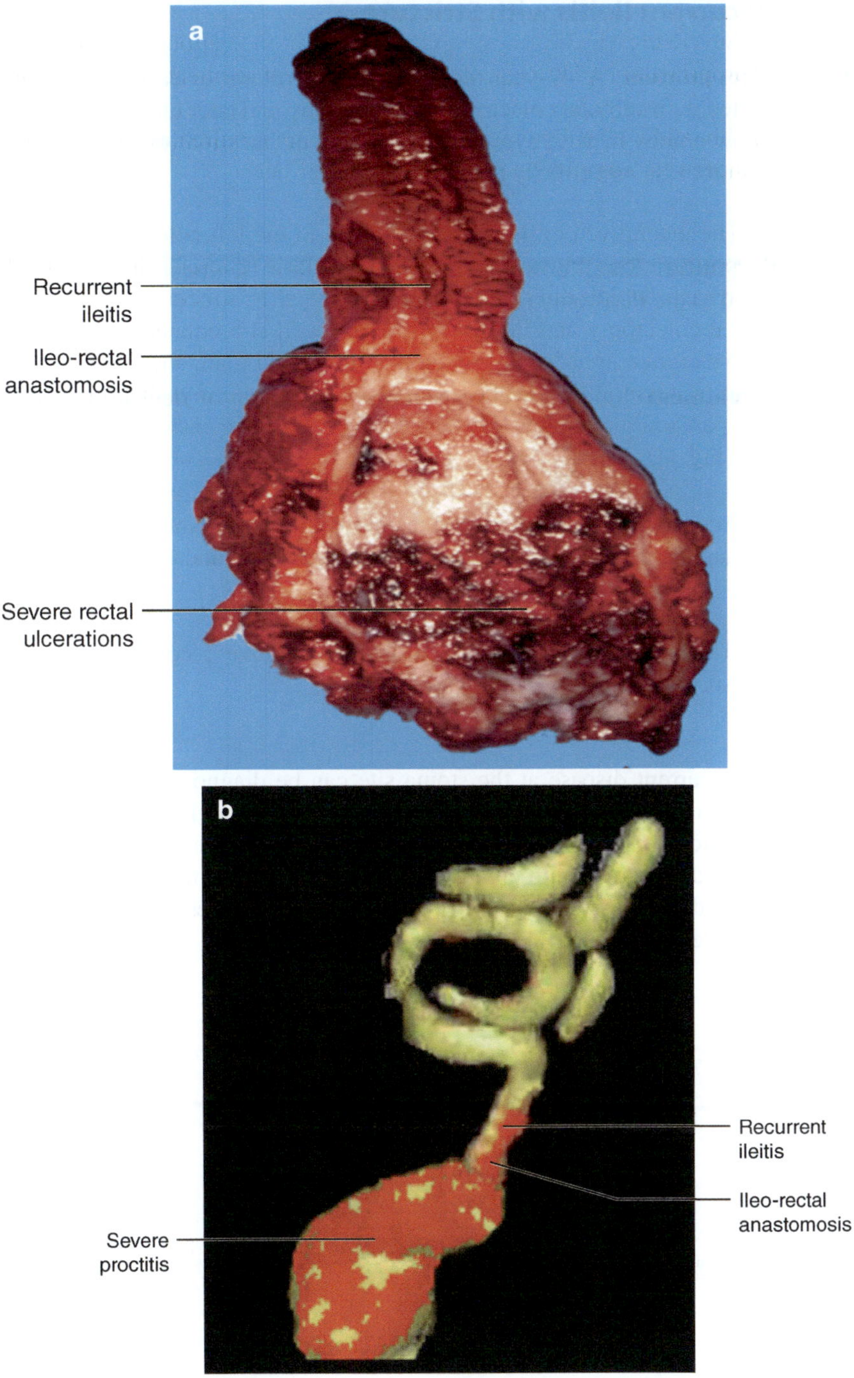

Fig. 8.10 Recurrent ileitis with stricture

8.11 Recurrent Ileitis with Stricture

Clinical Presentation A 47-year-old male with Crohn's disease for 30 years. Initially treated with subtotal colectomy and ileostomy and later underwent proctectomy. He now comes in with symptoms of recurrent intestinal obstruction manifested by weight loss and colicky abdominal pain.

Diagnostic Studies Small bowel series showed a short segment of recurrent disease proximal to the ileostomy (see Fig. 8.11c).

Surgical Treatment Small bowel resection with revision of ileostomy (see Fig. 8.11a, b).

Pathology Active Crohn's ileitis with transmural chronic inflammation and ulcerations. No granulomas are seen. The proximal margin is normal.

Follow-Up This patient had an uneventful postoperative recovery and is well 3 years after surgery.

Comment Recurrent disease at the stoma site can be diagnosed by small bowel series or endoscopy. When the symptoms become severe enough that the patient has recurrent symptoms of obstruction, then surgery becomes necessary. Most patients require a limited resection with creation of a new ileostomy in the same location. When compared to intestinal anastomosis, ileostomies are less likely to develop recurrent disease (Fig. 8.11).

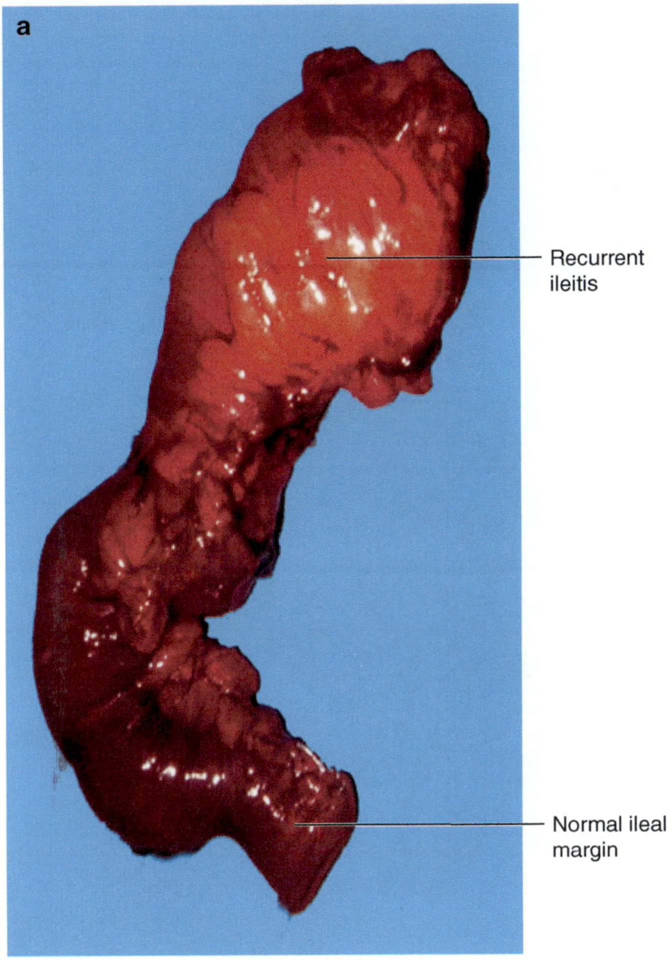

Fig. 8.11 Recurrent ileitis with stricture

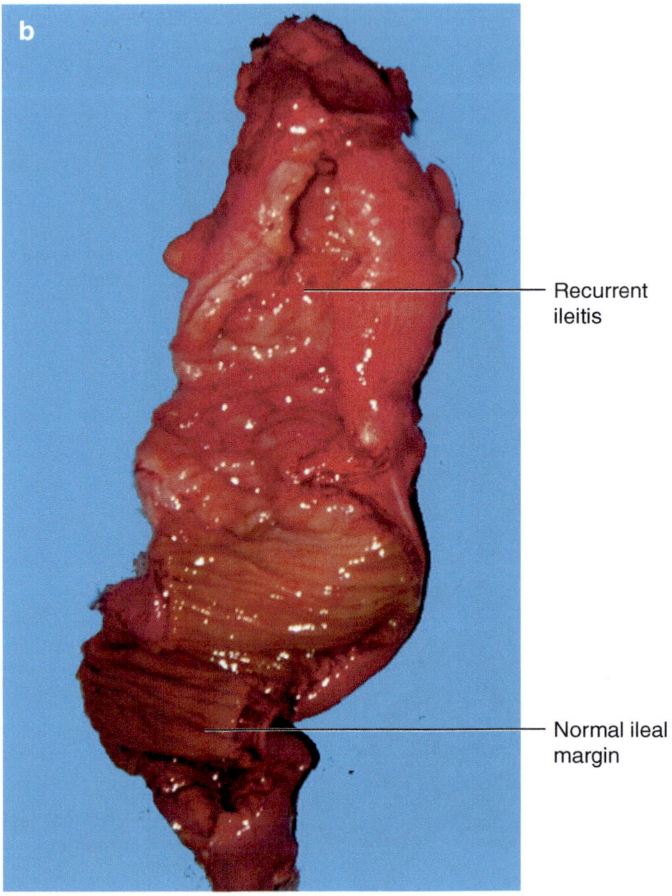

Fig. 8.11 (continued)

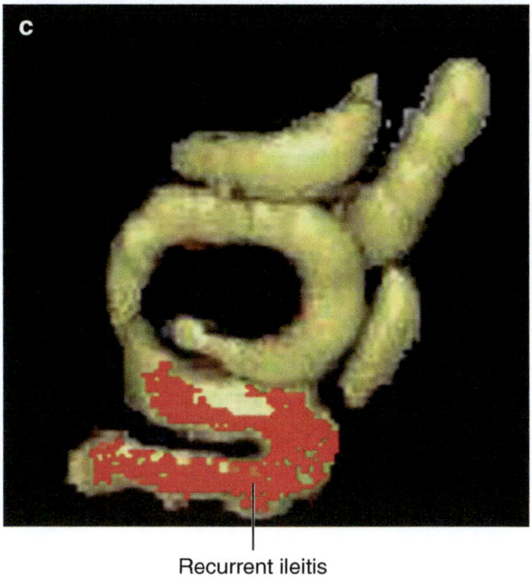

Fig. 8.11 (continued)

Further Reading

Heimann TM, Aufses AH Jr. Prediction of recurrence in Crohn's disease: the role of peripheral lymphocytes. Surg Gynecol Obstet. 1985;160:295–8.

Heimann TM, Bolnick K, Aufses AH Jr. Correlation of preoperative lymphocytopenia and postoperative recurrence in Crohn's disease. Surg Forum. 1984;XXXV:150–3.

Heimann TM, Greenstein AJ, Lewis B, Kaufman D, Heimann DM, Aufses AH Jr. Comparison of primary and reoperative surgery in patients with Crohn's disease. Ann Surg. 1998;227:492–5.

9 Recurrent Ileitis with Penetrating Sinuses and Recurrent Ileitis with Fistula

Tomas M. Heimann and Robert J. Kurtz

Recurrence of Crohn's disease in the small intestine after surgical resection usually presents with some degree of thickening of the bowel wall and narrowing of the lumen. In some patients, however, this is not the main cause of symptoms. Penetrating sinuses resulting in abscess and fistula formation are responsible for the presenting symptoms and the need for reoperation. If the sinuses do not penetrate the bowel wall, then the symptoms of obstruction may predominate, while deeply penetrating sinuses will give rise mesenteric and retroperitoneal abscesses and fistulas to adjacent organs.

9.1 Recurrent Ileocolitis with Fistula

Clinical Presentation A 47-year-old female with Crohn's disease for 21 years with five previous resections who now comes in with multiple recurrent enterocutaneous fistulas.

Diagnostic Studies CT scan, fistulogram, and small bowel study showed recurrent disease at the iloetransverse anastomosis with multiple sinus tracts (see Fig. 9.1c, d).

Surgical Treatment She underwent a tertiary ileocolic resection with end ileostomy and closure of the colon (see Fig. 9.1a, b).

T. M. Heimann (✉) · R. J. Kurtz
Department of Surgery, Icahn School of Medicine at Mount Sinai, New York, NY, USA
e-mail: Tomas.Heimann@mountsinai.org; Robert.Kurtz@mountsinai.org

T. M. Heimann (ed.), *Atlas of Surgical Treatment of Inflammatory Bowel Disease*, https://doi.org/10.1007/978-3-031-62431-5_9

Pathology Ileocolic segment with transmural chronic inflammation and multiple sinus tracts.

Follow-Up This patient had only 5 ft. of residual small bowel and was discharged on chronic intravenous hyperalimentation at night to supplement her oral feedings. She returned 1 year later with duodenal obstruction from Crohn's disease and required a gastroenterostomy. She remains on intravenous supplementation.

Comment This patient has aggressive Crohn's disease requiring multiple frequent operations. Her symptoms have frequently manifested with the onset of multiple fistulas. Due to many previous small bowel resections, she is unable to maintain a normal nutritional status without intravenous supplementation of fluids and calories. Attempts at restoration of intestinal continuity have always resulted in early recurrence and intractable fistulas. She is currently addicted to pain medication and requires a tincture of opium to control the enterostomy output. Her quality of life is poor, and since her family is unable to cope with her medical requirements, she is currently living in a chronic care facility (Fig. 9.1).

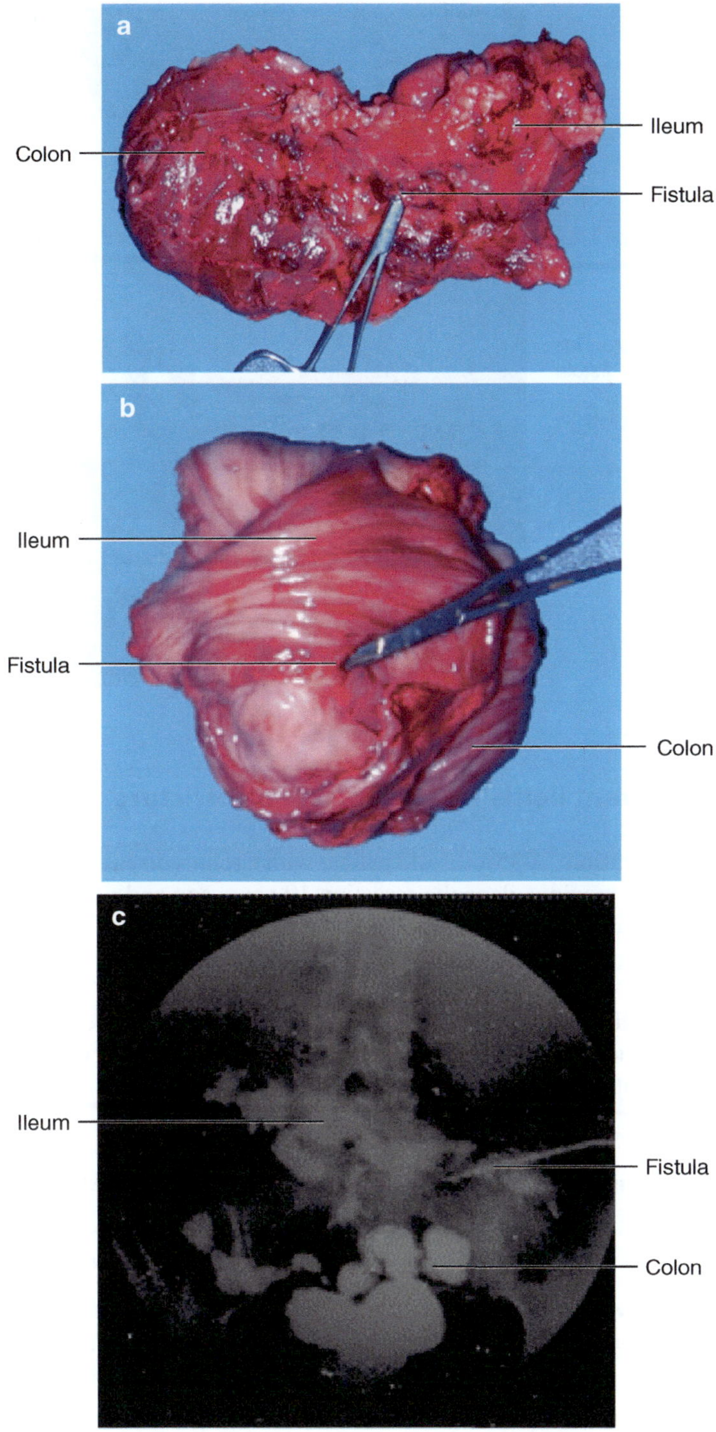

Fig. 9.1 (**a**–**d**) Recurrent ileocolitis with fistula

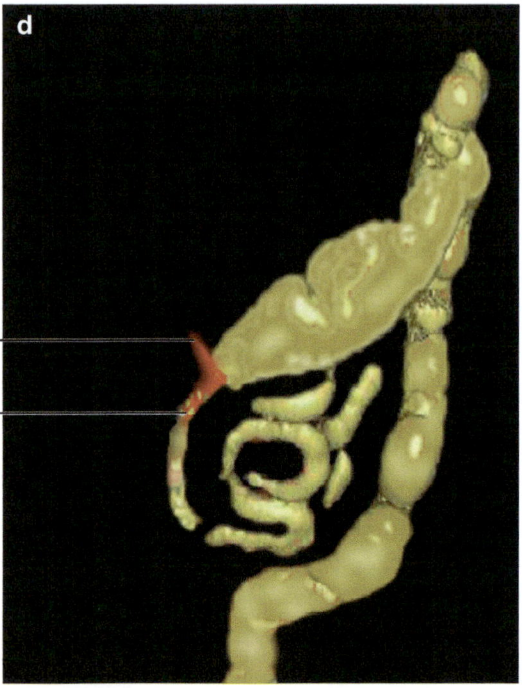

Fig. 9.1 (continued)

9.2 Recurrent Ileitis + Sinus Tracts and Stricture

Clinical Presentation A 35-year-old patient with Crohn's disease since age 12. He had undergone a previous ileocolic resection 10 years ago and now comes in with increasing symptoms of recurrent abdominal pain and weight loss.

Diagnostic Studies Colonoscopy showed a normal colon with severe stricture at the ileocolonic anastomosis. Small bowel series demonstrated recurrent disease in the neoterminal ileum with severe stricture (see Fig. 9.2c, d).

Surgical Treatment Secondary ileocolic resection with ileotransverse anastomosis (see Fig. 9.2a, b).

Pathology Active Crohn's disease with inflammatory stricture at the anastomosis with ulcerations and sinus tracts. No granulomas are seen. Margins of resection are unremarkable.

Follow-Up He recovered following surgery and continues to do well 4 years later.

Comment This is an example of a limited recurrence in the neoterminal ileum with a severe stricture causing obstructive symptoms. There is evidence that wide side-side anastomosis makes this problem less likely to occur. This patient underwent a secondary ileocolic resection with side-side ileotransverse anastomosis and has now done well for several years (Fig. 9.2).

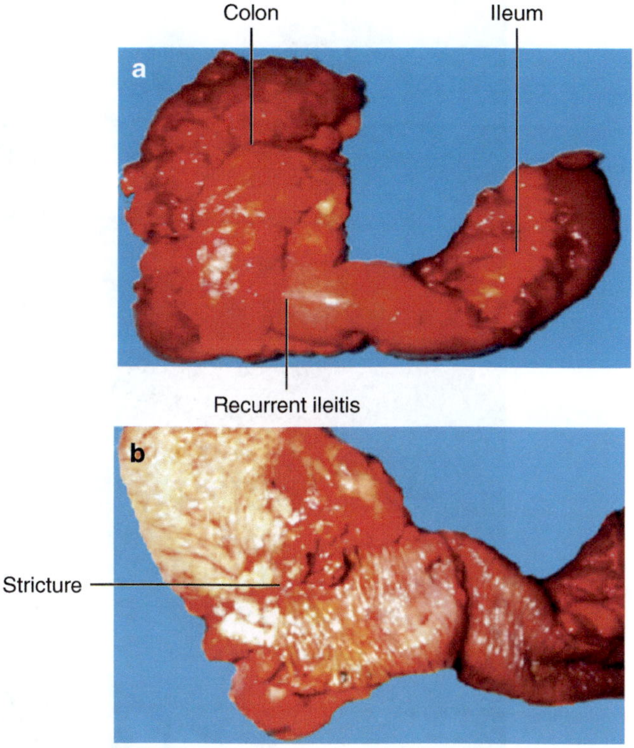

Fig. 9.2 (**a**–**d**) Recurrent ileitis + sinus tracts and stricture

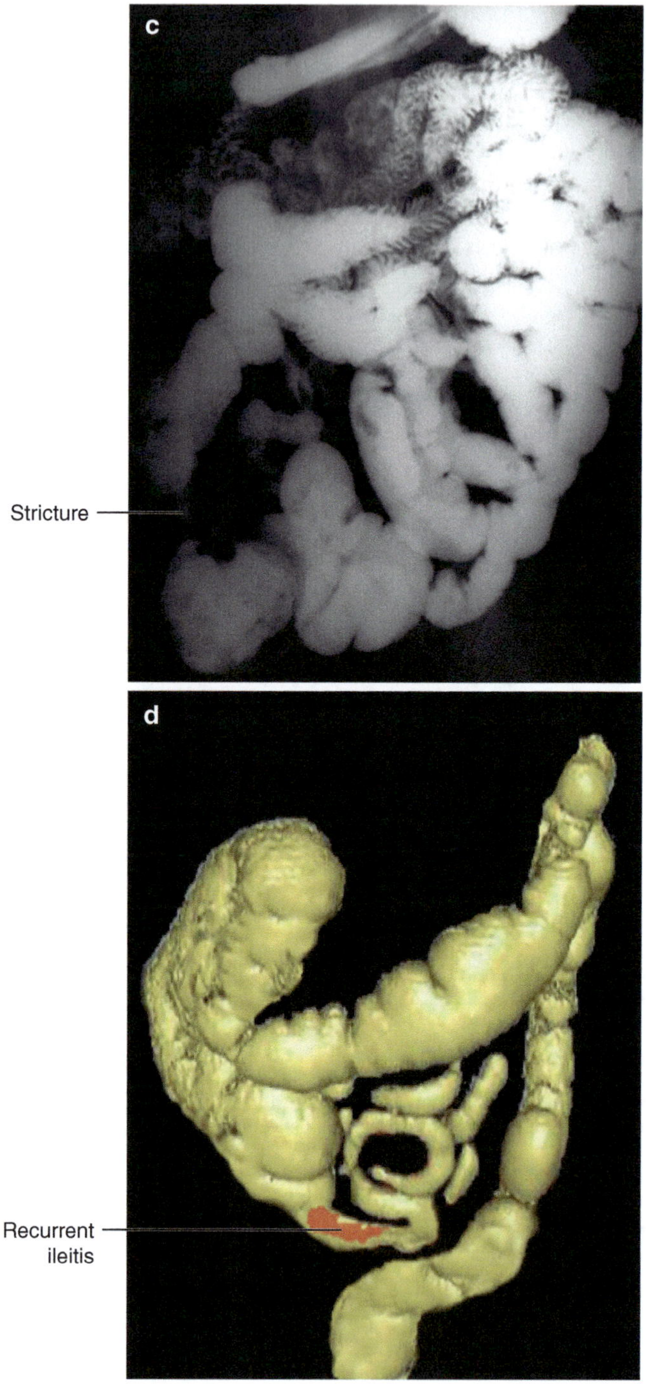

Fig. 9.2 (continued)

9.3 Recurrent Ileitis + Sinus Tracts and Stricture

Clinical Findings A 64-year-old woman with a long-standing history of Crohn's disease. She had a previous ileocolic resection 6 years ago and now has increasing symptoms of partial intestinal obstruction with recurrent colicky abdominal pain and abdominal distention.

Diagnostic Tests Small bowel series showed recurrent disease in the neoterminal ileum with severe narrowing. Colonoscopy showed mild colitis in the ascending colon (see Fig. 9.3b, c).

Surgical Treatment Secondary ileocolic resection with anastomosis. There was some thickening of the sigmoid colon consistent with mild colitis (see Fig. 9.3a).

Pathology Crohn's ileocolitis with severe transmural inflammation of the ileum with penetrating sinus tracts and acute serositis. Occasional granulomas are present. The colon shows patchy mild colitis. The resection margins are normal.

Follow-Up The patient recovered well after surgery. She continues on treatment for residual colitis.

Comment This patient has moderately severe Crohn's disease with a recurrence in the neoterminal ileum. The inflammation in the ascending and sigmoid colon is mild and can be controlled with medical treatment. Her symptoms are caused by severe narrowing proximal to the ileocolic anastomosis caused by recurrent disease. The ascending colon and the ileocolic anastomosis are distorted and drawn to the transverse colon; therefore, the ileocolic resection required extension to the right transverse colon. A fistula from the ileum to the transverse colon was not demonstrated. She has recovered since this operation and remains well 5 years later (Fig. 9.3).

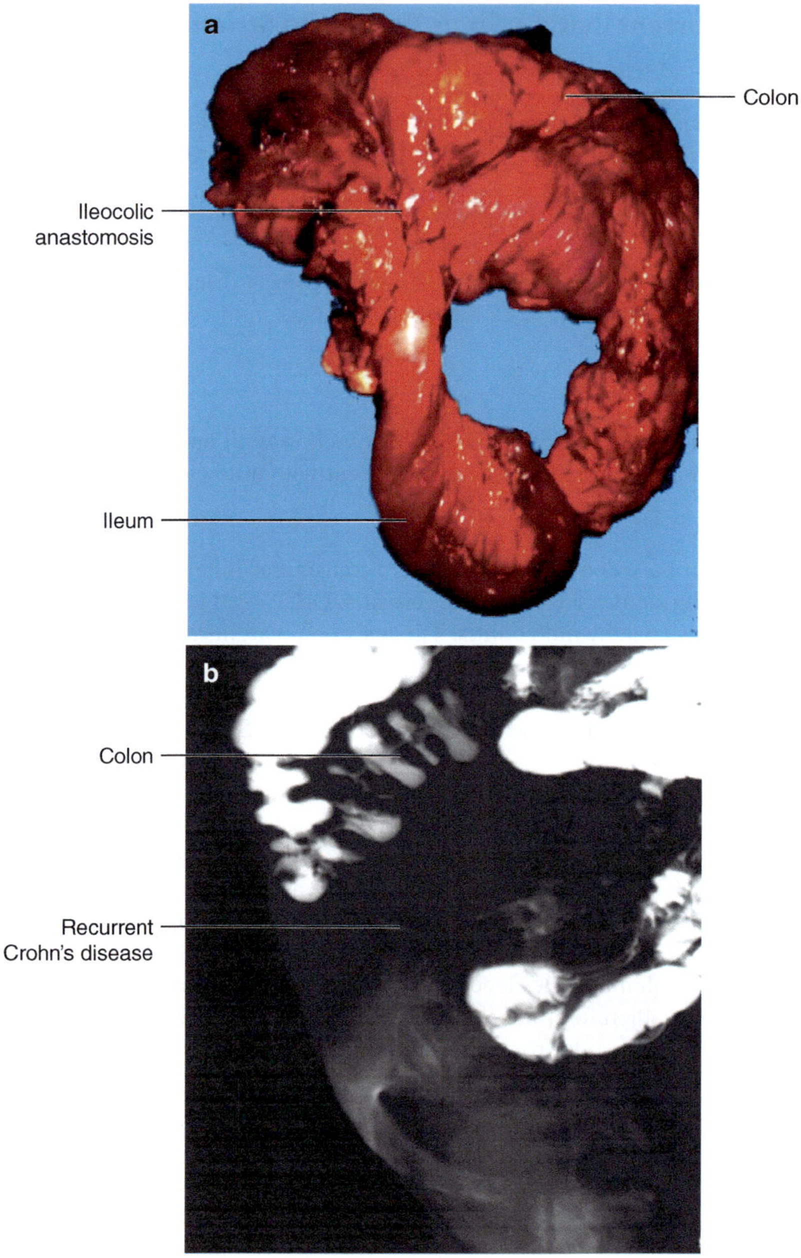

Fig. 9.3 (a–c) Recurrent ileitis + sinus tracts and stricture

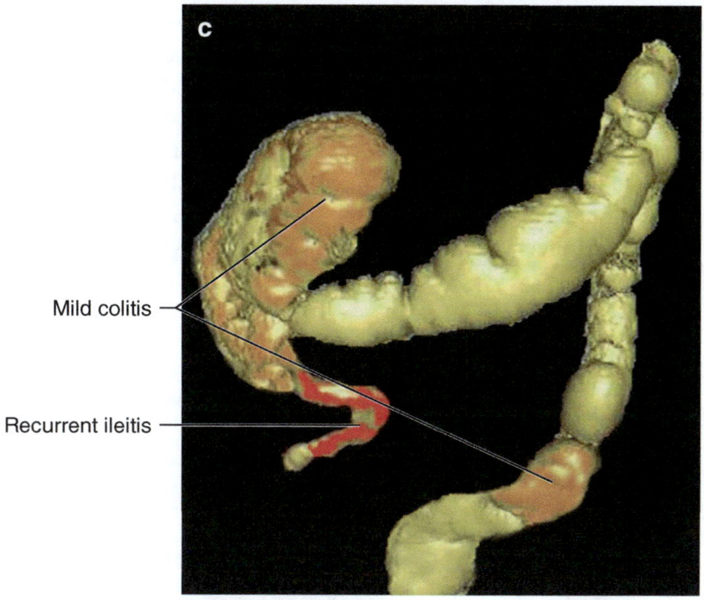

Fig. 9.3 (continued)

9.4 Recurrent Ileitis + Sinus Tracts and Stricture

Clinical Presentation A 34-year-old woman with Crohn's disease for 13 years. This patient had multiple previous operations with a subtotal colectomy and ileorectal anastomosis 4 years ago. She has recently developed increasing symptoms of intestinal obstruction.

Diagnostic Studies Small bowel series and CT scan show a short segment of recurrent disease at the ileorectal anastomosis with severe narrowing. Colonoscopy revealed normal rectal mucosa with marked narrowing at the anastomosis (see Fig. 9.4a, b, c).

Surgical Treatment Resection of the distal ileum and upper rectum with secondary ileorectal anastomosis.

Pathology Active Crohn's ileitis with transmural chronic inflammation, inflammatory stricture, penetrating sinus tracts, and acute and chronic serositis. No granulomas were seen. The rectal margin was normal, and the ileal margin showed mild inflammation.

Follow-Up This patient had an uneventful postoperative recovery. She had some initial difficulty with frequent bowel movements which gradually improved with antidiarrheal medication.

Comment This patient developed recurrent disease with a stricture at the previous ileorectal anastomosis. The segment with recurrent disease in the ileum was short, the rectum was normal, and there was no perianal disease. Resection of the diseased segment with secondary ileorectal anastomosis eliminates the obstructive symptoms. This patient is likely to develop recurrent disease in the same area again at some time in the future and may even eventually require an ileostomy. Most young patients, however, will opt for an ileorectal anastomosis with a higher risk of recurrence and loose bowel movements as opposed to a permanent ileostomy (Fig. 9.4).

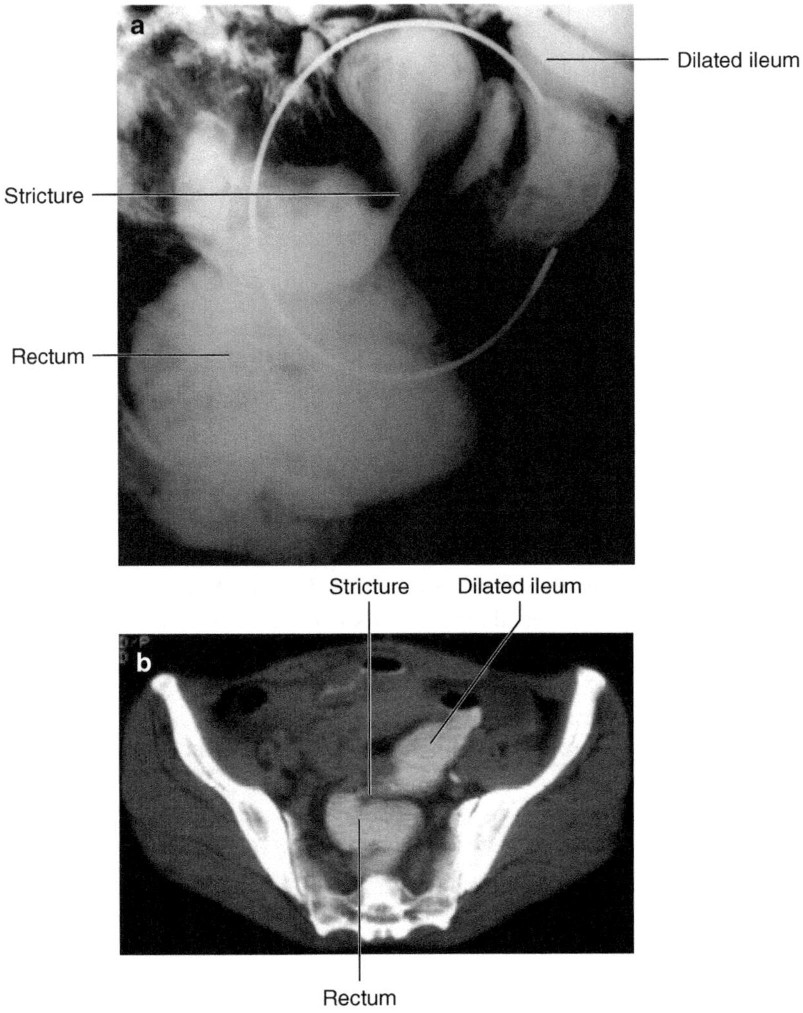

Fig. 9.4 (**a–c**) Recurrent ileitis + sinus tracts and stricture

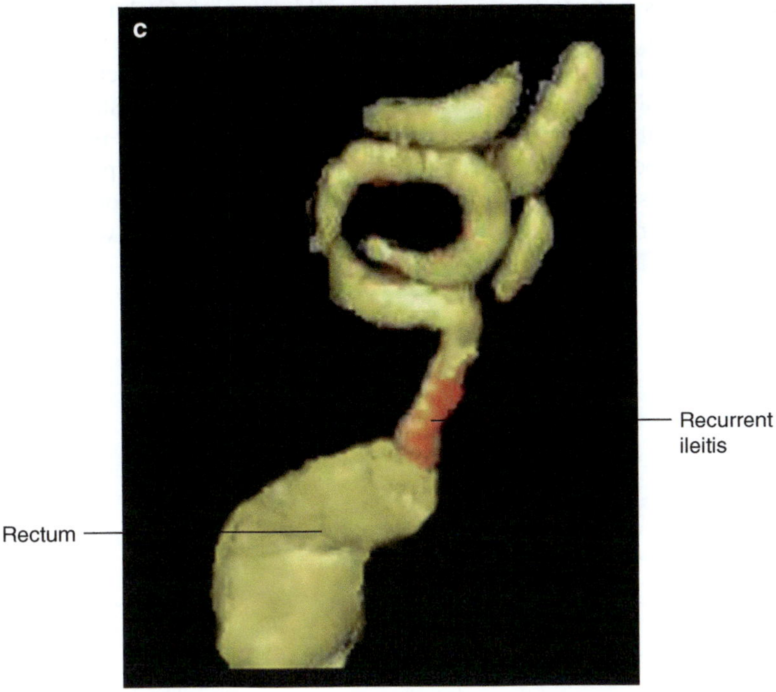

Fig. 9.4 (continued)

9.5 Recurrent Ileitis + Sinus Tracts and Stricture

Clinical Presentation A 37-year-old woman with Crohn's disease for 14 years. Previous ileocolic resection 11 years ago. She has recently developed symptoms of intestinal obstruction with weight loss, abdominal distention, and colicky abdominal pain.

Diagnostic Studies Small bowel series showed recurrent disease in the neoterminal ileum. Colonoscopy showed a normal colon with a severe stricture at the ileocolic anastomosis (see Fig. 9.5b, c).

Surgical Treatment This patient underwent a secondary ileocolic resection with anastomosis (see Fig. 9.5a).

Pathology Crohn's ileitis with transmural inflammation, multiple sinus tracts, and a perforating anastomotic fistula. Occasional granulomas are present. The margins are normal.

Follow-Up This patient did well following surgery. She was reoperated 1 year later for intestinal obstruction due to a single adhesive band. There was no recurrent disease at reoperation.

Comment This patient has a relatively mild form of Crohn's disease. The inflammation is limited to the terminal ileum, and she was well for nearly 11 years after having an ileocolic resection. She now has a stricture in the neo-terminal ileum and symptoms of obstruction. The rest of the small bowel and colon are normal, and she required a limited secondary ileocolic resection with a side-to-side ileocolic anastomosis to the ascending colon. We prefer the wider side-to-side anastomosis in Crohn's disease since the anastomotic site is often likely to stricture especially when the EEA stapler is used, which creates a smaller circular anastomosis (Fig. 9.5).

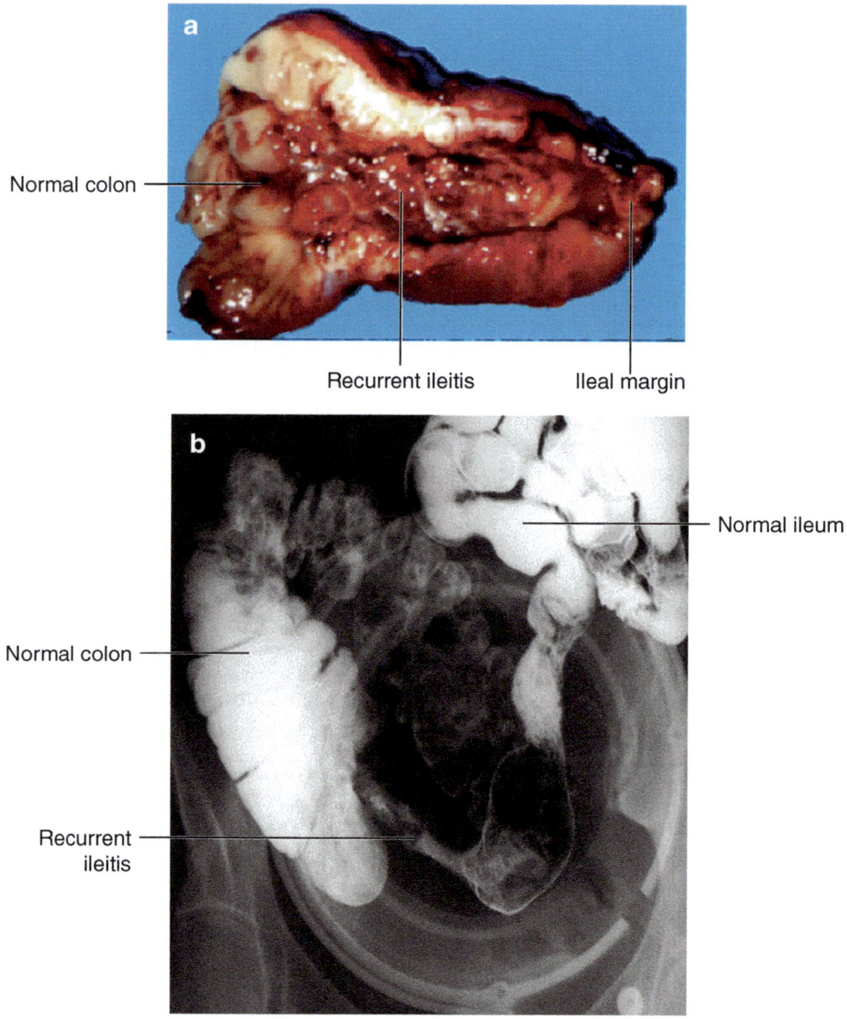

Fig. 9.5 (a–c) Recurrent ileitis + sinus tracts and stricture

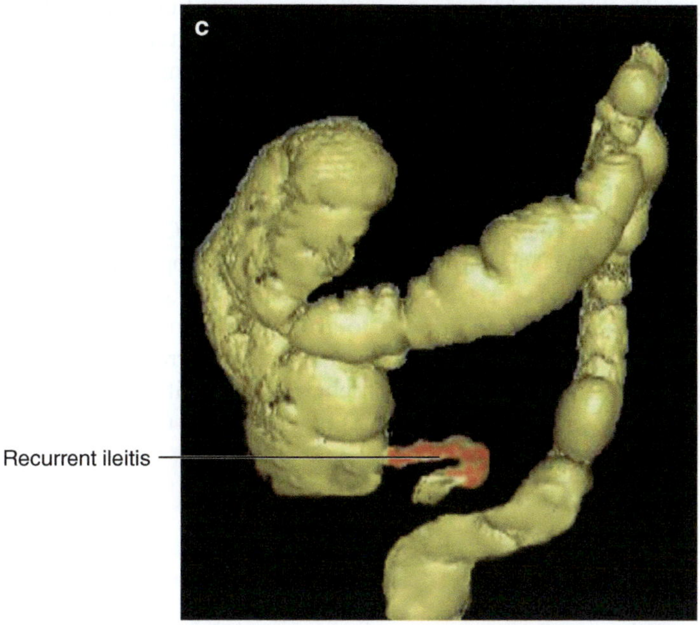

Fig. 9.5 (continued)

9.6 Extensive Recurrent Ileitis with Fistula

Clinical Presentation A 27-year-old male with a 15-year history of Crohn's disease. Previous small bowel resection 5 years ago. Now has recurrent symptoms of intestinal obstruction with colicky abdominal pain and weight loss not responsive to steroid treatment. His father and two siblings have inflammatory bowel disease.

Radiographic Studies Showed diffuse small bowel involvement with multiple strictures. The colon was normal on colonoscopy (see Fig. 9.6b, c, d).

Surgical Treatment The patient underwent multiple strictureplasties of the jejunum and ileum. A 10 cm mass at the site of previous anastomosis was resected, and he also required a limited ileocolic resection (see Fig. 9.6a).

Pathology Active Crohn's ileitis with ulceration, granulomas, and fistula tract. Margins of resection show mild inflammation.

Follow-Up This patient had an uneventful recovery after surgery. He was taken off steroid medication and returned to his normal weight, and the abdominal distention was no longer present. He did well for 4 years and then required reoperation for a new mid small bowel stricture, which caused near-complete intestinal obstruction.

Comment This is a young patient with very aggressive Crohn's disease. He has a strong family history, onset at age 12, and rapid postoperative recurrence with extensive small bowel disease. This is an ideal patient for strictureplasty. Resection should be kept to a minimum in order to avoid further loss of bowel. The limited resections at the site of a mesenteric mass and at the recurrent disease in the neoterminal ileum were unavoidable since strictureplasty is difficult at these locations. Prophylactic treatment is important in this type of patient (Fig. 9.6).

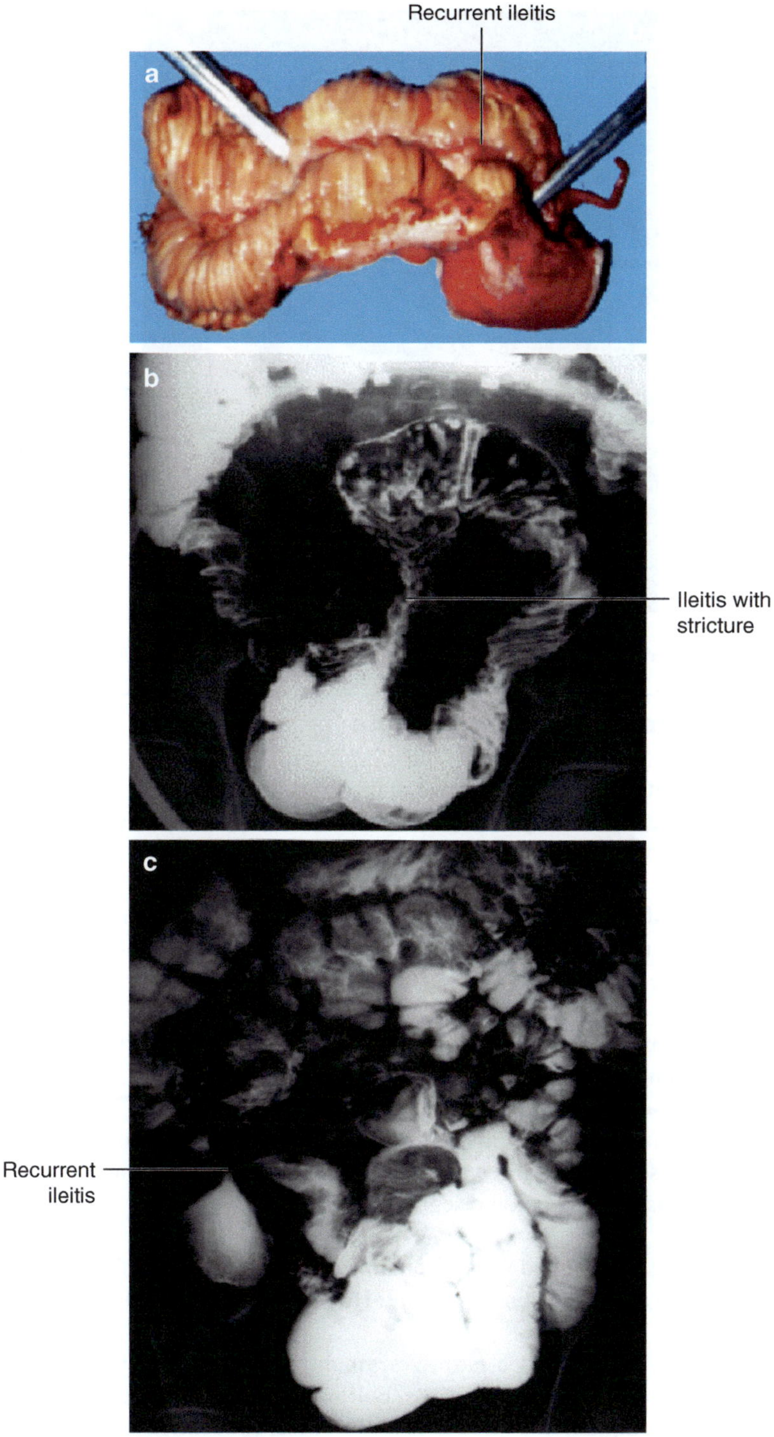

Fig. 9.6 (**a**–**d**) Extensive recurrent ileitis with fistula

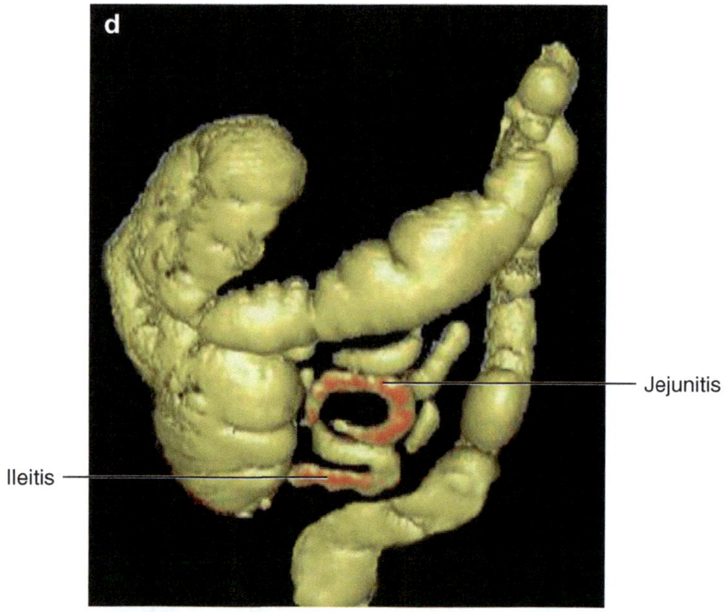

Fig. 9.6 (continued)

9.7 Recurrent Ileitis with Fistula

Clinical Presentation A 45-year-old man with Crohn's disease since age 20. He had a previous resection 13 years ago and now returns with colicky abdominal pain, abdominal distention, and 15 lb. weight loss.

Diagnostic Studies Small bowel series showed recurrent Crohn's disease in the neoterminal ileum with significant stricture and a fistula. Colonoscopy showed a normal colon (see Fig. 9.7c, d).

Surgical Treatment He underwent a secondary ileocolic resection with excision of a small mesenteric abscess and ileocolic anastomosis (see Fig. 9.7a, b).

Pathology Active Crohn's ileitis with transmural chronic inflammation, multiple fissures, and mesenteric fistulas with a mesenteric abscess. No granulomas are seen. The proximal margin and colonic segment are normal.

Follow-Up This patient had 9 ft. of remaining small bowel. He did well following surgery and was able to regain his weight. He remains on prophylactic therapy.

Comment This patient had a narrow segment of recurrent disease in the distal ileum with a chronic mesenteric abscess. Following surgery, he was able to maintain his weight but complained of frequent loose bowel movements requiring tincture of opium. It is interesting to note that he still has 9 ft. of small bowel and most of the colon is intact. With early onset, two operations, and fistulizing disease, the risk of early recurrence is high in this patient (Fig. 9.7).

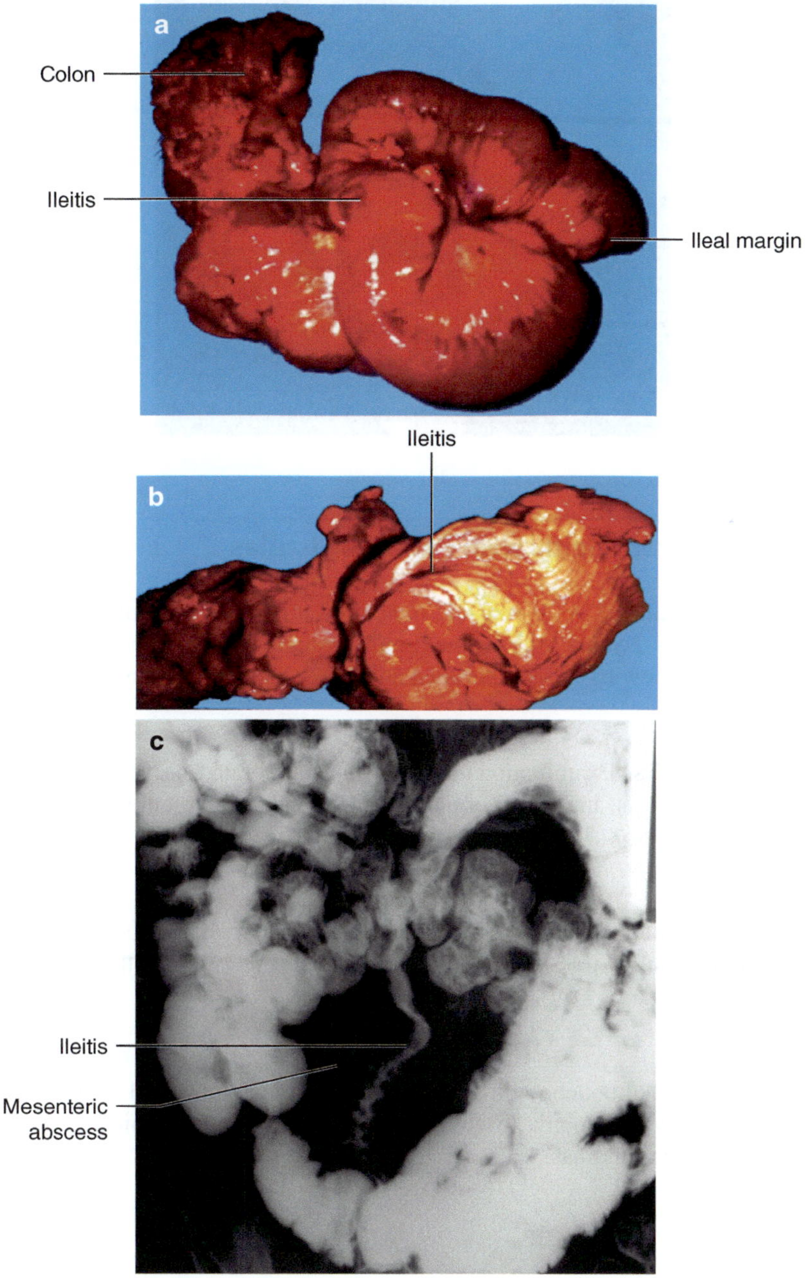

Fig. 9.7 (**a**–**d**) Recurrent ileitis with fistula

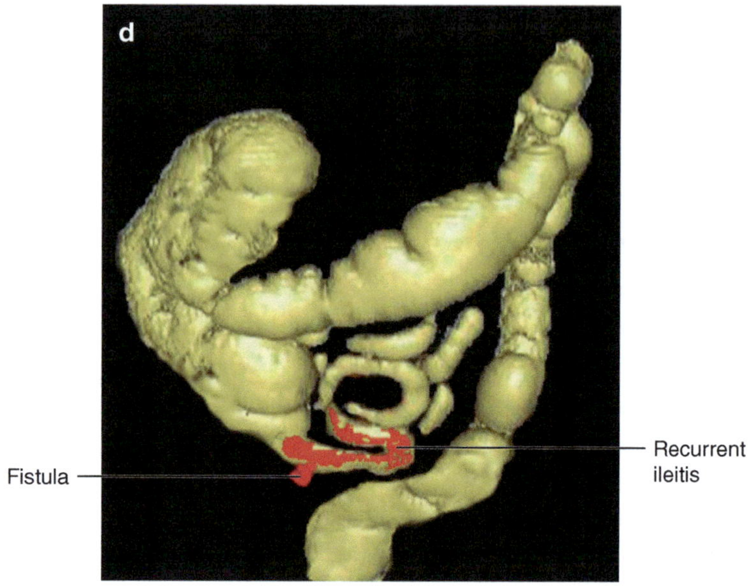

Fig. 9.7 (continued)

9.8 Recurrent Ileitis with Perianal Fistulas

Clinical Presentation A 29-year-old male presenting with multiple perianal fistulas and abscesses 2 years after ileoanal pull-through operation for apparent ulcerative colitis. He now has severe perianal and lower abdominal pain.

Diagnostic Studies Examination under anesthesia revealed a severe stricture at the ileoanal anastomosis, multiple perianal fistulas, and inflammation of the ileoanal pouch (see Fig. 9.8b).

Surgical Treatment Abdominoperineal resection of pelvic pouch with Brooke ileostomy. The inflow tract of the pouch showed severe inflammation and stricture (see Fig. 9.8a).

Pathology Ileoanal pouch, with active chronic inflammation, and neoterminal ileitis, consistent with Crohn's disease. There is transmural chronic inflammation, ulceration, and granulomas.

Follow-Up This patient had an uneventful recovery after surgery. The perineal wound healed well, and he is asymptomatic 6 months later.

Comment This patient was originally thought to have intractable ulcerative colitis and therefore underwent an ileoanal pull-through operation. He subsequently developed multiple perianal fistulas, a severe stricture at the ileoanal anastomosis, and inflammation of the J-pouch. The presence of inflammation at the inflow of the pouch helped confirm the diagnosis of recurrent Crohn's disease. This patient required excision of the pouch, including the anorectal canal with an end ileostomy. The risk of developing Crohn's disease in patients with the diagnosis of ulcerative colitis at the time of colectomy is under 3% in our series (Fig. 9.8).

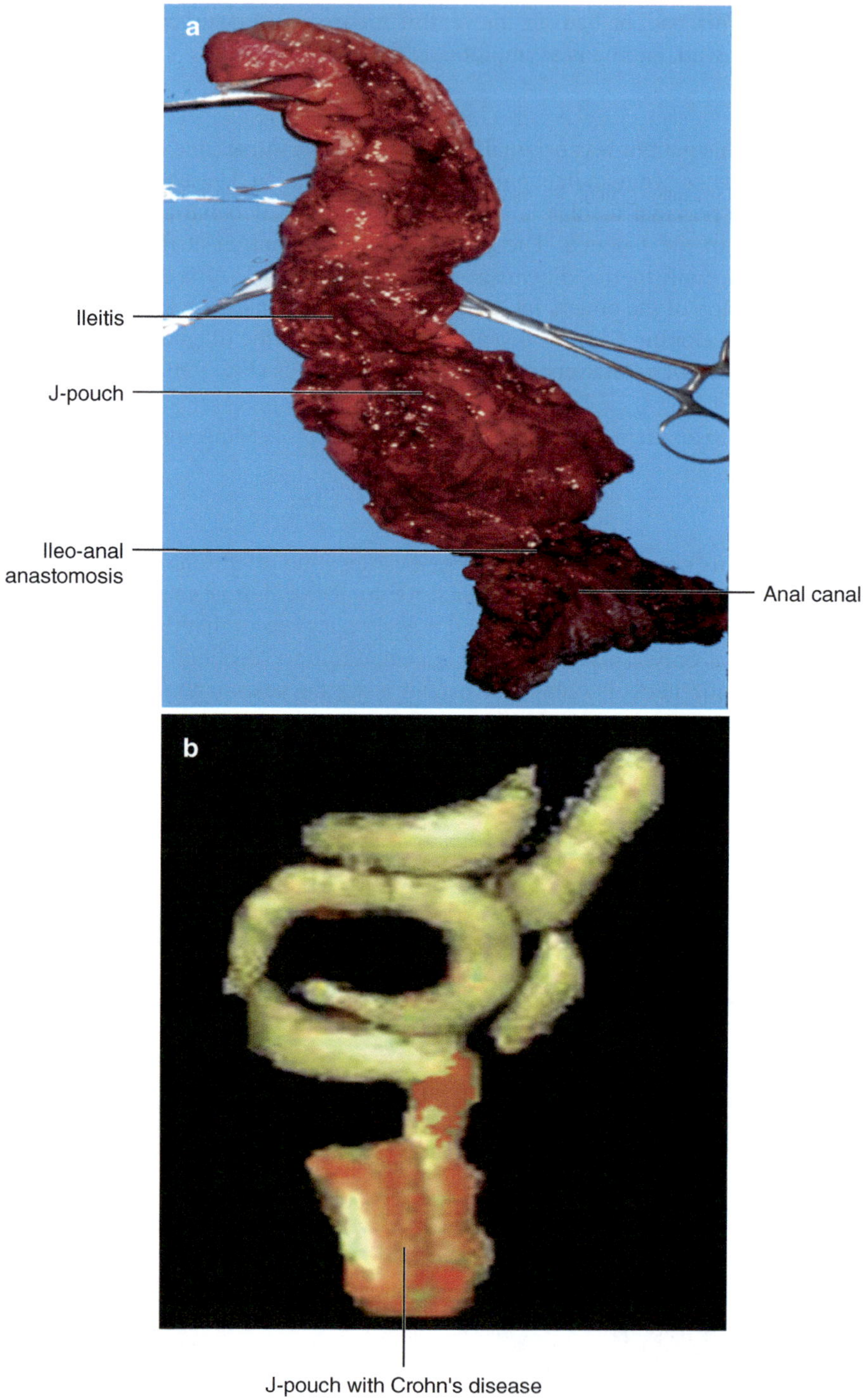

Fig. 9.8 (**a** and **b**) Recurrent ileitis with perianal fistulas

Further Reading

Greenstein AJ, Lachman P, Sachar DB, Springhorn J, Heimann TM, Janowitz HD, Aufses AH Jr. Perforating and non-perforating indications for repeated operations in Crohn's disease: evidence for two clinical forms. Gut. 1988;29:588–92.

Heimann TM, Greenstein AJ, Lewis B, Kaufman D, Heimann DM, Aufses AH Jr. Prediction of early symptomatic recurrence following intestinal resection in Crohn's disease. Ann Surg. 1993;218:294–9.

Part II

Ulcerative Colitis

Severe Ulcerative Colitis

10

Tomas M. Heimann and Robert J. Kurtz

The indications for surgery in ulcerative colitis are intractability and colorectal cancer risk. Ninety percent of patients in our series undergo surgery for intractability, while 10% are operated for dysplasia. The vast majority of patients with ulcerative colitis undergoing surgery opt to have an ileoanal pull-through procedure. Elderly patients and those with sphincter problems usually are not good candidates for this operation and most undergo proctocolectomy and Brooke ileostomy. We may perform a mucosectomy and hand-sewn ileoanal anastomosis since this operation removes all diseased mucosa or in patients with short mesentery, a stapled ileoanal anastomosis is performed instead.

Patients with severe ulcerative colitis can be divided into two categories. One group consists of patients with severe disease, responsive only to high-dose intensive medical treatment. In this category, the side effects of treatment contribute to the indications for surgery. The other group consists of patients with fulminant colitis, where the disease does not respond to medical treatment and surgery must be performed in an urgent setting. Patients with fulminant colitis are initially treated with subtotal colectomy and Brooke ileostomy. Patients with severe colitis may require initial subtotal colectomy and ileostomy, depending on their physical condition. Most patients in both groups are candidates for ileoanal pull-through operation at a later date.

10.1 Severe Ulcerative Colitis

Clinical Presentation A 37-year-old man with ulcerative colitis for 31/2 years. In the past 18 months, the symptoms have increased in severity and he has required increasing doses of steroids.

T. M. Heimann (✉) · R. J. Kurtz
Department of Surgery, Icahn School of Medicine at Mount Sinai, New York, NY, USA
e-mail: Tomas.Heimann@mountsinai.org; Robert.Kurtz@mountsinai.org

T. M. Heimann (ed.), *Atlas of Surgical Treatment of Inflammatory Bowel Disease*, https://doi.org/10.1007/978-3-031-62431-5_10

Diagnostic Studies Normal small bowel study. Colonoscopy showed moderately severe pancolitis.

Surgical Findings This patient had a subtotal colectomy and Brooke ileostomy. The entire colon showed severe colitis (see Fig. 10.1a, b).

Pathology Severely active ulcerative colitis with deep mucosal ulcerations extending retrograde from the sigmoid colon to the ascending colon. The distal sigmoid shows inactive chronic colitis. The ileal segment is unremarkable.

Follow-Up He did well following surgery. The steroids were gradually tapered off. He is still undecided whether to undergo ileoanal pull-through or have a completion proctectomy and keep the ileostomy.

Comment The indication for surgery in this patient was exacerbation of his symptoms requiring higher doses of steroids. At this dose, side effects of prednisone become a problem. Although he was well enough to undergo colectomy and ileoanal pull-through, this patient opted for a subtotal colectomy and ileostomy instead since he was concerned about the frequency of bowel movements. Decision as to further surgery is pending. He will require completion proctectomy if he decides to keep the ileostomy (Fig. 10.1).

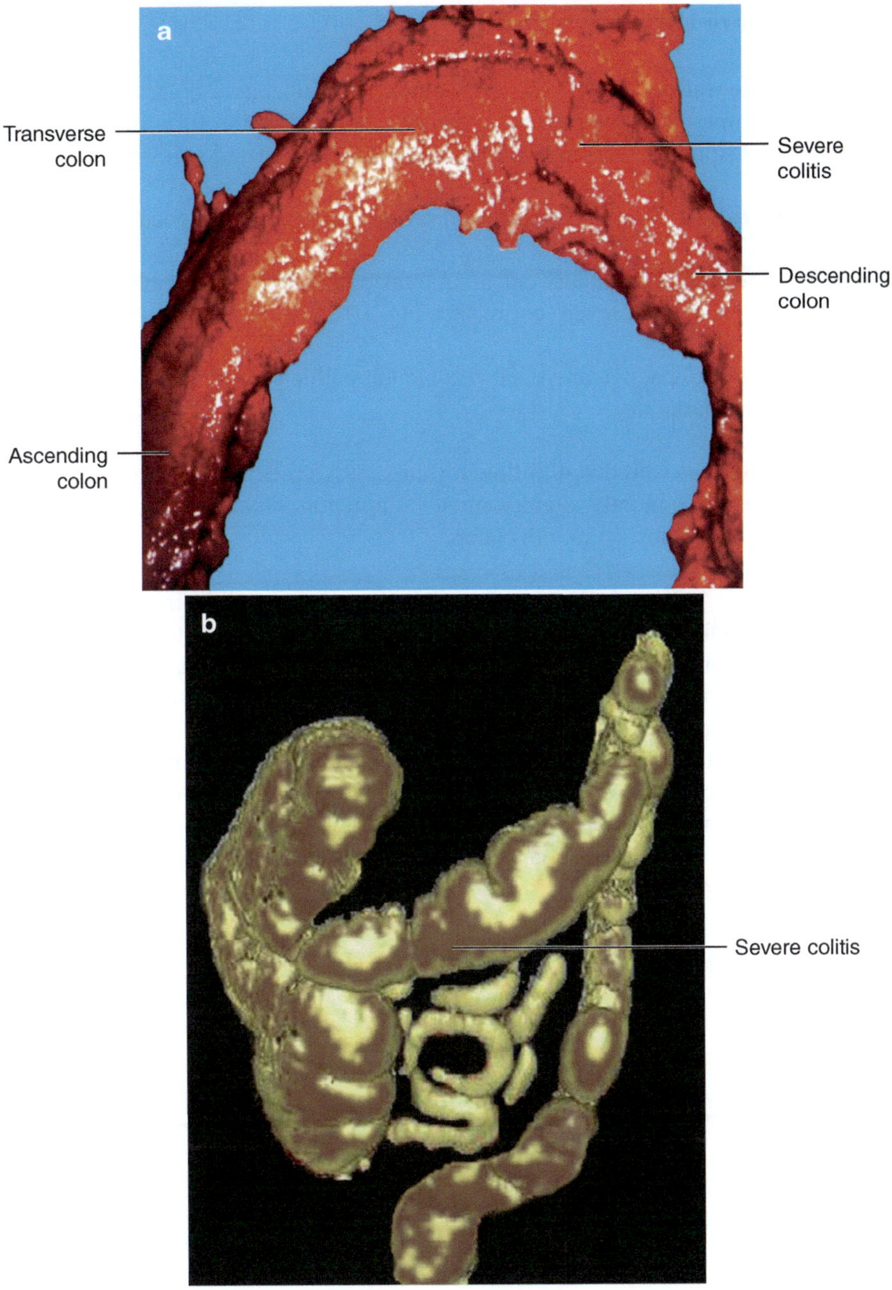

Fig. 10.1 (**a** and **b**) Severe ulcerative colitis

10.2 Severe Ulcerative Colitis

Clinical Presentation A 31-year-old woman with ulcerative colitis for 8 years. Increasing symptoms in the past year requiring hospitalization for intravenous steroids and cyclosporine. Currently on high-dose prednisone and still symptomatic.

Diagnostic Studies Normal small bowel series, colonoscopy showed pancolitis.

Surgical Findings She underwent a subtotal colectomy and Brooke ileostomy. The entire colon showed severe colitis (see Fig. 10.2a, b, c).

Pathology Severely active universal chronic idiopathic ulcerative colitis. The ileal segment is unremarkable.

Follow-Up She recovered well following surgery. All medications were discontinued, and she subsequently underwent a completion proctectomy with stapled J-pouch anal anastomosis 4 months later.

Comment This patient had severe exacerbation of her colitis in the past year, which became unresponsive to intensive medical treatment. Due to the severity of her disease combined with the immunosuppressive medications that she was taking, it was felt that performing a subtotal colectomy and ileostomy first would be safer. The completion proctectomy and ileoanal anastomosis was performed 4 months later after discontinuing all medication. Although we prefer to perform a mucosectomy and hand-sewn ileoanal anastomosis, this patient had a stapled ileoanal anastomosis without mucosectomy since her small bowel mesentery was too short to reach the dentate line (Fig. 10.2).

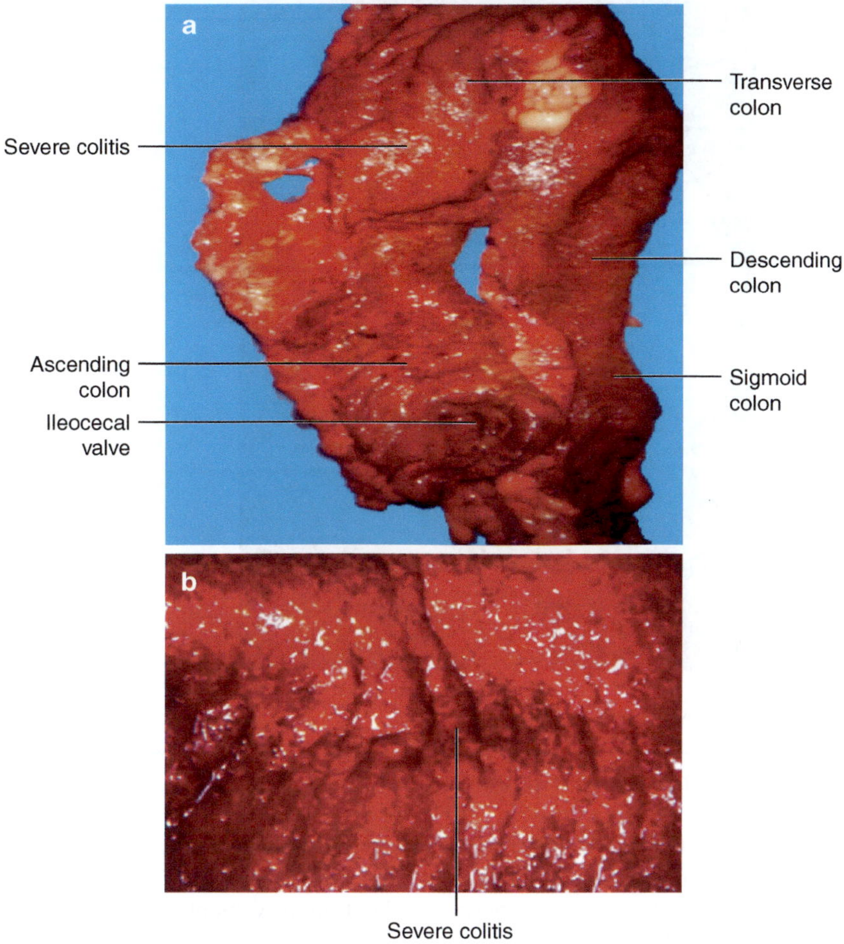

Fig. 10.2 (**a–c**) Severe ulcerative colitis

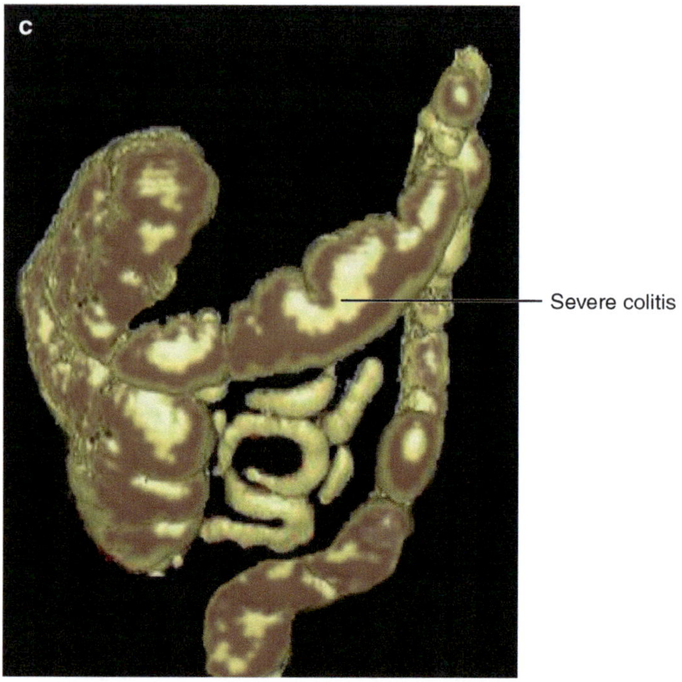

Fig. 10.2 (continued)

10.3 Fulminant Ulcerative Colitis

Clinical Presentation A 24-year-old man was admitted with a short history of fulminant ulcerative colitis. Patient was treated with high-dose intravenous steroids, followed by intravenous cyclosporine without improvement. He underwent an urgent subtotal colectomy and ileostomy for fulminant colitis.

Diagnostic Studies Flexible sigmoidoscopy showed severe colitis with ulcerations and pseudopolyps.

Surgical Findings Diffuse severe colitis. He underwent a subtotal colectomy with Hartmann's closure of the rectum and Brooke ileostomy (see Fig. 10.3a, b).

Pathology Universal fulminant chronic ulcerative colitis with extensive ulcerations and inflammatory polyposis. The ileal segment is unremarkable.

Follow-Up He recovered well following surgery and subsequently underwent completion proctectomy with mucosectomy and J-pouch anal anastomosis. He is well 2 years later.

Comment This patient is an example of severe fulminant ulcerative colitis. The duration of symptoms is short, but the entire colon is severely involved with mucosal destruction and secondary pseudopolyp formation. These patients are often refractory to medical therapy, including intravenous steroids and cyclosporine. Complications of this condition include the risk of colonic perforation and potential for sepsis exacerbated by severe weight and protein loss and the immunosuppressive effects of the medical therapy (Fig. 10.3).

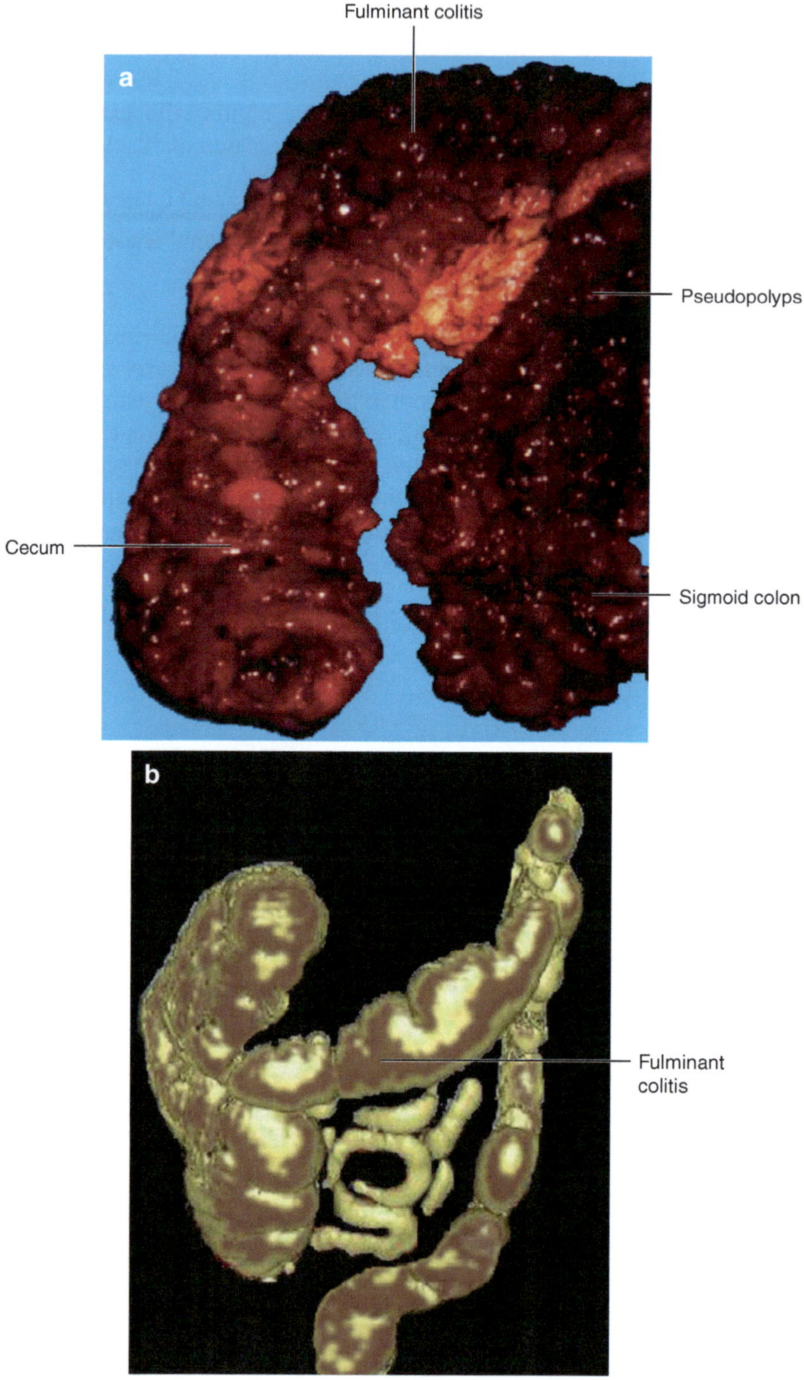

Fig. 10.3 (**a** and **b**) Fulminant ulcerative colitis

10.4 Fulminant Ulcerative Colitis

Clinical Presentation A 26-year-old man with a short history of severe ulcerative colitis unresponsive to high-dose intravenous steroids and intravenous cyclosporine.

Diagnostic Studies Severe ulcerative colitis on flexible endoscopy.

Surgical Findings Diffuse fulminant colitis. He underwent a subtotal colectomy and Brooke ileostomy (see Fig. 10.4a, b, c).

Pathology Severely active chronic ulcerative colitis with deep ulcerations and inflammatory polyps. The ileal segment is unremarkable.

Follow-Up He recovered well and 3 months later had completion proctectomy, mucosectomy, and J-pouch anal anastomosis with a loop ileostomy. The ileostomy was subsequently closed, and he is well 1 year later.

Comment This patient had a short history of symptoms with severe exacerbation requiring hospitalization. He was unresponsive to treatment with intravenous steroids and cyclosporine. Since his condition continued to deteriorate, he underwent an urgent total colectomy and ileostomy. After recovery from the colectomy, his weight returned to normal, the anemia improved, and steroids were discontinued. He subsequently had an ileoanal pull-through operation and did well. In severe fulminant colitis, colectomy is often a lifesaving procedure when all medical treatment modalities have been exhausted (Fig. 10.4).

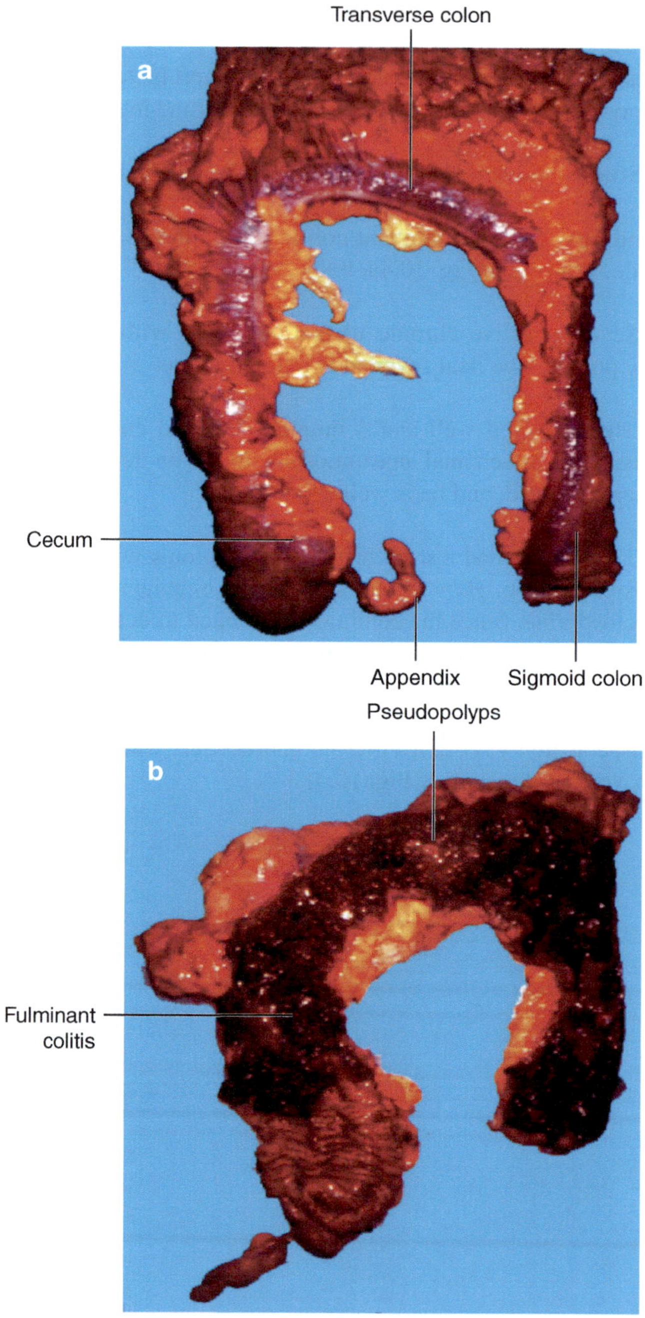

Fig. 10.4 (**a–c**) Fulminant ulcerative colitis

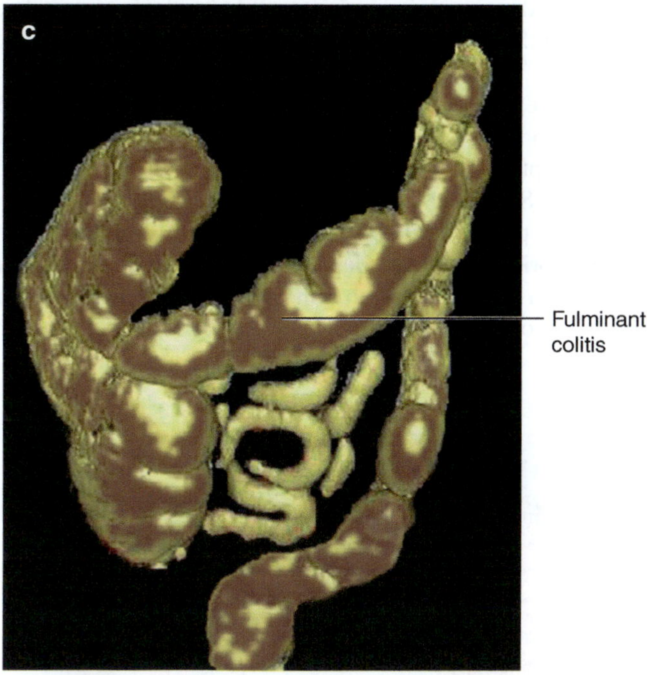

Fig. 10.4 (continued)

10.5 Fulminant Ulcerative Colitis

Clinical Presentation A 28-year-old man with ulcerative colitis for 10 years. Recent exacerbation not responsive to high dose oral and intravenous steroids.

Diagnostic Studies Flexible colonoscopy showed severe inflammation with deep ulcerations.

Surgical Findings He required urgent subtotal colectomy and Brooke ileostomy. The colon showed fulminant ulcerative colitis (see Fig. 10.5a, b, c, d).

Pathology Universal fulminant chronic ulcerative colitis with acute fissures and extensive ulcerations, some of which involve the muscularis propria. Multiple inflammatory polyps are present. The ileal segment is unremarkable.

Follow-Up He had an uneventful recovery and 4 months later had completion proctectomy, mucosectomy, and J-pouch anal anastomosis. He is well 1 year later.

He remained on low-dose prednisone for several months because of residual pyoderma gangrenosa in the lower extremities, which is now completely healed.

Comment This patient had a long-standing history of ulcerative colitis, which responded initially to medical therapy. Prior to admission, he developed a severe exacerbation of symptoms, which did not improve with high-dose oral and later intravenous steroids. Since the disease had already been present for 10 years, the decision was made to proceed with a subtotal colectomy and ileostomy and not use intravenous cyclosporine treatment. He recovered well after surgery but developed pyoderma gangrenosa of the lower extremities. The pyoderma finally healed about 6 months after the completion proctectomy and ileoanal pull-through operation (Fig. 10.5).

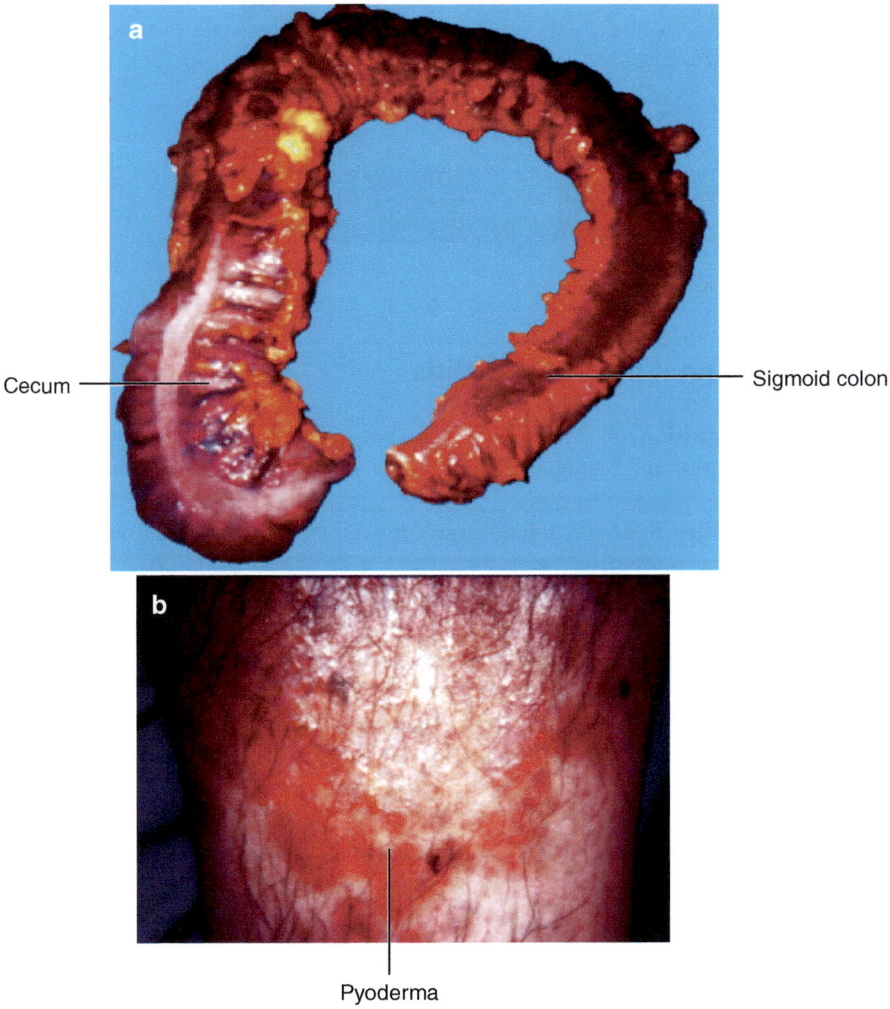

Fig. 10.5 (**a–d**) Fulminant ulcerative colitis

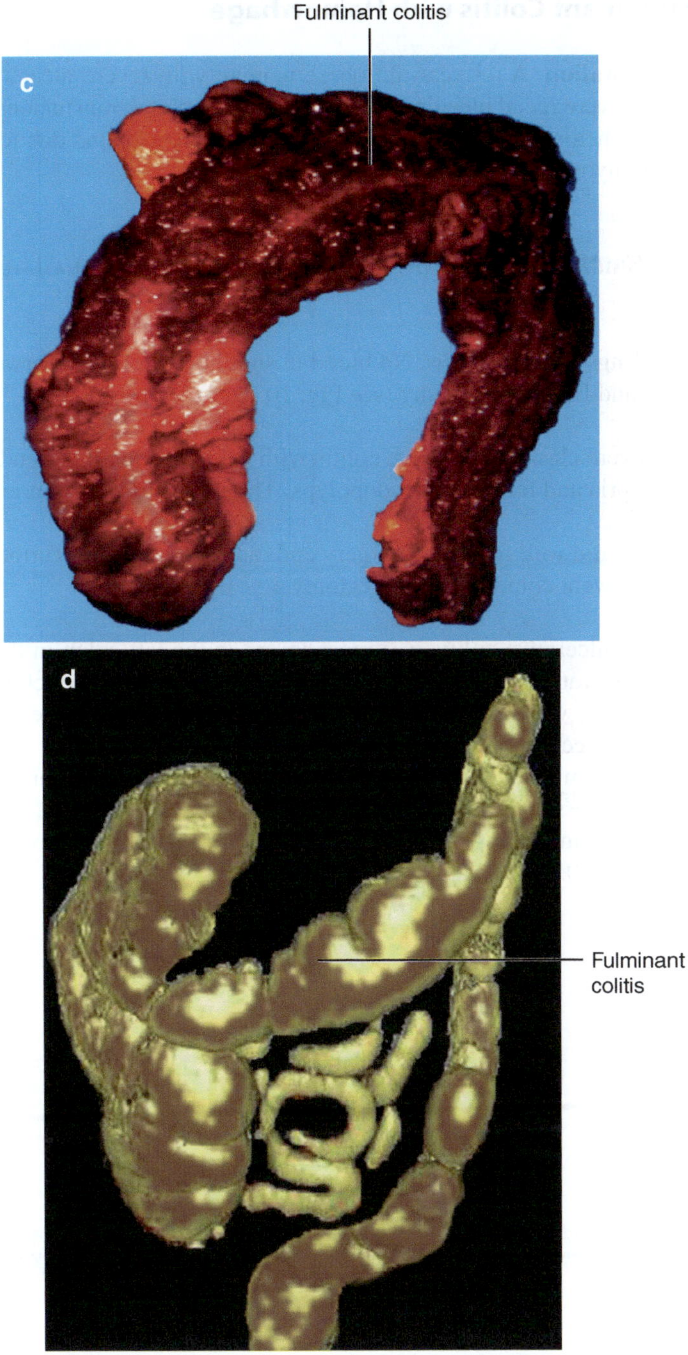

Fig. 10.5 (continued)

10.6 Fulminant Colitis with Hemorrhage

Clinical Presentation A 43-year-old obese woman with severe ulcerative colitis manifested by severe rectal bleeding requiring multiple blood transfusions. She was admitted with a hematocrit of 13%. She is also wheelchair bound due to the presence of severe myositis.

Diagnostic Studies Colonoscopy showed severe colitis. UGI endoscopy was normal.

Surgical Findings Severe colitis. No blood in small bowel. She underwent subtotal colectomy and Brooke ileostomy (see Fig. 10.6a, b).

Pathology Severe chronic ulcerative colitis with deep ulcerations extending to the muscularis propria and multiple pseudopolyps. The ileal segment is unremarkable.

Follow-Up She did well following surgery and did not require any further transfusions. She underwent completion proctectomy 1 year later.

Comment The ulcerative colitis was most severe in the left colon in this patient. She had deep ulcerations extending into the muscularis propria, which resulted in severe hemorrhage, which did not respond to medical treatment. She required an urgent subtotal colectomy and ileostomy and did well subsequently. The residual disease in the rectum responded to treatment with steroid foam and further transfusions were not necessary. Due to the presence of her severe myositis, the decision was made to perform a completion proctectomy 1 year later instead of an ileoanal anastomosis (Fig. 10.6).

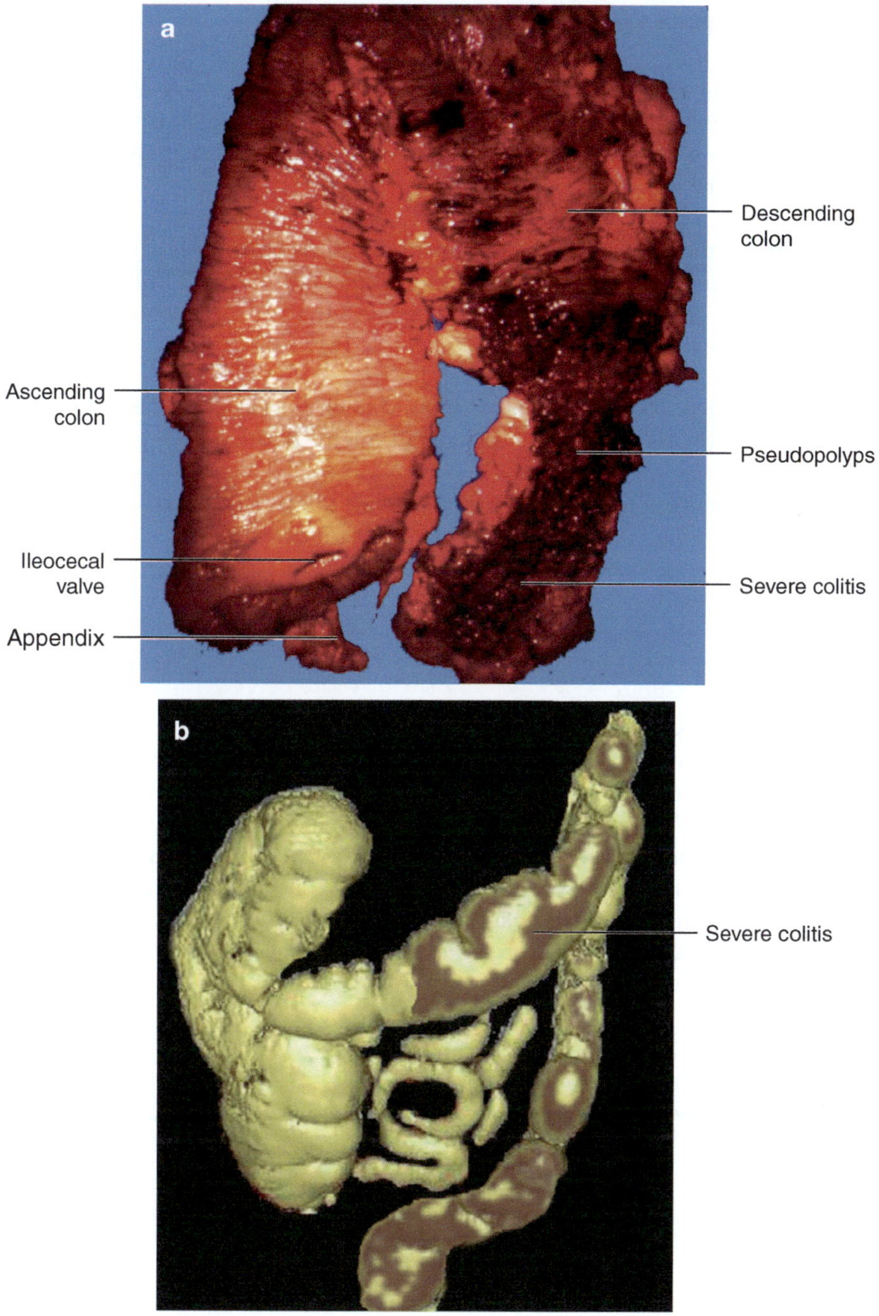

Fig. 10.6 (**a** and **b**) Fulminant colitis with hemorrhage

10.7 Toxic Megacolon

Clinical Presentation A 58-year-old man with severe coronary artery disease, chronic pulmonary disease, and now acute pneumonia who presents with a short history of severe ulcerative colitis unresponsive to intravenous steroids and intravenous cyclosporine.

Diagnostic Studies On physical examination, his abdomen is distended and diffusely tender. His serum albumin is 2.6 and hematocrit is 25%. Obstructive series showed colonic dilatation consistent with increasing toxic megacolon, and endoscopy of the rectum showed fulminant colitis (see Fig. 10.7b, c).

Surgical Findings He underwent urgent subtotal colectomy and Brooke ileostomy. A small abscess was present around the splenic flexure (see Fig. 10.7a).

Pathology Fulminant ulcerative colitis with toxic dilatation. Ulcerations and acute fissures extending into the muscularis propria. The ileal segment is unremarkable.

Follow-Up Following surgery, he developed candida sepsis, renal failure, and polyneuropathy. He required long-term respiratory support and was eventually transferred to a chronic care facility.

Comment This is an example of delay in surgical treatment caused by patient refusal. He was severely ill at another hospital for nearly 1 month prior to transfer. He had been on intravenous hyperalimentation, steroids, and cyclosporine without any improvement. The presence of acute pneumonia before surgery is an ominous problem in an immunosuppressed patient. At surgery, he had toxic megacolon and a walled off perforation at the splenic flexure. His postoperative recovery was stormy mostly due to pulmonary sepsis, resulting in secondary renal failure. All these problems could have been prevented if he had agreed to have surgery 2 weeks earlier (Fig. 10.7).

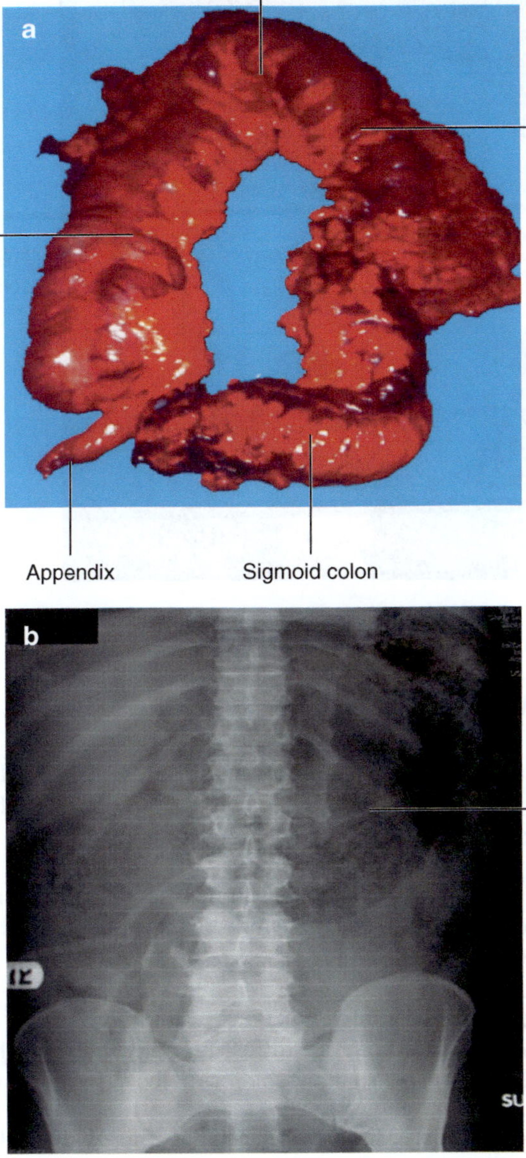

Fig. 10.7 (**a–c**) Toxic megacolon

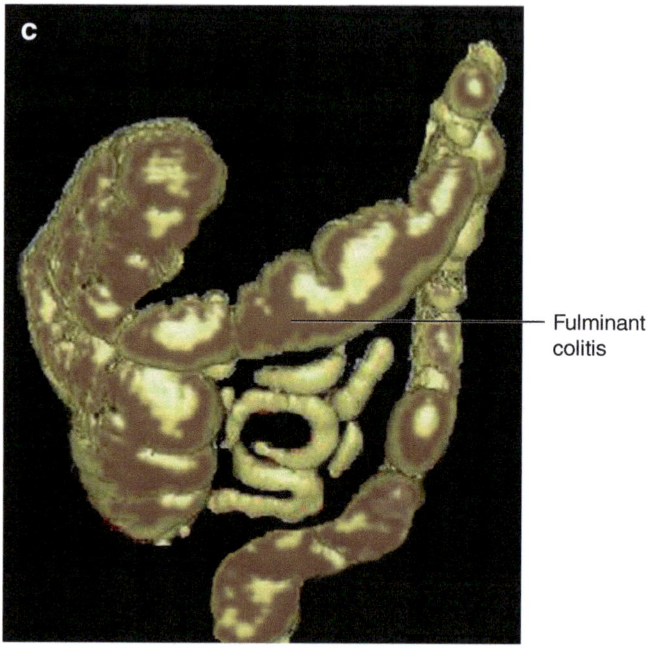

Fig. 10.7 (continued)

10.8 Toxic Megacolon with Perforation

Clinical Presentation An 82-year-old man with a recent onset of severe ulcerative colitis. He has recently required multiple hospital admissions and has not responded to treatment with high-dose oral and intravenous steroids.

Diagnostic Studies Physical exam showed diffuse abdominal distention and tenderness. Obstructive series showed toxic megacolon and upright chest x-ray showed free air under the diaphragm (see Fig. 10.8b, c, d).

Surgical Findings He underwent an emergency subtotal colectomy and Brooke ileostomy. The surgical findings were severe diffuse ulcerative colitis with toxic megacolon and a colonic perforation in the sigmoid colon with fecal peritonitis (see Fig. 10.8a).

Pathology Severely active chronic ulcerative colitis with perforating fissuring ulcerations in the sigmoid colon and multiple inflammatory polyps. The ileal segment is unremarkable.

Follow-Up He had a difficult postoperative recovery requiring long-term respiratory support. His mental status never recovered completely, and he expired about 3 months later.

Comment Ulcerative colitis in the elderly can be fulminant with a very short duration of symptoms. Older patients deteriorate rapidly and do not respond well to high dose steroids. Early surgery is essential to avoid severe complications, which are poorly tolerated. Reluctance by the patient and his family to allow a colectomy with ileostomy resulted in multiple readmissions to the hospital and ultimately colonic perforation with severe peritonitis. Although he survived the surgery, his pulmonary function deteriorated to the point that he remained respirator-dependent and eventually expired from respiratory failure (Fig. 10.8).

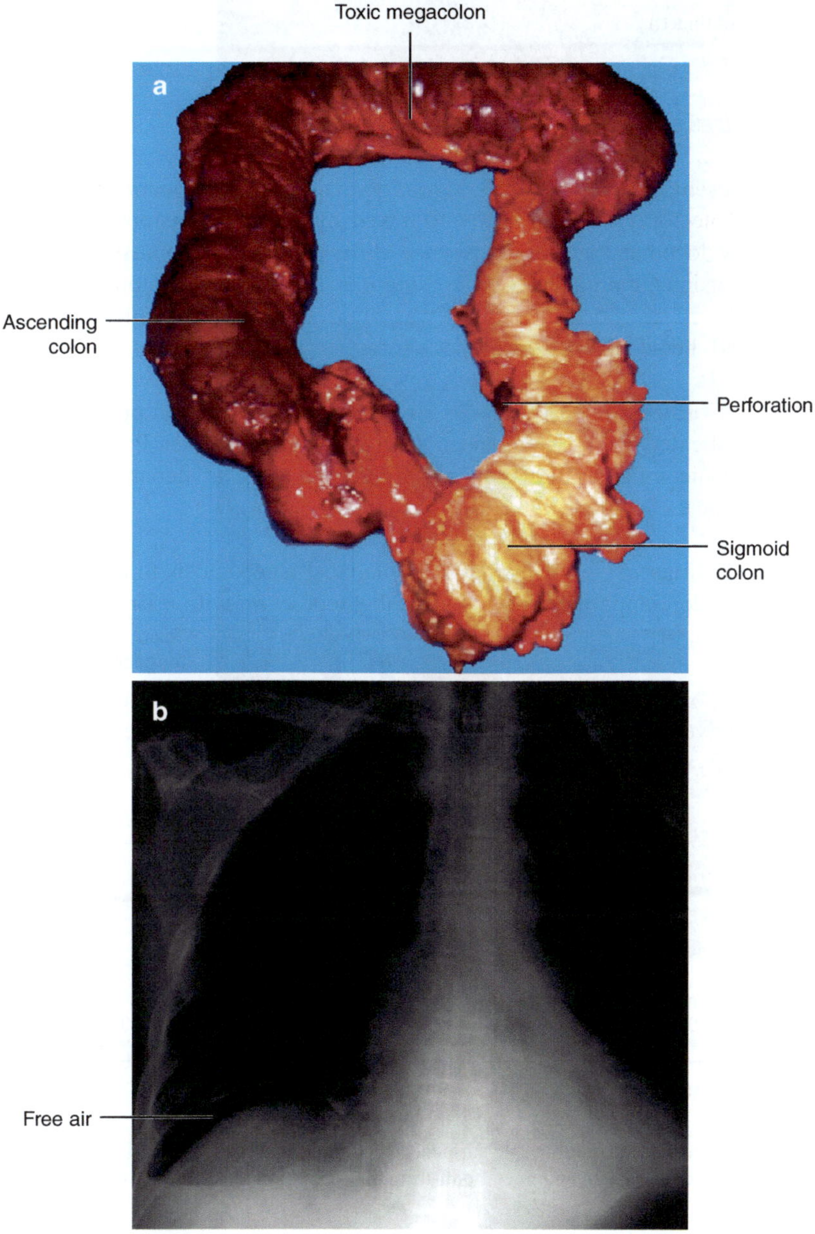

Fig. 10.8 (**a–d**) Toxic megacolon with perforation

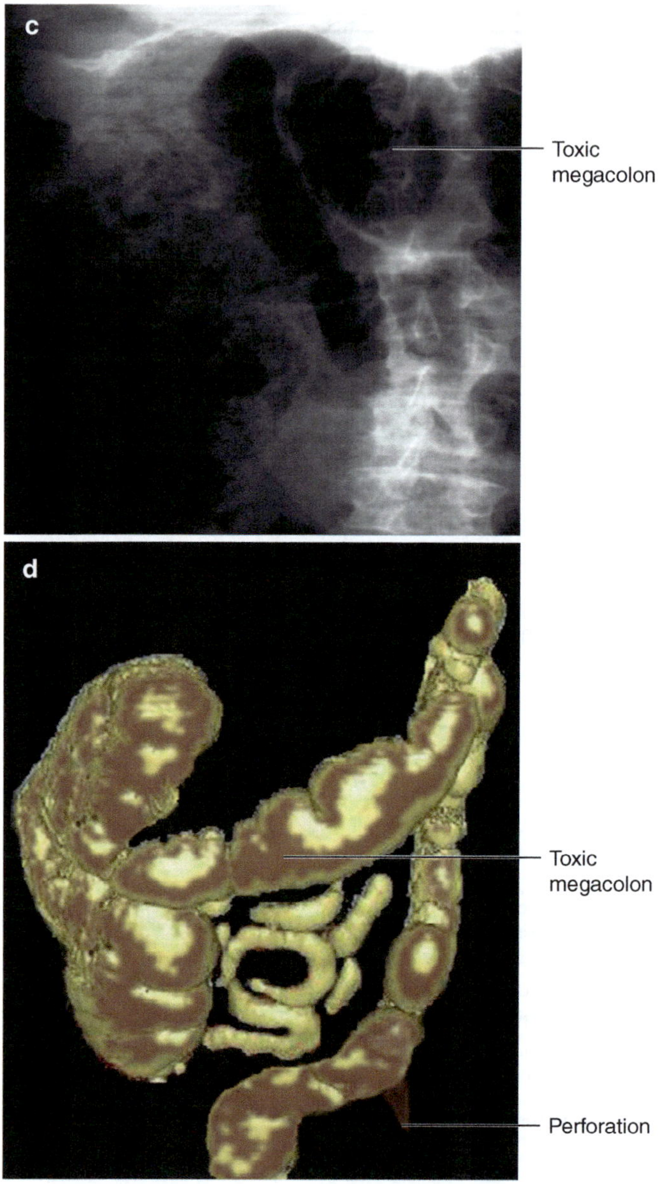

Fig. 10.8 (continued)

Further Reading

Heimann T. The endorectal pullthrough: surgical considerations. Mt. Sinai J Med. 1980;47:606–11.
Heimann TM. Symposium on endorectal pull-through operations. Contemp Surg. 1988;33:41–66.

Intractable Ulcerative Colitis

11

Tomas M. Heimann and Robert J. Kurtz

Patients with intractable ulcerative colitis requiring surgical treatment can have a variety of problems. This chapter reviews some of the problems faced by these patients, including those related to outcomes of surgical treatment. Since the advent of ileoanal pull-through operations, very few patients undergo continent ileostomies, partly because of problems related to these procedures. While the vast majority of patients undergoing proctocolectomy with ileostomy and those having ileoanal pull-through operations do well, some of the problems related to these operations are also presented here.

11.1 Intractable Colitis with Pyoderma

Clinical Presentation A 57-year-old woman with a 6-year history of ulcerative colitis. She recently developed pyoderma gangrenosa throughout her body, which has not responded to high-dose steroids (see Fig. 11.1a).

Diagnostic Studies Colonoscopy revealed moderately severe pancolitis.

Surgical Findings Moderately severe ulcerative colitis involving the entire colon and rectum. She underwent total proctocolectomy with mucosal proctectomy and sphincter preservation (see Fig. 11.1b).

Pathology Active chronic ulcerative colitis. The ileal segment is unremarkable.

T. M. Heimann (✉) · R. J. Kurtz
Department of Surgery, Icahn School of Medicine at Mount Sinai, New York, NY, USA
e-mail: Tomas.Heimann@mountsinai.org; Robert.Kurtz@mountsinai.org

T. M. Heimann (ed.), *Atlas of Surgical Treatment of Inflammatory Bowel Disease*, https://doi.org/10.1007/978-3-031-62431-5_11

Follow-Up The pyoderma gangrenosa gradually resolved following surgical treatment. She is well with the Brooke ileostomy and has decided not to undergo an ileoanal pull-through operation.

Comment Severe pyoderma gangrenosum is one of the most difficult complications of ulcerative colitis. It often will not respond to medical treatment, and proctocolectomy with removal of all diseased colorectal mucosa is the only treatment that can cure the problem. This patient underwent a proctocolectomy with distal mucosectomy and preservation of the sphincter muscles. These patients can undergo an ileoanal anastomosis at a later date by dilating the sphincter muscles and performing an ileoanal anastomosis. This patient opted to keep the ileostomy and avoid further surgery (Fig. 11.1).

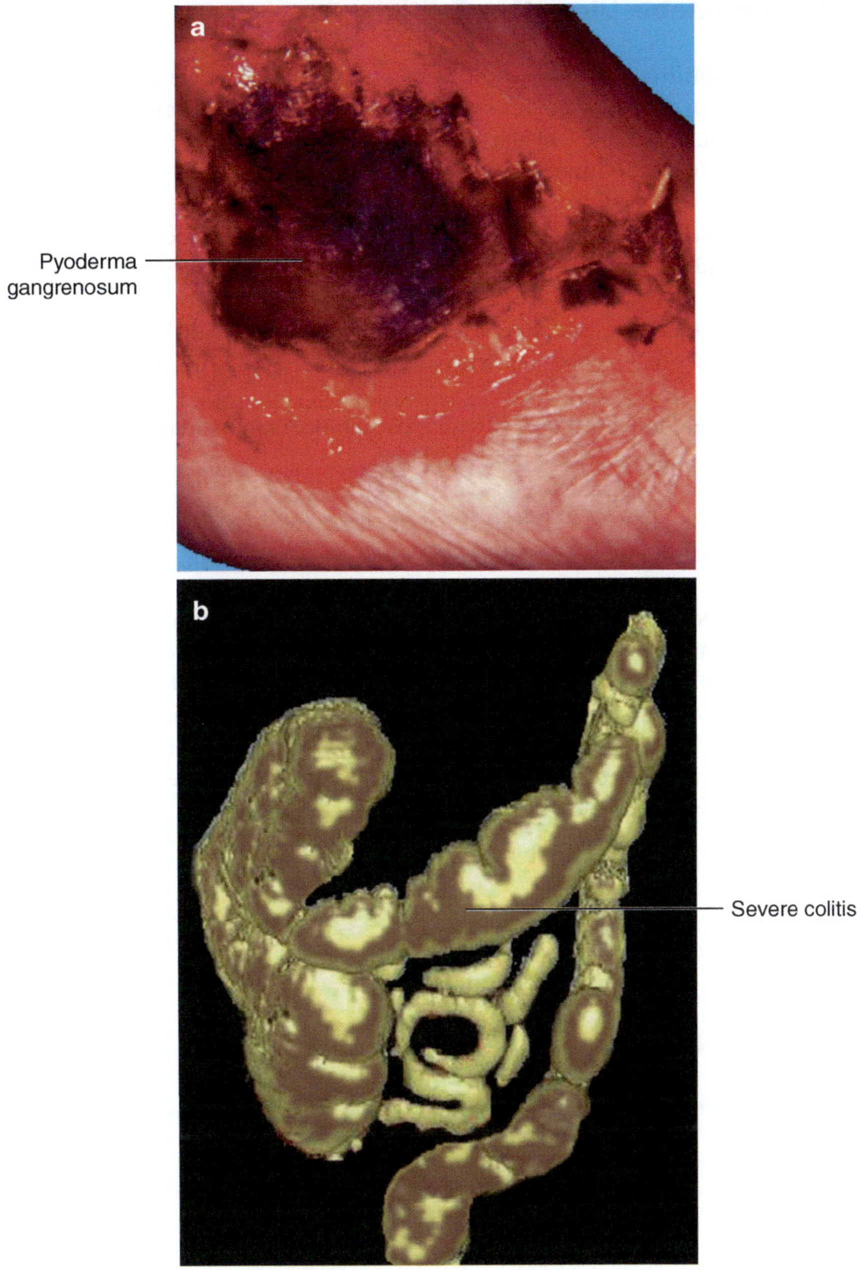

Fig. 11.1 (**a** and **b**) Intractable colitis with pyoderma

11.2 Intractable Ulcerative Colitis

Clinical Presentation A 68-year-old man with intractable ulcerative colitis present for 7 years. In the past year, his symptoms have increased in severity, and he has required high-dose steroids in the range of 40 mg of prednisone daily without improvement. He has continued to lose weight and is anemic.

Diagnostic Studies Recent colonoscopy showed severe pancolitis with most severe disease in the rectum (see Fig. 11.2c).

Surgical Treatment He underwent a subtotal colectomy with Brooke ileostomy and 9 months later had a completion proctectomy (see Fig. 11.2a, b).

Pathology Severe universal colitis with mucosal ulceration and inflammatory polyps. The rectum showed severe proctitis.

Follow-Up This patient is doing well 2 years later. He regained his normal weight and is off steroids.

Comment This patient had a late onset of ulcerative colitis with severe symptoms and poor response to steroids. At the time of initial surgery, he required a subtotal colectomy because of his poor nutritional status and the side effects of being on high-dose steroids for several years. Nine months later, a completion proctectomy was performed. He was not a good candidate for an ileoanal pull-through because of his age and his frail health. He has done well with the Brooke ileostomy as his health and nutrition have slowly returned to normal (Fig. 11.2).

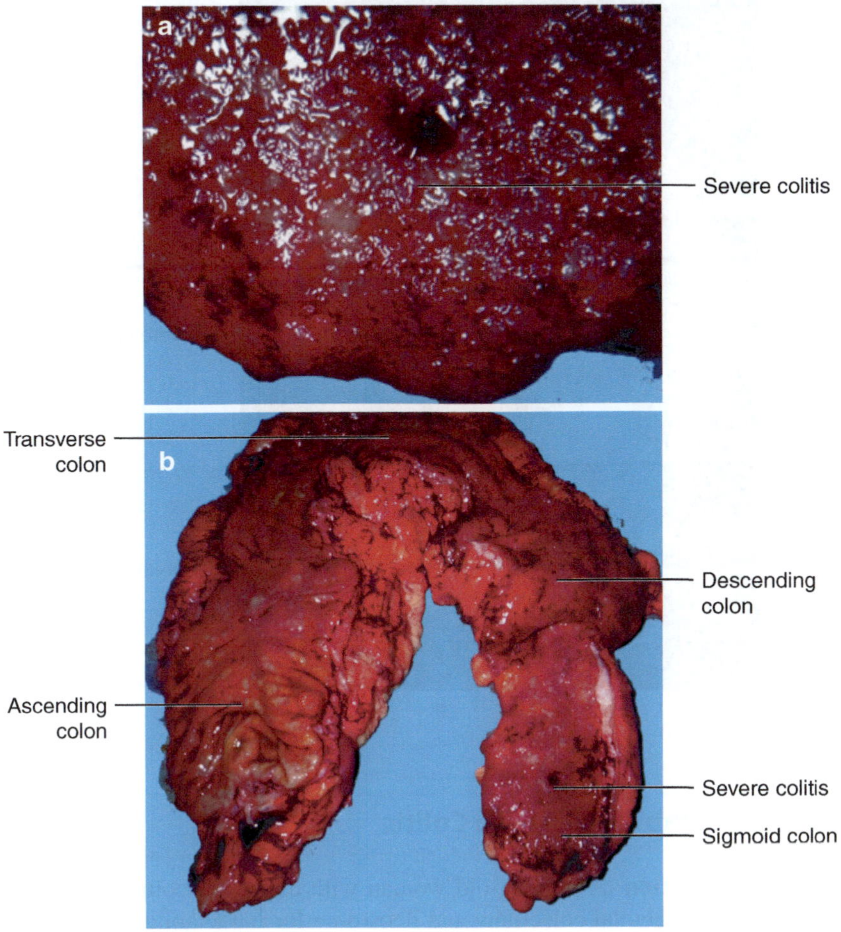

Fig. 11.2 (**a**–**c**) Intractable ulcerative colitis

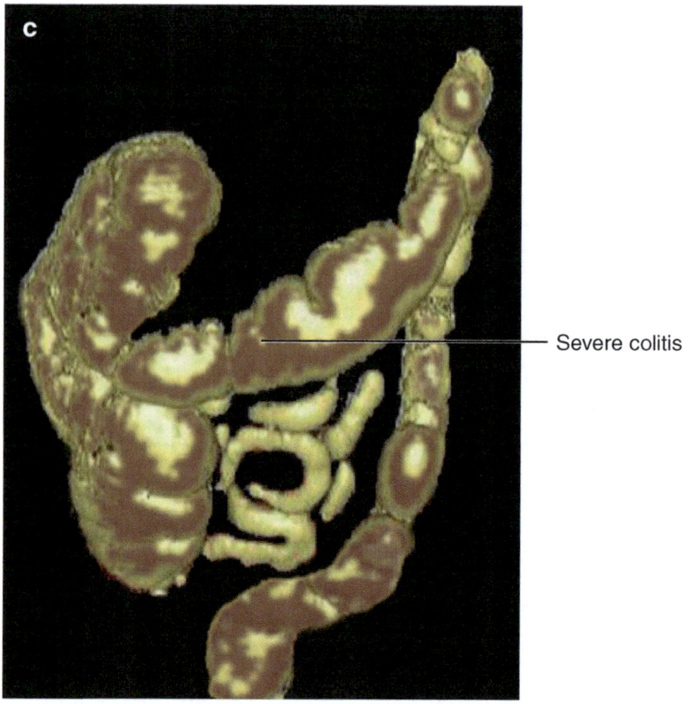

Fig. 11.2 (continued)

11.3 Intractable Ulcerative Colitis

Clinical Presentation A 47-year-old woman with ulcerative colitis for 10 years. She underwent a subtotal colectomy and ileostomy for intractability 4 months ago and now comes in for ileoanal anastomosis.

Diagnostic Studies Endoscopy showed moderately severe residual proctitis (see Fig. 11.3b).

Surgical Findings Moderate residual proctitis. She underwent completion proctectomy, mucosectomy, and J-pouch anal anastomosis (see Fig. 11.3a).

Pathology Chronic idiopathic ulcerative colitis. Ileal segment is unremarkable.

Follow-Up She had an uneventful recovery and is well 18 months later.

Comment This patient had severe intractable colitis and underwent subtotal colectomy with ileostomy elsewhere. She was referred 4 months later for ileoanal pull-through. Preservation of the blood supply to the terminal ileum in order to allow for a sufficient length to perform an ileoanal anastomosis is critical during subtotal colectomy in patients having subsequent ileoanal pull-through operation. The length of the mesentery in this patient was sufficient to perform a mucosectomy and subsequent hand-sewn J-pouch anal anastomosis (Fig. 11.3).

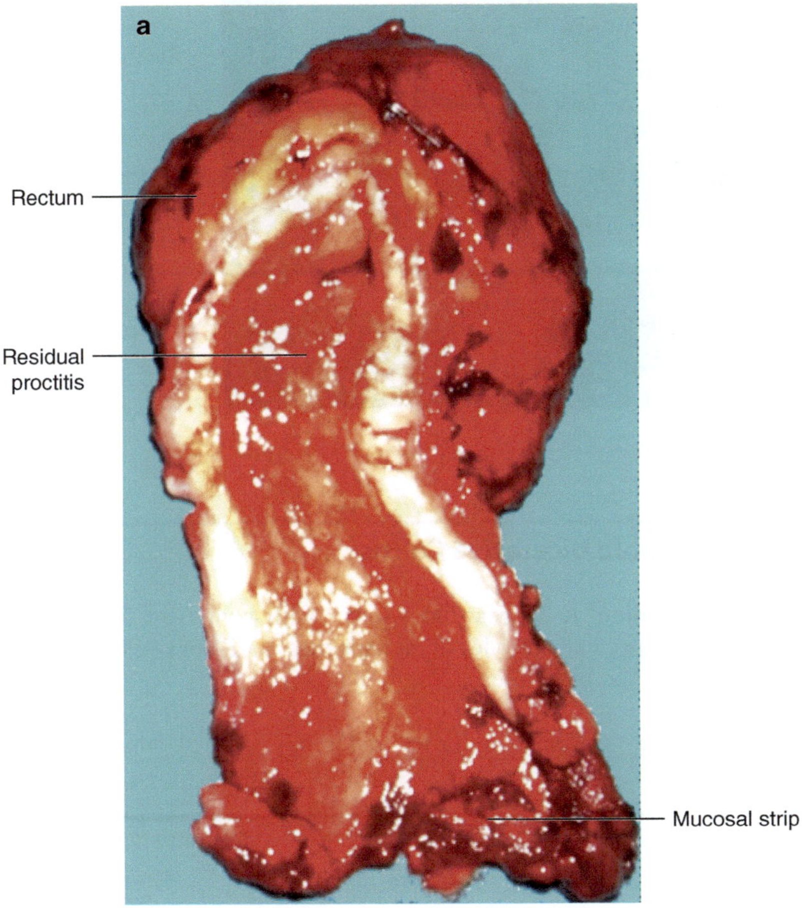

Fig. 11.3 (**a** and **b**) Intractable ulcerative colitis

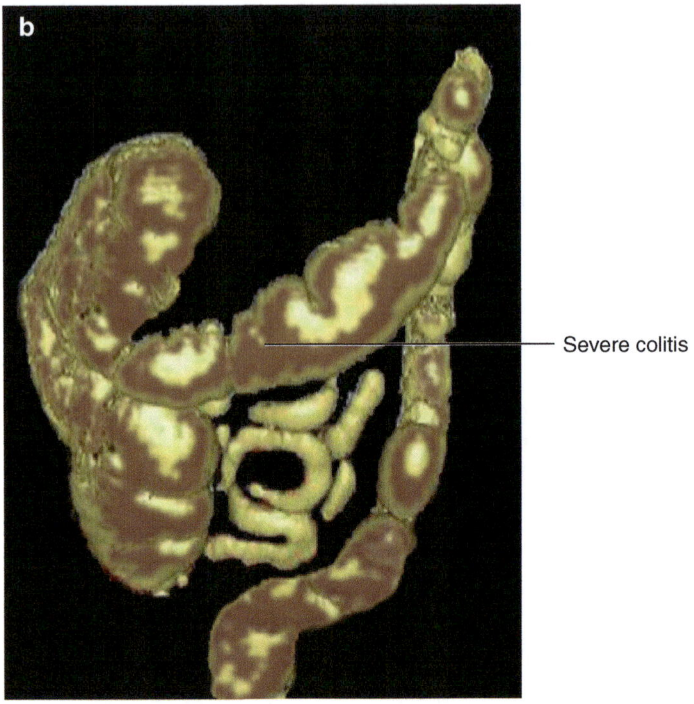

Fig. 11.3 (continued)

11.4 Intractable Ulcerative Colitis

Clinical Presentation A 53-year-old woman with colitis for 7 years. Recent increase in symptoms with episodes of incontinence, unresponsive to medical treatment. No history of perianal disease.

Diagnostic Studies Chronic colitis on endoscopy, normal small bowel study (see Fig. 11.4c).

Surgical Findings Moderately severe colitis. She underwent subtotal colectomy with Brooke ileostomy (see Fig. 11.4a, b).

Pathology Severely active indeterminate colitis with several areas showing transmural chronic inflammation and mild subserosal fibrosis. The ileal segment is unremarkable.

Follow-Up She had an uneventful recovery. One year later, she decided to keep the ileostomy and returned for completion proctectomy. The pathology report from the rectal segment was consistent with ulcerative colitis.

Comment This patient's age, features of indeterminate colitis, and history of incontinence all contributed to her decision not to undergo an ileoanal pull-through operation. She was satisfied living with the Brooke ileostomy and did not want to undergo a surgical procedure, which may result in incontinence. After living with the ileostomy for 1 year, she underwent completion proctectomy and has done well. Patients with indeterminate features without perianal disease, in general, are not at high risk to have poor results after ileoanal pull-through operations (Fig. 11.4).

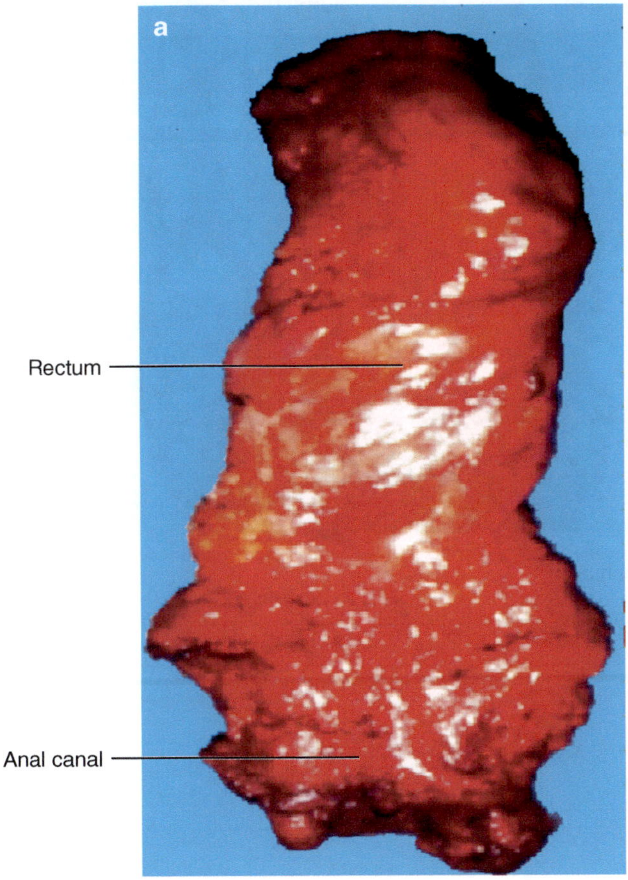

Fig. 11.4 (a–c) Intractable ulcerative colitis

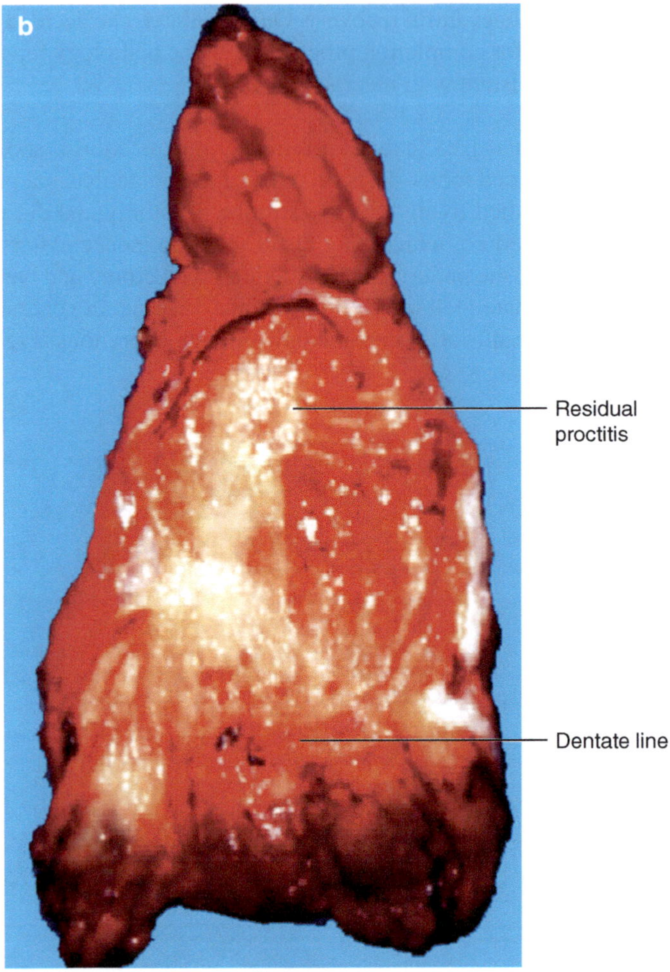

Fig. 11.4 (continued)

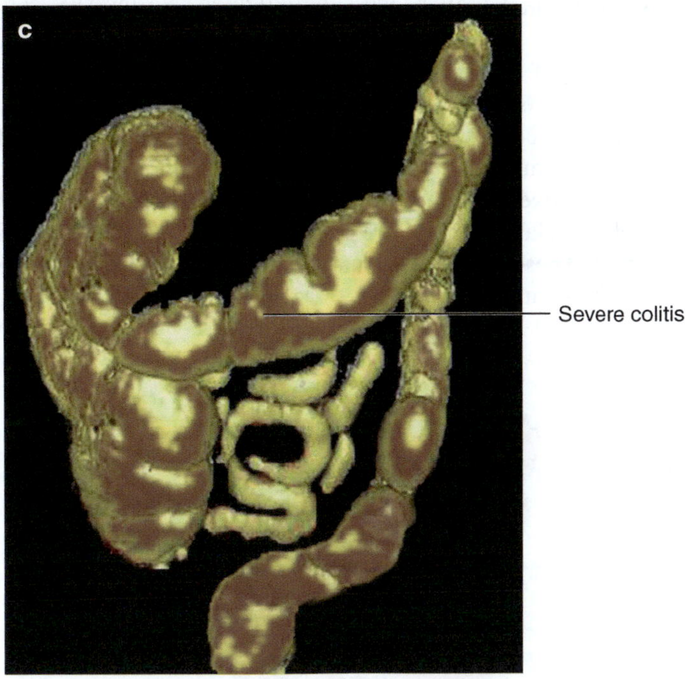

Fig. 11.4 (continued)

11.5 Ulcerative Colitis with Pouch Dysfunction

Clinical Presentation A 48-year-old woman with ulcerative colitis for 23 years. Recently, she required a subtotal colectomy and ileostomy because of increased symptoms and less response to steroids (see Fig. 11.5c). She subsequently had completion proctectomy, mucosectomy, and J-pouch anal anastomosis 4 months later. She now returns complaining of frequent bowel movements and frequent episodes of incontinence, worse at night.

Diagnostic Studies Pouch endoscopy showed well-healed ileoanal anastomosis and J-pouch. No evidence of Crohn's disease.

Surgical Findings Well-healed J-pouch and ileoanal anastomosis. No evidence of pouchitis. She had abdominoperineal excision of the neorectum with Brooke ileostomy (see Fig. 11.5a, b).

Pathology Subtotal colectomy showing chronic ulcerative colitis. Unremarkable J-pouch and ileoanal anastomosis.

Follow-Up She recovered well after surgery and is asymptomatic 1 year later.

Comment Removal of the neorectum following ileoanal anastomosis is unusual when the anastomosis is well healed. In this case, problems with incontinence, worse at night, convinced this patient to have the neorectum removed. She had no improvement in her symptoms with constipating medication and after 2 years felt that living with a Brooke ileostomy would improve her quality of life. Episodes of seepage of stool especially at night are not uncommon, and some patients wear a pad when sleeping. These symptoms usually tend to improve with time, which was not the case with this patient (Fig. 11.5).

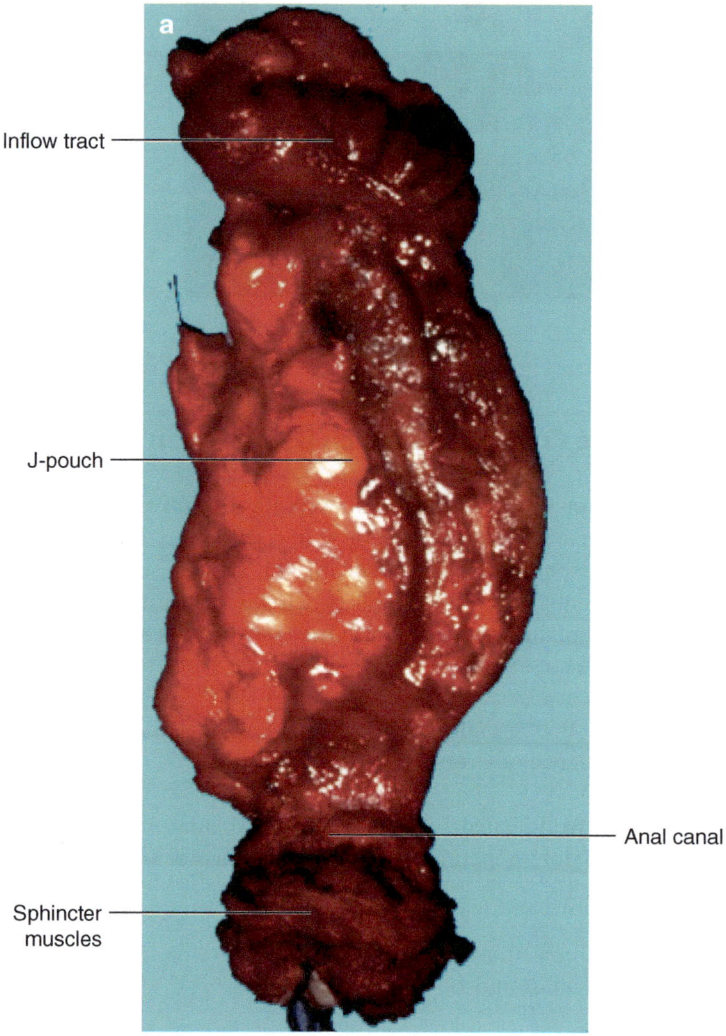

Fig. 11.5 (**a–c**) Ulcerative colitis + pouch dysfunction

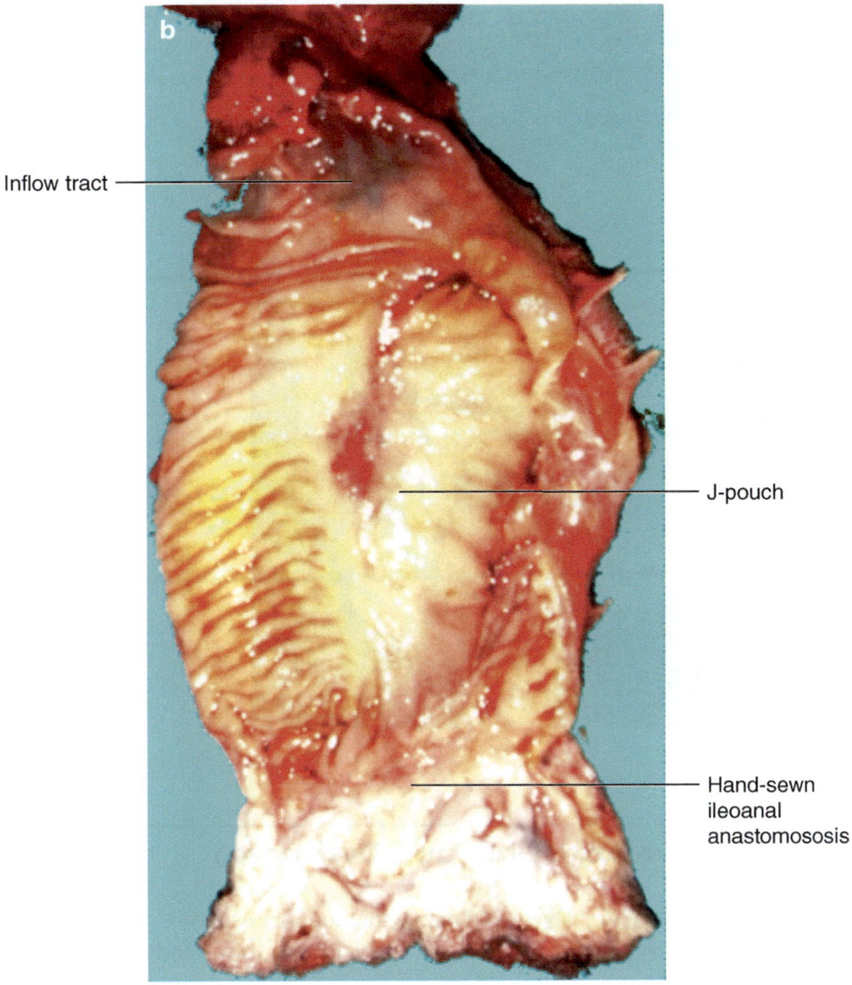

Fig. 11.5 (continued)

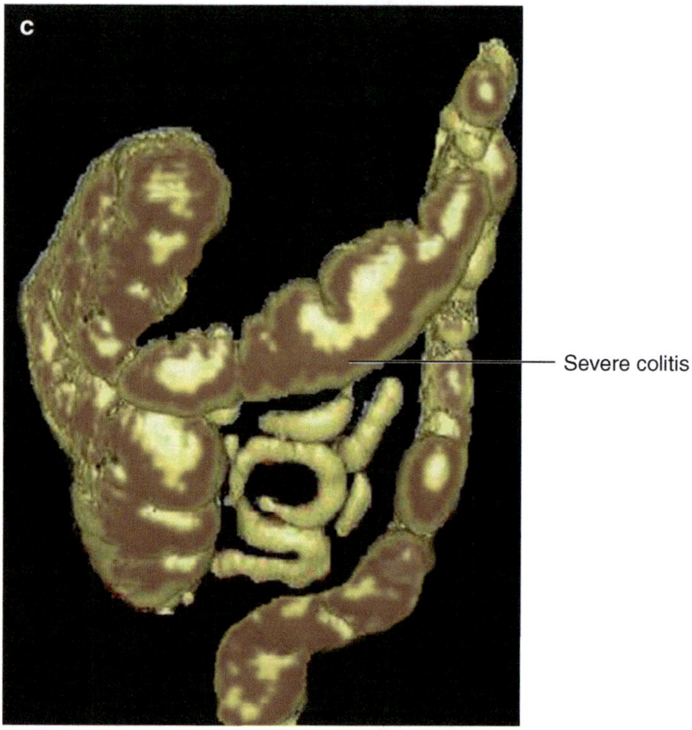

Fig. 11.5 (continued)

11.6 Ulcerative Colitis with Pouch Dysfunction

Clinical Presentation A 32-year-old man with moderately severe ulcerative colitis (see Fig. 11.6c) who underwent total colectomy, proctectomy, and stapled J-pouch anal anastomosis 18 months ago. He required percutaneous drainage of a suprapubic abscess 3 weeks later and subsequently did well. He now returns with a chronic history of pelvic pain, worse during bowel movements, and requiring narcotic medication.

Diagnostic Studies Pouch endoscopy showed a short segment of residual rectum with mild colitis and a well-healed ileoanal anastomosis and normal J-pouch. CT scan of the pelvis showed a well-healed pouch and no residual abscess or fistulas.

Surgical Findings This patient underwent excision of the neorectum and Brooke ileostomy. Severe adhesions were found around the ileoanal anastomosis (see Fig. 11.6a, b).

Pathology The colectomy specimen showed chronic ulcerative colitis with an unremarkable ileum.

J-pouch and anorectum showed mild residual proctitis. No evidence of Crohn's disease. Pouch mucosa appears unremarkable.

Follow-Up He is doing well 2 years after surgery with a Brooke ileostomy.

Comment This patient had a short mesentery and underwent a stapled ileoanal anastomosis. He subsequently developed a pelvic abscess that responded to percutaneous-guided drainage, and no leak was demonstrated. He subsequently complained of chronic pelvic pain, which ultimately required excision of the neorectum and Brooke ileostomy. The etiology of the pelvic pain is unclear but most likely is related to scarring caused by the pelvic abscess (Fig. 11.6).

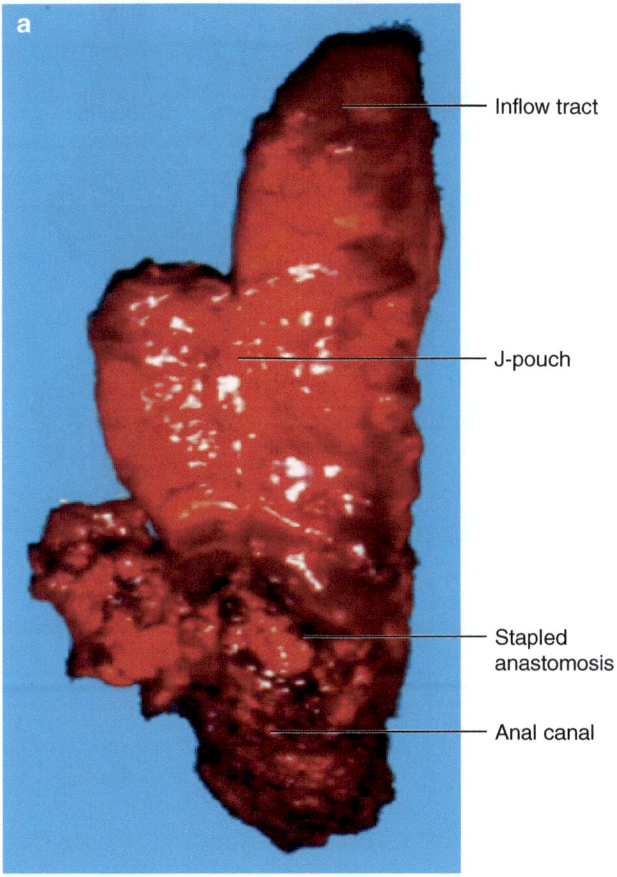

Fig. 11.6 (**a–c**) Ulcerative colitis + pouch dysfunction

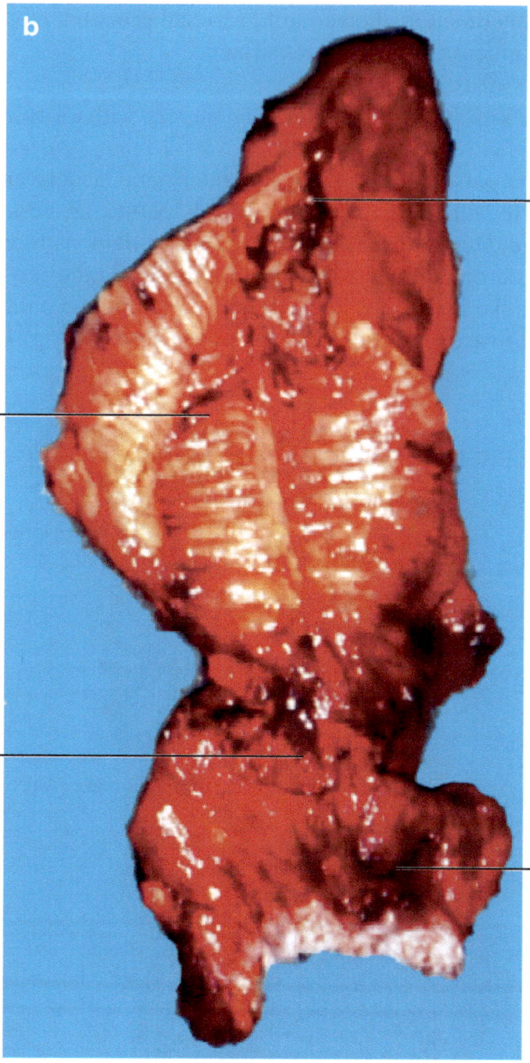

Fig. 11.6 (continued)

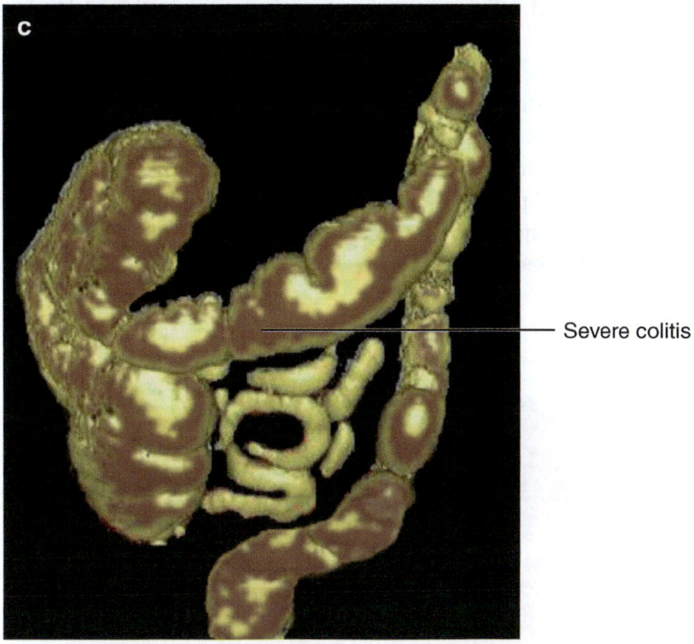

Fig. 11.6 (continued)

11.7 Continent Ileostomy Dysfunction

Clinical Presentation 52 year old man with ulcerative colitis for 18 years. He underwent a total proctocolectomy with a Barnett continent ileostomy. He required reoperation 2 years later for valve prolapse with difficulty intubating. Following this revision he developed an enterocutaneous fistula originating from the pouch which failed to heal with intravenous hyperalimentation.

Diagnostic Studies Fistulogram showed enterocutaneous fistula from pouch to midline incision.

Surgical Findings He underwent excision of the continent ileostomy and conversion to a Brooke ileostomy. An enterocutaneous fistula was present arising from the pouch suture line (see Fig. 11.7a, b).

Pathology Continent ileostomy with mild active pouchitis (see Fig. 11.7c).

Follow-Up He did well following excision of the pouch and Brooke ileostomy.

Comment Continent ileostomies were performed with some frequency until ileo-anal pull-through operations became popular. Problems with the outflow tract are the Achilles' heel of this operation. Nipple valve prolapse causes incontinence and difficulty with intubation. Although revision of the valve is possible, the potential for further valve-related problems increases with each revision. In general, patients with ulcerative colitis not undergoing ileoanal pull-through operations are best treated with a Brooke ileostomy (Fig. 11.7).

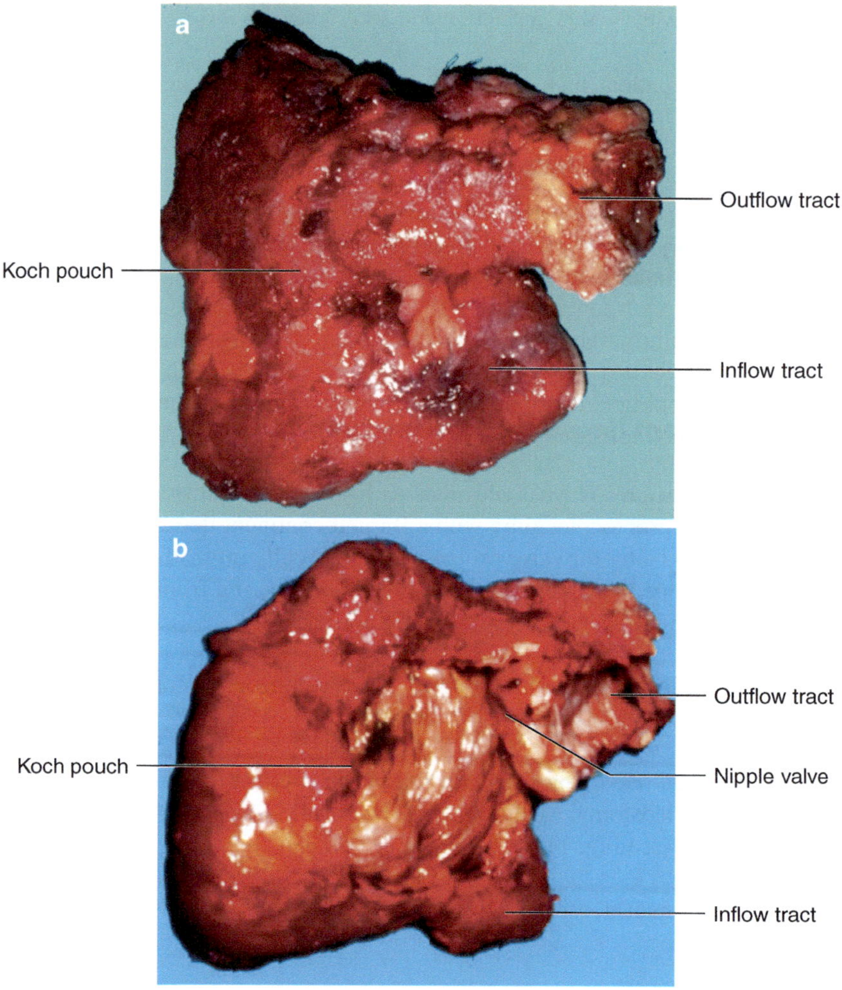

Fig. 11.7 (**a–c**) Continent ileostomy dysfunction

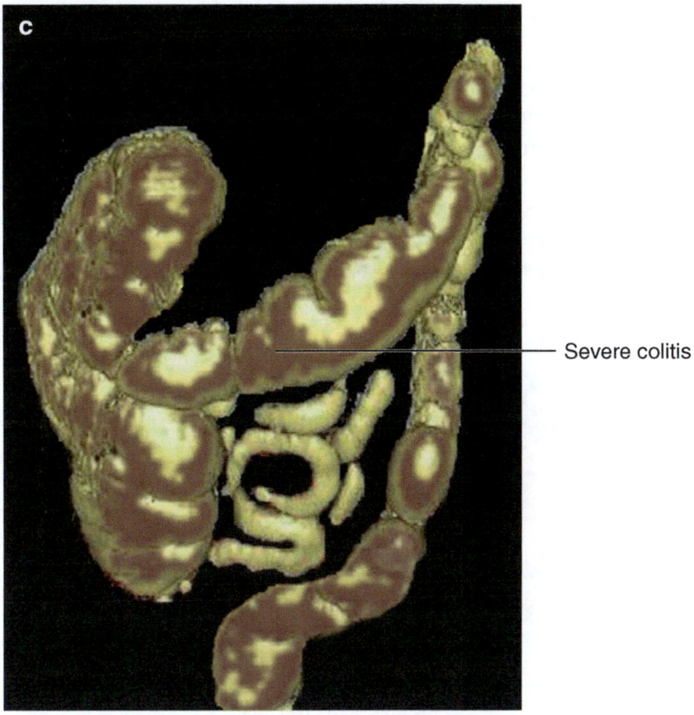

Fig. 11.7 (continued)

11.8 Continent Ileostomy Dysfunction

Clinical Presentation A 32-year-old man with moderately severe ulcerative colitis (see Fig. 11.8c), who underwent total colectomy, proctectomy, and stapled J-pouch anal anastomosis 18 months ago. He required percutaneous drainage of a suprapubic abscess 3 weeks later and subsequently did well. He now returns with a chronic history of pelvic pain, worse during bowel movements and requiring narcotic medication.

Diagnostic Studies Pouch endoscopy showed a short segment of residual rectum with mild colitis, a well-healed ileoanal anastomosis, and a normal J-pouch. CT scan of the pelvis showed a well-healed pouch and no residual abscess or fistulas.

Surgical Findings This patient underwent excision of the neorectum and Brooke ileostomy. Severe adhesions were found around the ileoanal anastomosis (see Fig. 11.8a, b).

Pathology The colectomy specimen showed chronic ulcerative colitis with an unremarkable ileum. J-pouch and anorectum showed mild residual proctitis. No evidence of Crohn's disease. Pouch mucosa appears unremarkable.

Follow-Up He is doing well 2 years after surgery with a Brooke ileostomy.

Comment Fistula from the pouch suture line or from the nipple valve is one of the complications of continent ileostomies. Valve prolapse with incontinence is another. The enterocutaneous fistula in this patient failed to heal after months of intravenous hyperalimentation and pouch decompression. In these situations, pouch excision and Brooke ileostomy are the most reliable operation to return to good health again (Fig. 11.8).

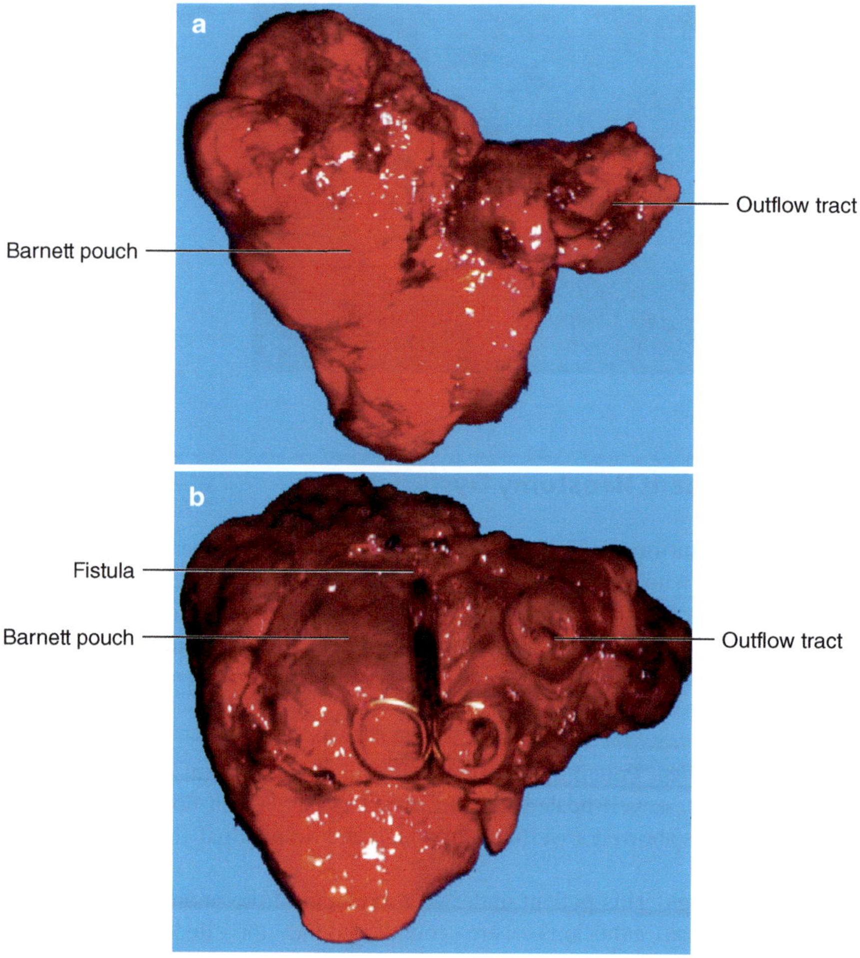

Fig. 11.8 (**a–c**) Continent ileostomy dysfunction

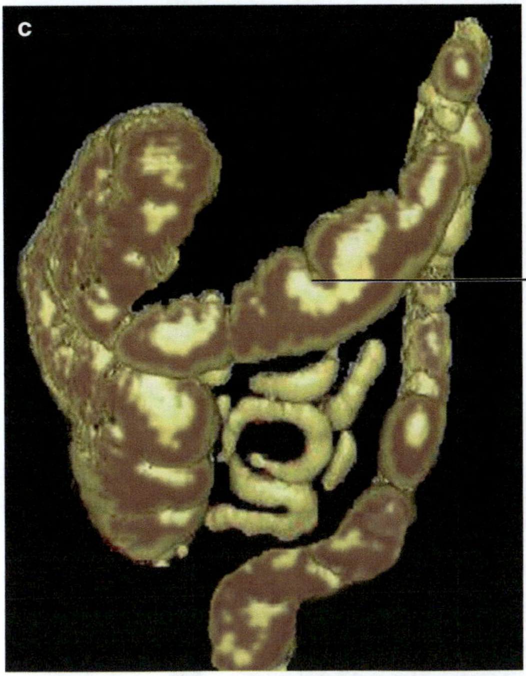

Fig. 11.8 (continued)

11.9 Ileostomy Prolapse

Clinical Presentation A 68-year-old woman who underwent proctocolectomy and ileostomy nearly 50 years ago for ulcerative colitis (see Fig. 11.9b). She now returns for evaluation of a markedly prolapsed Brooke ileostomy.

Diagnostic Studies Severe prolapse of Brooke ileostomy seen on physical exam.

Surgical Findings Ileostomy prolapsed nearly one foot with very lax mesentery. The prolapsed segment was resected, and the ileostomy was resited to the opposite side of the abdomen (see Fig. 11.9a).

Pathology Ileostomy stoma with inflammatory polyp.

Follow-Up She did well following surgery except for a superficial wound infection which healed within 1 month.

Comment Retraction of the Brooke ileostomy is more common than prolapse. Retraction usually occurs in obese patients and when the blood supply is borderline. Minor degrees of prolapse are also common and usually do not require revision. Major prolapse as seen in this patient creates problems with the appliance and can cause ulceration. Correction of this problem usually requires resection and may involve resiting of the stoma (Fig. 11.9).

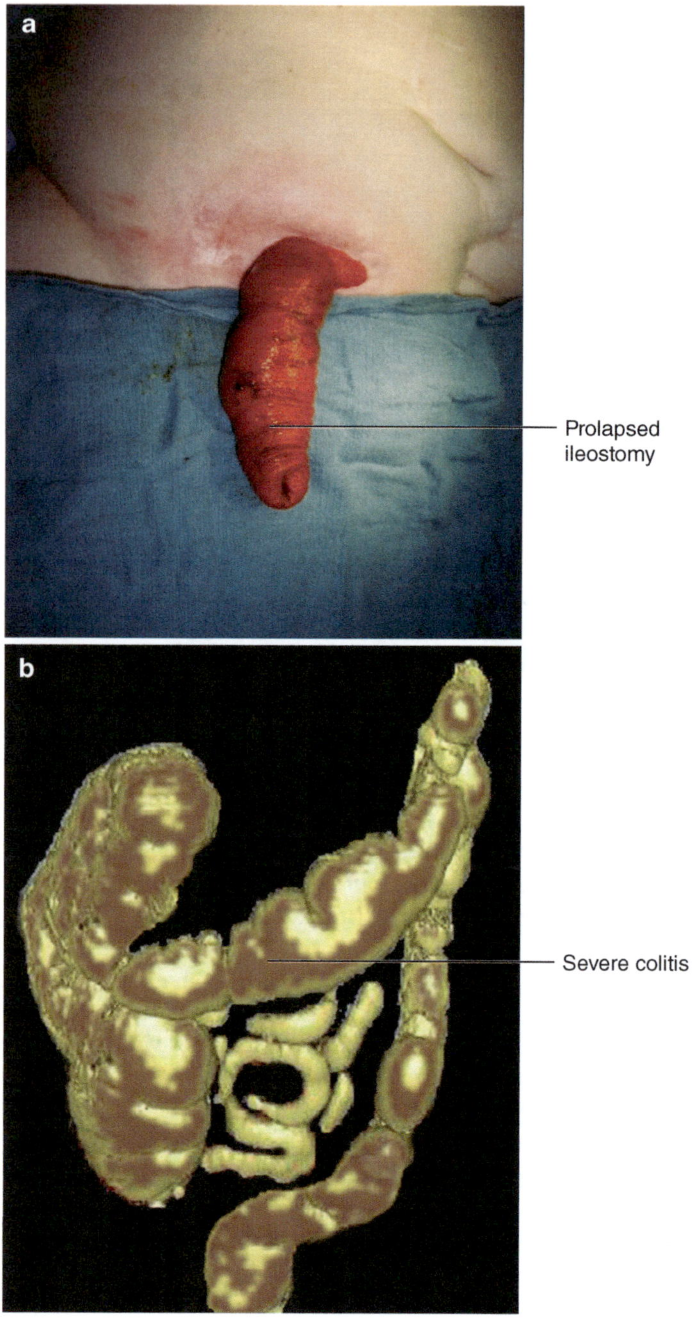

Fig. 11.9 (**a** and **b**) Ileostomy prolapse

Further Reading

Blam M, Bari M, Brauer C, Heimann T, Gorfine S, Weiss A. Health related quality of life (HRQOL) in patients after Ileo-anal pull-through procedure (IAPT). Gastroenterology. 1998;01:114.

Slater G, Heimann T. Colectomy and Ileoanal-pouch anastomosis. Surg Rounds. 1993;16:733–9.

Stey AM, Brook RH, Keeler E, Harris MT, Heimann TM, Steinhagen RM. Outcomes and cost of diverted versus undiverted restorative proctocolectomy. J Gastrointest Surg. 2014;18:995–1002.

Part III

Indeterminate Colitis

12 Indeterminate Colitis

Tomas M. Heimann and Robert J. Kurtz

Indeterminate colitis creates problems when surgical treatment of patients with colitis is being contemplated. Total colectomy with ileoanal pull-through is the operation of choice for most patients with ulcerative colitis. This same operation is contraindicated in patients with Crohn's disease. Patients with indeterminate colitis without perianal disease and without small bowel involvement may do well with an ileoanal pull-through operation, while most patients with indeterminate colitis and perianal disease are likely to have problems with this operation. Sometimes the colon has typical features of ulcerative colitis, and later the patient may be found to have Crohn's disease. Most patients in this category have small bowel recurrence or onset of severe perianal disease. The majority ultimately require excision of the neorectum and Brooke ileostomy.

12.1 Indeterminate Colitis

Clinical Presentation A 59-year-old man with colitis for 4 years, who underwent a subtotal colectomy and ileostomy for intractability.

Diagnostic Studies Sigmoidoscopy showed severe residual proctitis.

Surgical Findings He underwent completion proctectomy with mucosectomy and sphincter muscle preservation. The distal small bowel showed creeping of the mesenteric fat consistent with Crohn's disease. Similar findings were seen in the rectal segment (see Fig. 12.1a, b).

T. M. Heimann (✉) · R. J. Kurtz
Department of Surgery, Icahn School of Medicine at Mount Sinai, New York, NY, USA
e-mail: Tomas.Heimann@mountsinai.org; Robert.Kurtz@mountsinai.org

T. M. Heimann (ed.), *Atlas of Surgical Treatment of Inflammatory Bowel Disease*, https://doi.org/10.1007/978-3-031-62431-5_12

Pathology Colectomy specimen showing severely active chronic colitis and pan diverticulitis. Ileal segment is unremarkable. Proctectomy specimen with chronic proctitis and inflammatory polyps consistent with ulcerative colitis. Ileal segment shows no evidence of inflammation (see Fig. 12.1c).

Follow-Up This patient had an uneventful recovery and is well 4 years later.

Comment This patient was nearly 60 years old at the time of surgery and had severe colitis. The findings of diverticulitis make the differentiation from Crohn's disease more difficult, and the small bowel appearance at the time of surgery had features seen in Crohn's disease. Since the patient already had an ileostomy and was satisfied with it, the decision was made to perform a completion proctectomy with mucosectomy and preservation of the sphincter muscles. If necessary, an ileoanal pull-through operation could be performed at a later date (Fig. 12.1).

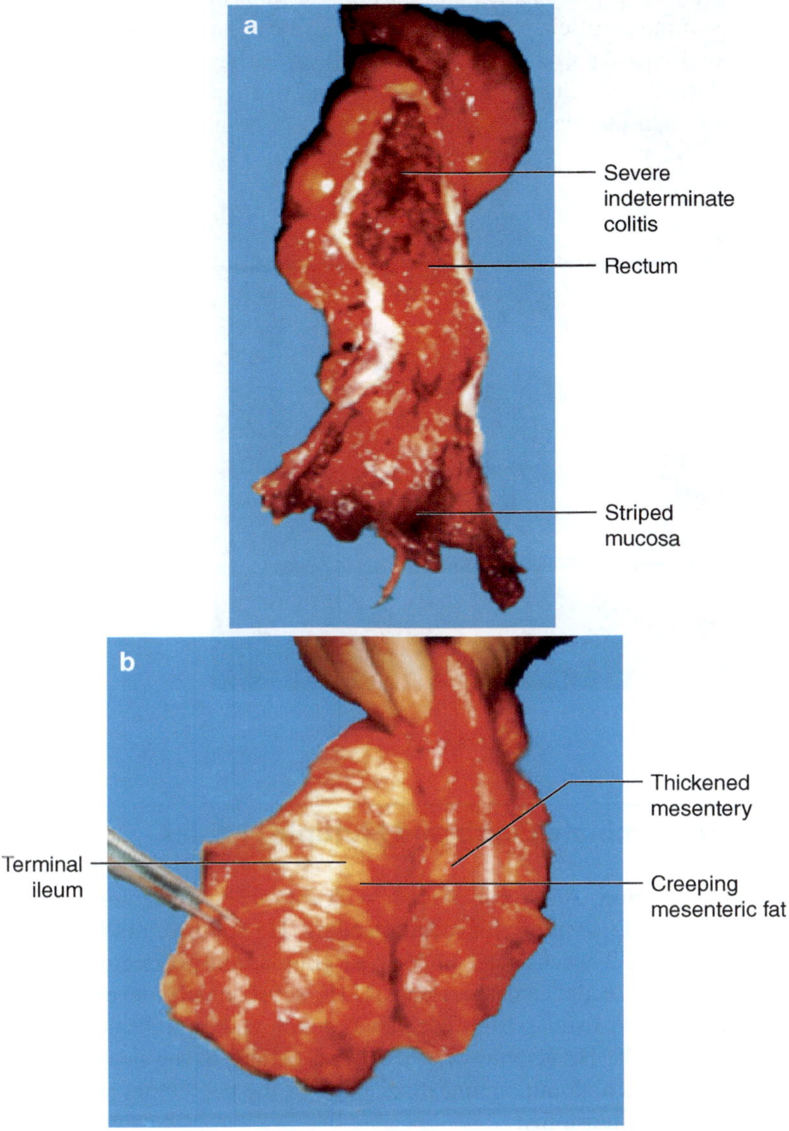

Fig. 12.1 (**a–c**) Indeterminate colitis

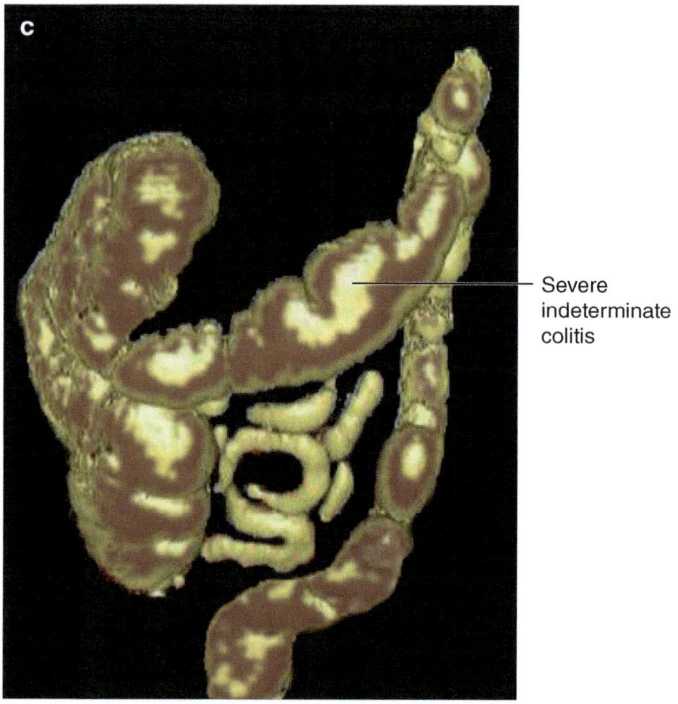

Fig. 12.1 (continued)

12.2 Indeterminate Colitis and Multiple Fistulas

Clinical Presentation A 38-year-old man with chronic colitis required urgent subtotal colectomy and ileostomy for rectal bleeding. He continued to bleed from the rectal segment and 2 weeks later underwent completion proctectomy, mucosectomy, and hand-sewn ileoanal anastomosis. He subsequently developed a pelvic abscess secondary to fistulas from the pelvic pouch and an unhealed sinus at the ileoanal anastomosis. He also developed several fistulas at the ileostomy site and 1 year later required abdominoperineal resection of the neorectum and distal small bowel with Brooke ileostomy.

Diagnostic Studies Barium enema of the pouch showed a fistula at the ileoanal anastomosis and multiple fistulas in the J-pouch. Endoscopy of the pouch showed chronic inflammation (see Fig. 12.2b, c).

Surgical Findings Severe inflammation of the J-pouch and inflow tract with multiple fistulas in the pelvis and adjacent to the ileostomy area (see Fig. 12.2a).

Pathology Colectomy specimen showing chronic active ulcerative colitis with extensive ulcerations and multiple pseudopolyps. The terminal ileum shows moderate nonspecific chronic inflammation. Excised neorectum with chronic inflammation and ulceration consistent with Crohn's disease. Multiple epithelioid granulomas are present.

Follow-Up The perineal wound healed slowly but he ultimately did well. There has been no further recurrence of Crohn's disease on follow-up of 14 years.

Comment This patient had the diagnosis of ulcerative colitis made on examination of the colon after subtotal colectomy. Review of the colonic histology showed no evidence of Crohn's disease, and his small bowel was normal at the time. Nevertheless, he has typical Crohn's disease of the small bowel with epithelioid granulomas. This case shows how difficult it is to differentiate ulcerative from Crohn's colitis and the potential catastrophic consequences of performing an ileoanal anastomosis in patients with Crohn's disease (Fig. 12.2).

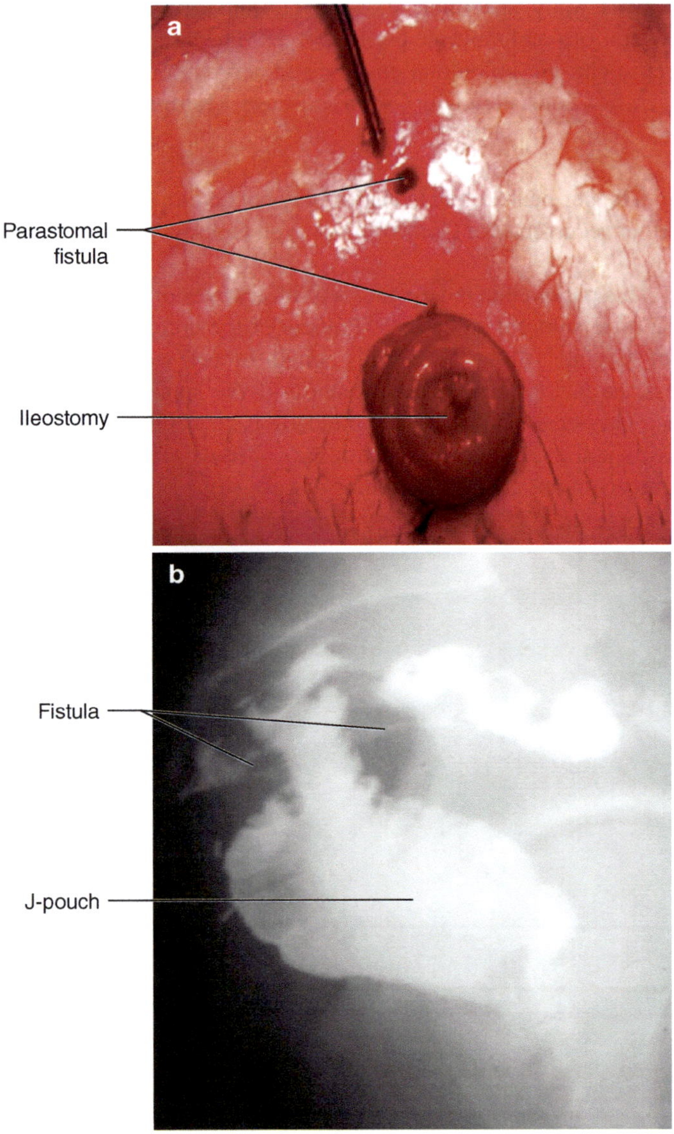

Fig. 12.2 (a–c) Indeterminate colitis and multiple fistulas

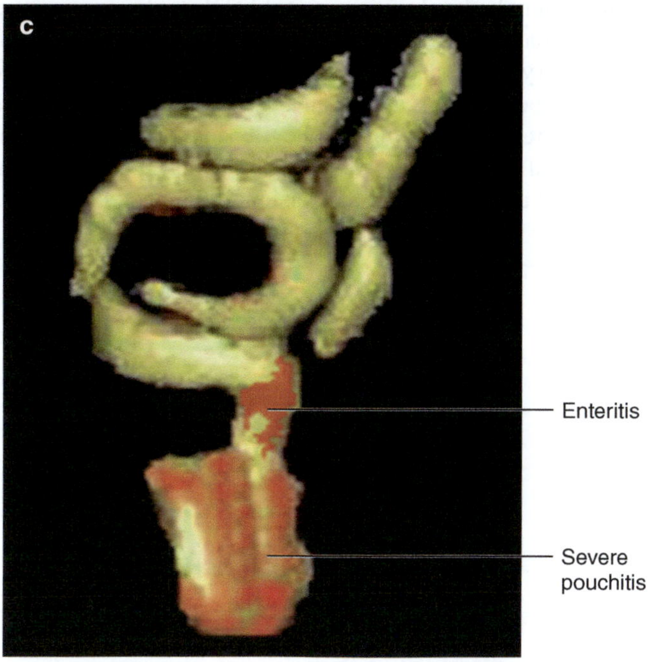

Fig. 12.2 (continued)

12.3 Indeterminate Colitis and Perianal Disease

Clinical Presentation A 39-year-old woman who required an urgent subtotal colectomy and ileostomy for fulminant colitis (see Fig. 12.3b). She returns 7 months later for completion proctectomy. The pathology of the colectomy specimen showed indeterminate colitis, and the patient decided to keep the Brooke ileostomy.

Diagnostic Studies Endoscopy showed universal colitis. A small perianal fistula was present (see Fig. 12.3a).

Surgical Findings Universal colitis. Small bowel was normal.

Pathology Colectomy specimen showing universal chronic fulminant colitis most consistent with idiopathic ulcerative colitis. There is extensive deep ulceration with involvement of the muscularis propria. The ileal segment is unremarkable. No granulomas are seen.

Follow-Up She had an uneventful recovery after both operations. The perineal wound and ileostomy healed well. There has been no evidence of recurrent disease in the small intestine.

Comment This patient had a chronic perianal fistula and was concerned about the possibility that she may have Crohn's disease. In general, regardless of the pathology report, we are very concerned about performing an ileoanal pull-through operation in a patient with perianal disease. Even an asymptomatic fistula present prior to surgery may interfere with healing of the ileoanal anastomosis, and in some instances, the perianal disease may worsen with the development of multiple fistulas and abscesses and ultimately lead to excision of the neorectum (Fig. 12.3).

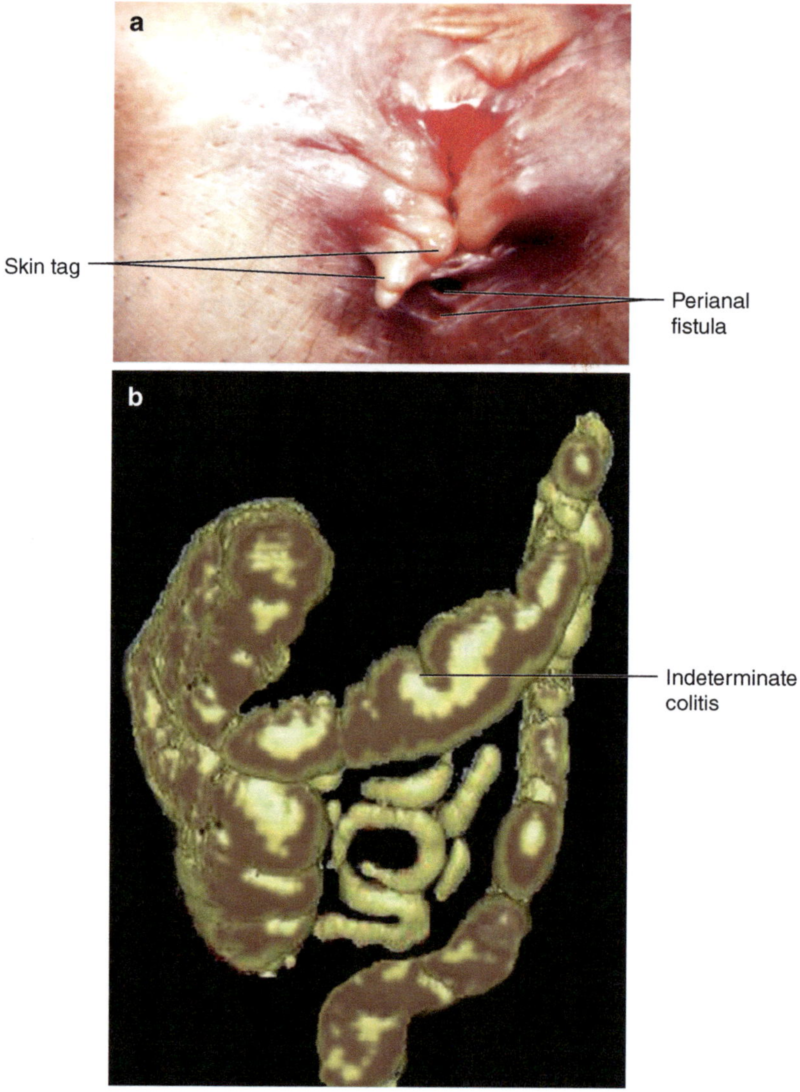

Fig. 12.3 (**a** and **b**) Indeterminate colitis and perianal disease

12.4 Indeterminate Colitis and Perianal Disease

Clinical Presentation A 23-year-old patient who previously underwent a subtotal colectomy and Brooke ileostomy for intractable colitis. He subsequently developed a perianal fistula which healed spontaneously. This patient underwent completion proctectomy with mucosectomy and sphincter preservation. Three years later, he was seen again with multiple perianal fistulas.

Diagnostic Studies Physical exam revealed multiple perianal fistulas. Residual anal stump otherwise unremarkable.

Surgical Findings He underwent perineal excision of the remaining anorectal area with gracilis muscle flap reconstruction (see Fig. 12.4a, b).

Pathology Subtotal colectomy with indeterminate colitis (see Fig. 12.4c). Proctectomy with mucosectomy showing chronic ulcerative colitis. Anal tissue with chronic nonspecific inflammation and sinus tracts. Multiple small granulomatous foci around the sinus tracts.

Follow-Up Within the next 12 months, the perineal wound improved but did not heal, and he subsequently required a second revision. Currently, the perineal wound is still not completely healed.

Comment This patient had histologic features of indeterminate colitis and a history of a perianal fistula. After initial subtotal colectomy and Brooke ileostomy, he underwent completion proctectomy with mucosectomy and sphincter preservation. He subsequently developed severe exacerbation of his perianal disease with multiple perianal fistulas and abscesses and eventually required a completion proctectomy and still has an unhealed perineal wound. Perianal Crohn's disease is one of the most troublesome problems in patients with Crohn's colitis. It can continue to cause severe problems even after proctectomy requiring multiple revisions of the perineal wound (Fig. 12.4).

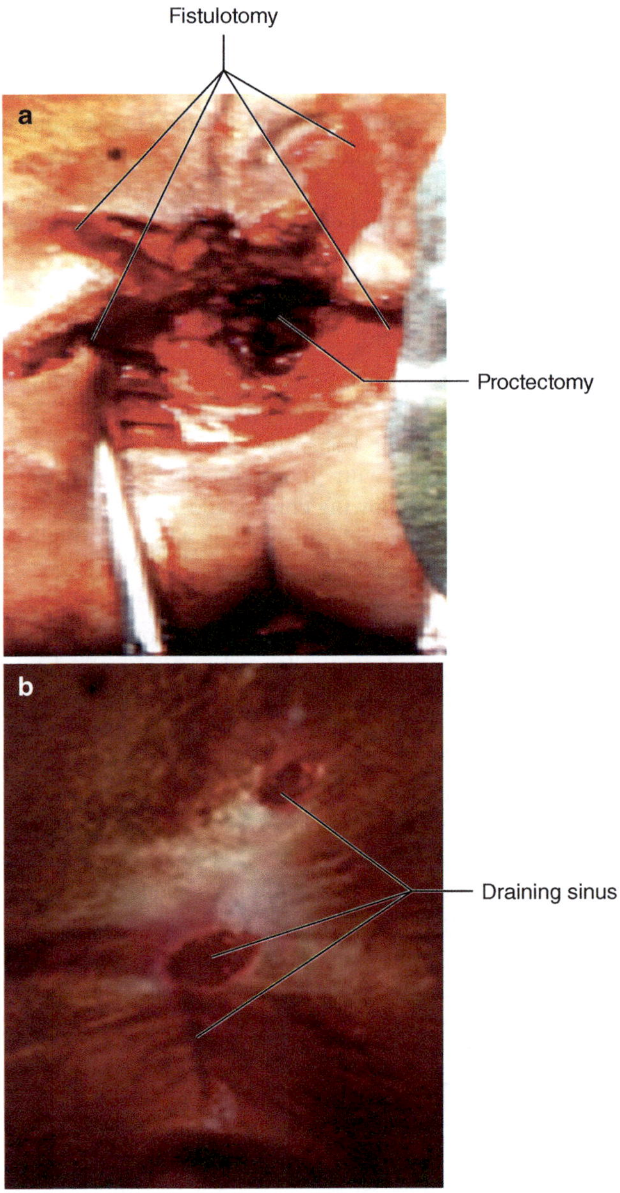

Fig. 12.4 (a–c) Indeterminate colitis and perianal disease

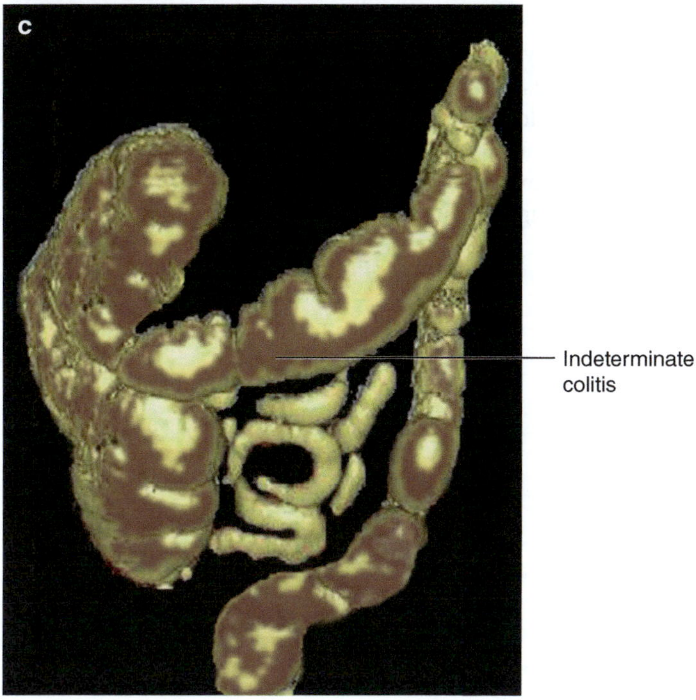

Fig. 12.4 (continued)

12.5 Indeterminate Colitis and Perianal Disease

Clinical Presentation An 18-year-old woman who required subtotal colectomy and ileostomy for intractable colitis. She subsequently underwent completion proctectomy and J-pouch anal anastomosis. Two years later, she presented with recurrent symptoms of pouchitis and a significant stricture at the ileoanal anastomosis. Several months later, she developed multiple perianal fistulas.

Diagnostic Studies Pouch endoscopy revealed erythema and ulcerations throughout the pouch and into the inflow tract for a distance of about 10 cm (see Fig. 12.5b).

Surgical Findings Stricture of ileoanal anastomosis multiple perianal fistulas. Dilatation of the stricture and fistulotomy were performed under general anesthesia (see Fig. 12.5a).

Pathology Colectomy specimen showed severely active chronic ulcerative colitis. Endoscopic biopsies of the pouch showed severely active nonspecific inflammation.

Follow-Up She is currently on ciprofloxacin and metronidazole antibiotics with some improvement.

Comment This patient had the diagnosis of ulcerative colitis made based on the findings of the colectomy specimen but the disease is behaving like Crohn's disease. The ileoanal anastomosis, which initially healed well, now is strictured and edematous, and she has developed multiple perianal fistulas. The presence of chronic inflammation in the J-pouch in this setting is not usually nonspecific pouchitis but Crohn's disease. In our experience, most patients with late onset of perianal disease after ileoanal pull-through eventually require excision on the pouch and Brooke ileostomy (Fig. 12.5).

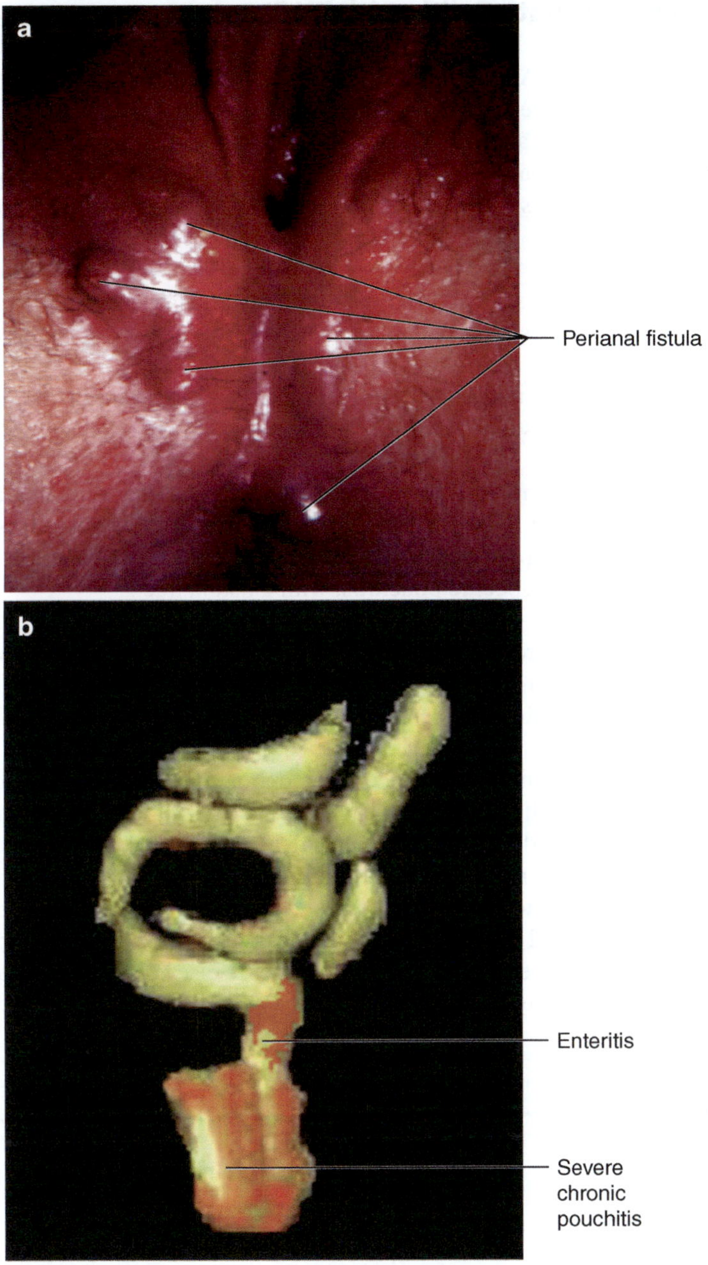

Fig. 12.5 (**a** and **b**) Indeterminate colitis and perianal disease

12.6 Indeterminate Colitis with RV Fistula

Clinical Presentation A 58-year-old woman with a history of total colectomy and ileoanal anastomosis 8 years ago for intractable colitis. She developed a stricture of the ileoanal anastomosis and required multiple dilatations and intubation of the neorectum in order to evacuate. She subsequently developed a rectovaginal fistula and recurrent perianal abscesses requiring multiple hospital admissions for antibiotic treatment.

Diagnostic Studies CT scan showed inflammatory changes around the neorectum and air in the vagina consistent with a rectovaginal fistula (see Fig. 12.6a, c).

Surgical Findings She underwent abdominoperineal resection of the neorectum with Brooke ileostomy (see Fig. 12.6b).

Pathology The colectomy specimen showed universal chronic inflammation and mucosal ulceration. The inflammatory process extends to the muscularis propria. The terminal ileum is unremarkable. There are no granulomas. The excised neorectum showed chronic nonspecific pouchitis, with a fistula tract.

Follow-Up She recovered well following surgery. The perineal wound healed without difficulty, and 5 months later, she underwent a revision of the ileostomy due to superficial stricture. She has been well for over 5 years.

Comment Differentiating severe ulcerative colitis with deep ulcerations from Crohn's colitis is difficult. This patient had poor healing of the ileoanal anastomosis with severe stricture and late development of a rectovaginal fistula. The excised neorectum also showed nonspecific chronic inflammation. Her problems may be attributed to indeterminate colitis and recurrent Crohn's disease in the pouch or may be secondary to surgical problems, such as tension and poor blood supply at the ileoanal anastomosis. There is no evidence of disease elsewhere in the small bowel. Further follow-up is necessary to clarify the possibility that she may have Crohn's disease (Fig. 12.6).

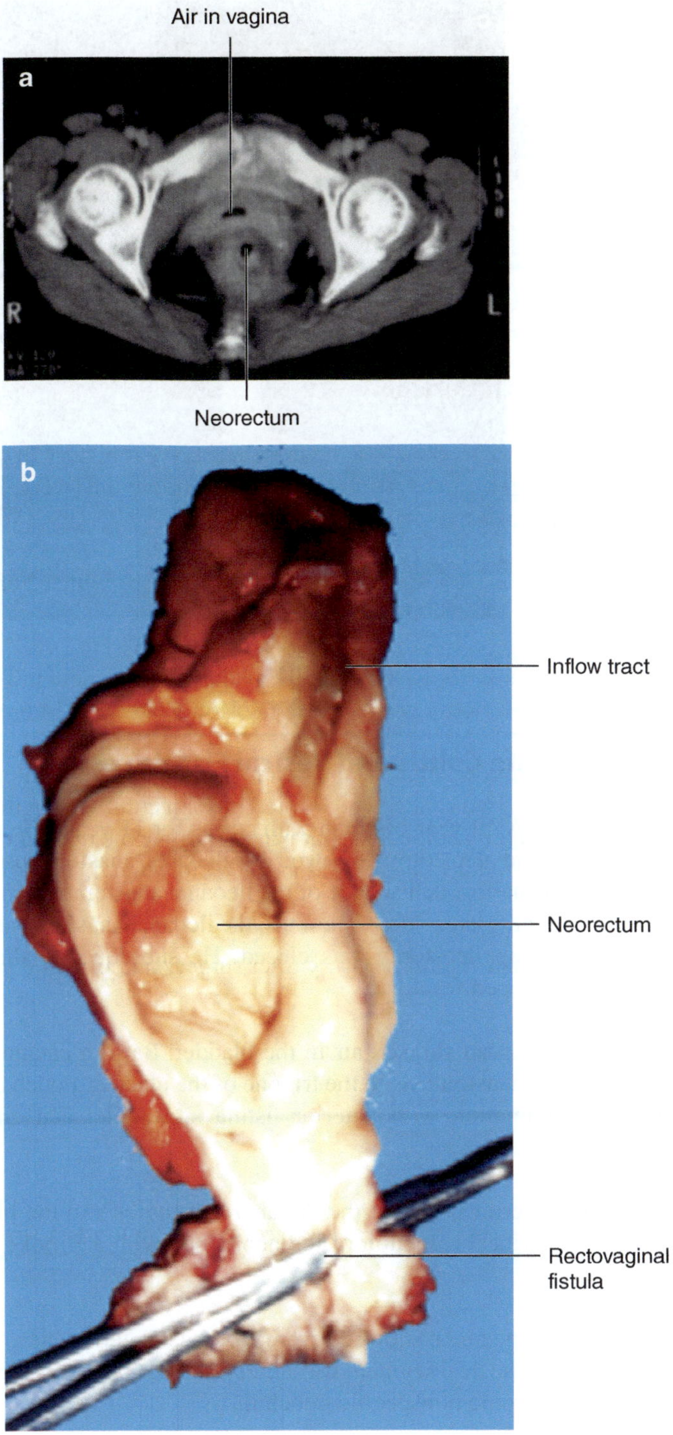

Fig. 12.6 (**a–c**) Indeterminate colitis with RV fistula

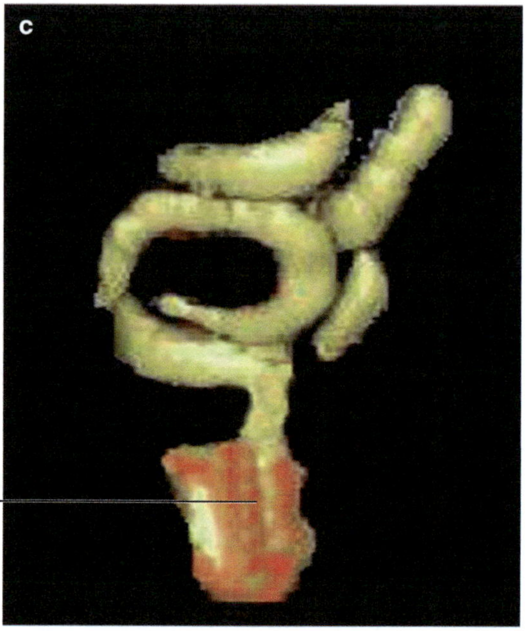

Fig. 12.6 (continued)

12.7 Indeterminate Colitis and Vesical Fistula

Clinical Presentation A 49-year-old man with colitis for 11 years. He underwent a subtotal colectomy and ileostomy followed by ileoanal anastomosis 5 months later. He developed an anterior dehiscence of the ileoanal anastomosis and required transanal revision 6 months later. After 3 months, the ileoanal anastomosis appeared well-healed, and the loop ileostomy was closed. He subsequently did well for 2.5 years and then developed fecaluria.

Diagnostic Studies CT scan showed air in the bladder. Barium enema showed a fistula from the ileoanal anastomosis to the trigone of the bladder. Pouch endoscopy showed chronic inflammation with anterior fistula site at ileoanal anastomosis (see Fig. 12.7c).

Surgical Findings Anterior fistula at the ileoanal anastomosis to the bladder. He underwent abdominoperineal resection of the neorectum with a Brooke ileostomy (see Fig. 12.7a, b).

Pathology Colectomy specimen showed severe chronic indeterminate colitis, most likely ulcerative colitis. The ileal segment was unremarkable. The excised neorectum showed mildly active chronic nonspecific pouchitis.

Follow-Up He had an uneventful recovery and is well 3 years later.

Comment This patient demonstrates some of the difficulties differentiating Crohn's disease from ulcerative colitis in patients undergoing ileoanal pull-through operations. The colon showed indeterminate colitis, the ileoanal anastomosis was slow to heal, and eventually a late enterovesical fistula developed. The excised neorectum had nonspecific inflammation, which may well represent Crohn's disease. It is still unclear even after careful examination of the colon and the excised neorectum whether these problems were caused by failure of the ileoanal anastomosis to heal well or whether they are secondary to Crohn's disease (Fig. 12.7).

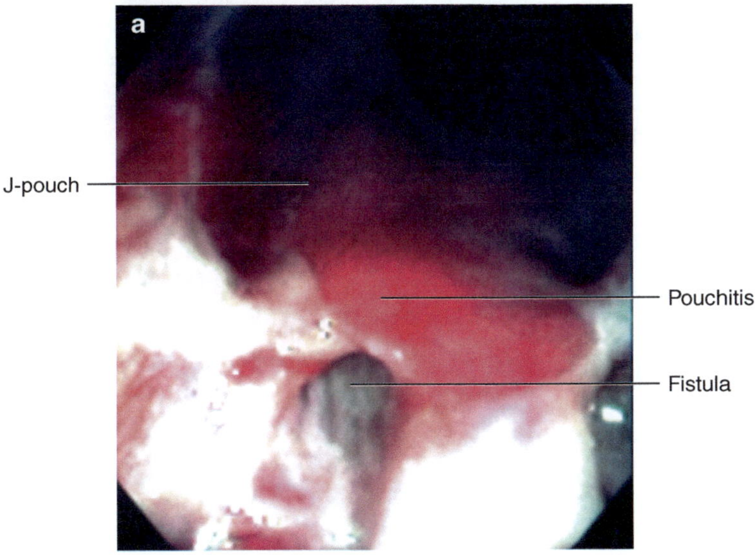

Fig. 12.7 (a–c) Indeterminate colitis and vesical fistula

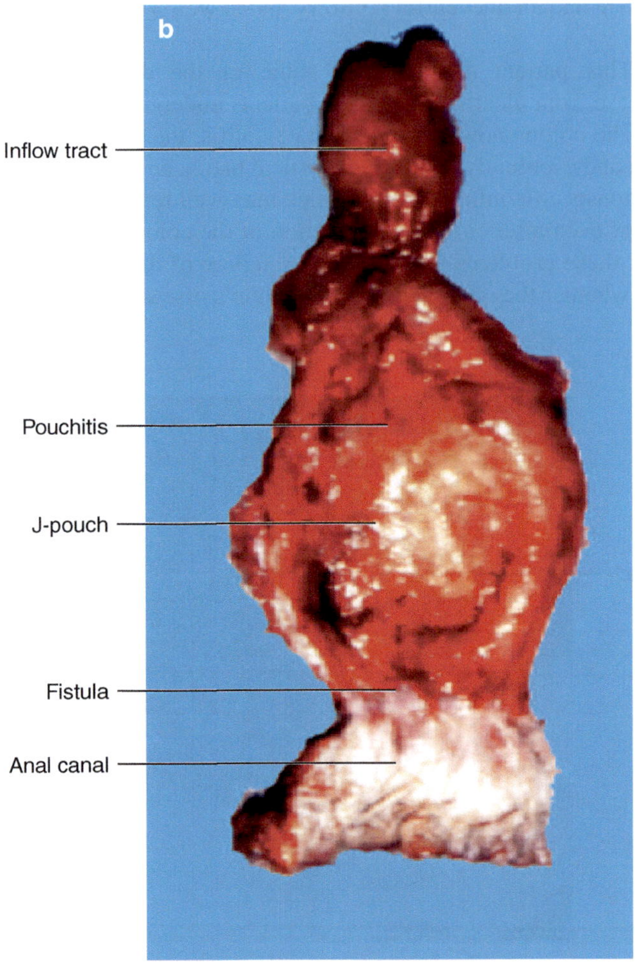

Fig. 12.7 (continued)

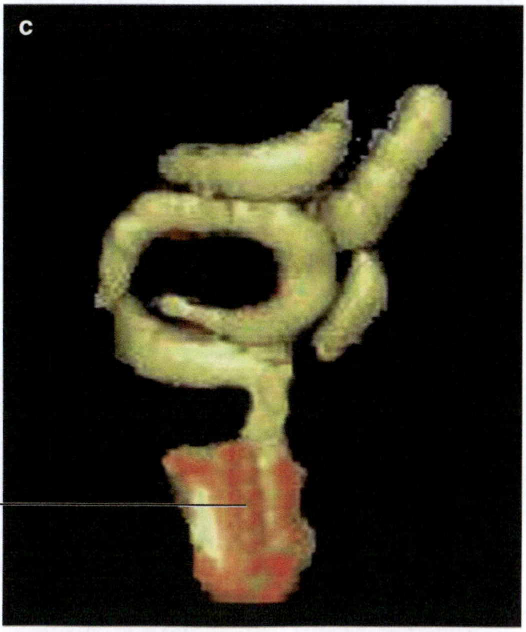

Fig. 12.7 (continued)

12.8 Indeterminate Colitis and RV Fistula

Clinical Presentation A 32-year-old woman with intractable colitis underwent subtotal colectomy and ileostomy followed by completion proctectomy, mucosectomy, and hand-sewn ileoanal anastomosis 5 months later. She developed a small sinus at the ileoanal anastomosis, which extended 2 cm on the left side and appeared unchanged after 6 months when the ileostomy was closed. Within several months, she had increasing narrowing of the ileoanal anastomosis and subsequently developed a rectovaginal fistula. A second labial fistula became present shortly thereafter. Eighteen months after closure of the ileostomy, she underwent abdominoperineal resection of the neorectum with Brooke ileostomy.

Diagnostic Studies Pouch endoscopy showed moderately severe pouchitis (see Fig. 12.8d).

Surgical Findings Inflamed neorectum with rectovaginal fistula (see Fig. 12.8a, b, c).

Pathology Colectomy specimen shows severe acute and chronic inflammation with focal areas of transmural inflammation. The terminal ileum is unremarkable. Neorectum shows severe chronic enteritis extending to the inflow tract. No granulomas are seen.

Follow-Up She did well following the excision of the neorectum. The perineal wound was slow to heal. There has been no further small bowel recurrence after follow-up of 9 years.

Comment This patient had some features of indeterminate colitis on examination of the colectomy specimen, mainly focal areas of transmural inflammation. The ileoanal anastomosis developed a small sinus, followed by subsequent stricture and multiple rectovaginal fistulas. There was severe chronic inflammation of the pouch and the inflow tract. These are all features seen in Crohn's disease. After removal of the neorectum, there is no further evidence of inflammation in the small bowel. The distinction between Crohn's and ulcerative colitis is very difficult to make in these patients after ileoanal pull-through operations until further small bowel disease develops (Fig. 12.8).

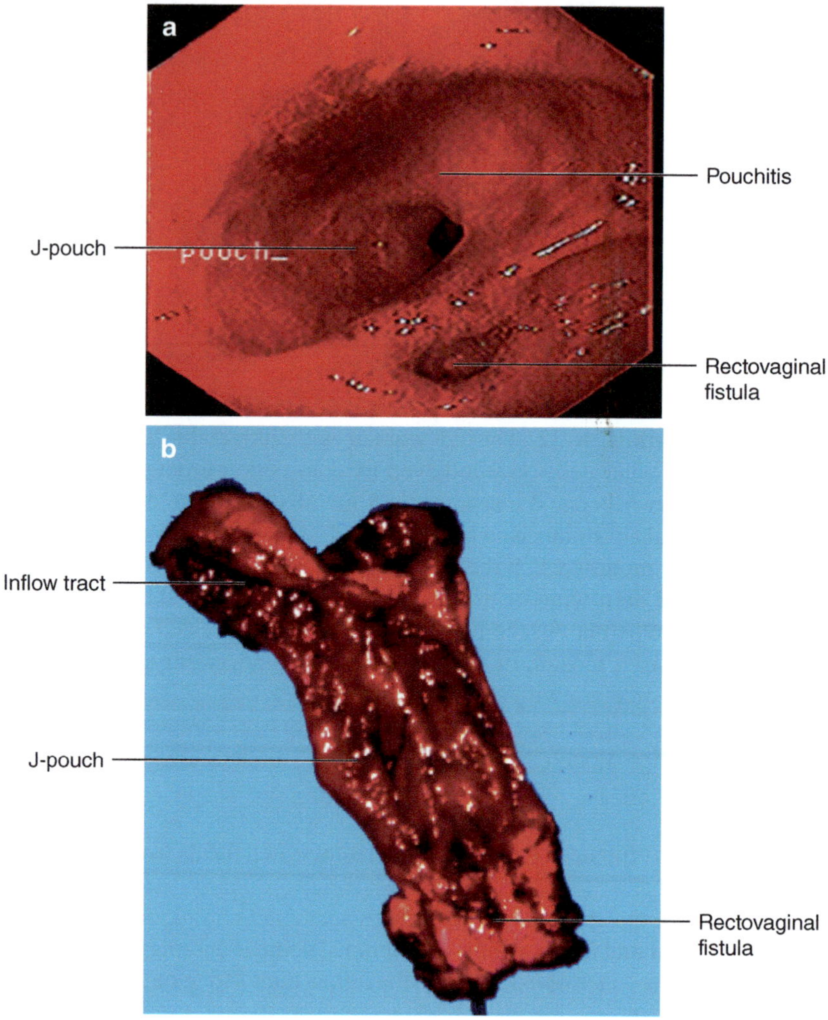

Fig. 12.8 (**a–d**) Indeterminate colitis with RV fistula

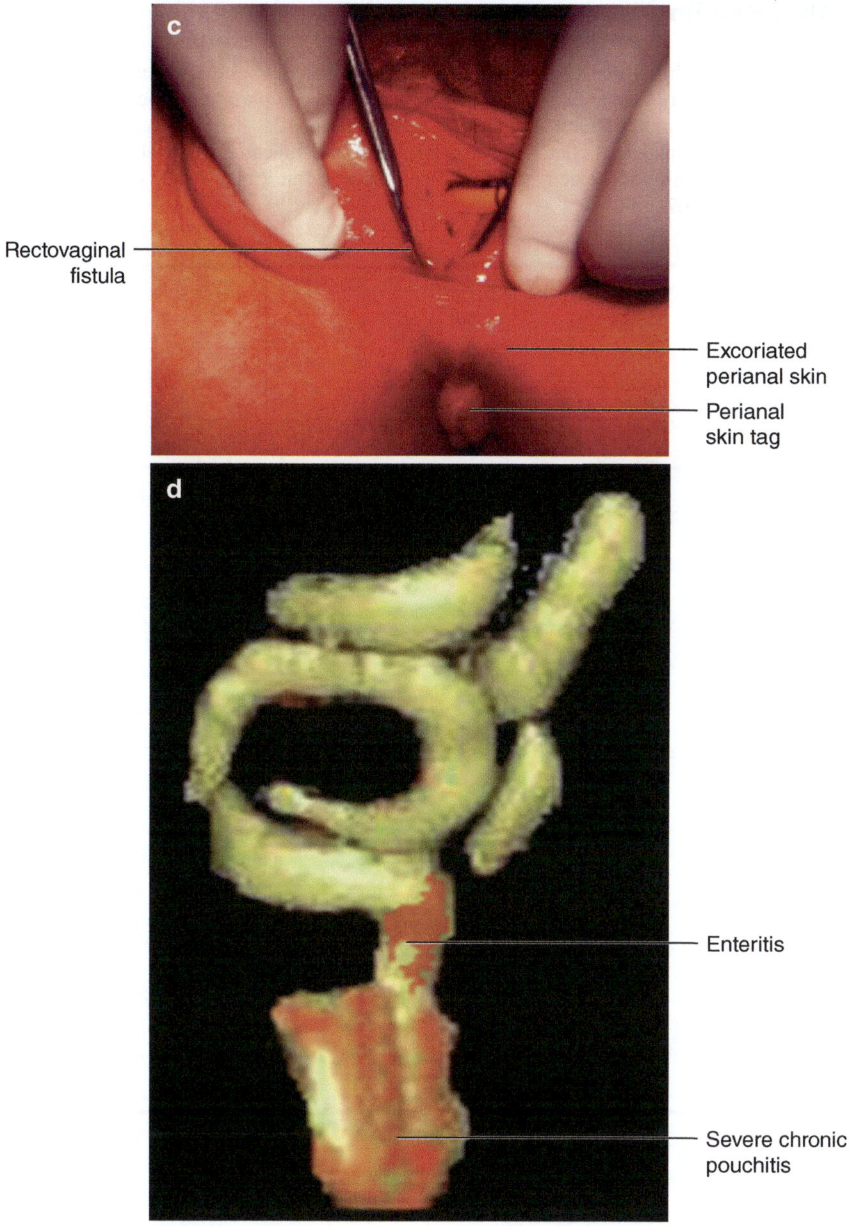

Fig. 12.8 (continued)

Further Reading

Aisenberg J, Wagreich J, Shim J, Almer S, Peen E, Heimann T, Gelernt IM, Greenstein A, Rubin P, Harpaz N, Mayer L, Sachar D. Pernuclear anti-neutrophil cytoplasmic antibody and refractory pouchitis (a case control study). Dig Dis Sci. 1996;9:1866–72.

Heimann TM, Swaminathan S, Slater G, Kurtz RJ. Perianal fistula after Ileoanal pouch in patients with ulcerative colitis: a review of 475 patients operated at a major IBD center. Dis Colon Rectum. 2022;65:76–82.

Part IV

Intestinal Cancer in Inflammatory Bowel Disease

13 Colorectal Cancer in Ulcerative Colitis

Tomas M. Heimann and Robert J. Kurtz

Colorectal cancer risk in ulcerative colitis is clearly recognized and in about 10% of our patients; the indication for colectomy is the presence of dysplasia on colonoscopic biopsies. In Crohn's disease, the risk of developing carcinoma of the small bowel has been well described. Although the percentage of patients developing jejunal or ileal cancer is small, the incidence is about 100-fold that of the general population. It is also clear that patients with Crohn's disease are at increased risk to develop colorectal cancer. It is likely that this risk is similar to that seen in patients with ulcerative colitis and that colonic surveillance with periodic colonoscopy is indicated in patients with Crohn's disease.

The incidence of colorectal cancer in patients with ulcerative colitis correlates with the extent and duration of the disease. Patients with early-onset ulcerative colitis also appear to be at increased risk. Periodic surveillance colonoscopy with multiple random biopsies is currently the best method to evaluate these patients for cancer risk. The presence of areas of dysplasia indicates a high risk for subsequent development of colorectal cancer and is an indication for surgery.

Patients with ulcerative colitis and dysplasia or cancer should undergo proctocolectomy, and, if possible, a restorative proctocolectomy may be performed. Patients with distal rectal cancer usually require proctocolectomy with Brooke ileostomy. The survival of patients with ulcerative colitis and cancer is similar to that seen with colorectal cancer in the general population.

T. M. Heimann (✉) · R. J. Kurtz
Department of Surgery, Icahn School of Medicine at Mount Sinai, New York, NY, USA
e-mail: Tomas.Heimann@mountsinai.org; Robert.Kurtz@mountsinai.org

T. M. Heimann (ed.), *Atlas of Surgical Treatment of Inflammatory Bowel Disease*, https://doi.org/10.1007/978-3-031-62431-5_13

13.1 Ulcerative Colitis with Dysplasia

Clinical Presentation A 66-year-old woman with ulcerative colitis for nearly 40 years. Recent colonoscopy showed an area of low-grade dysplasia in the cecum, hepatic flexure, and rectosigmoid. Her symptoms are well controlled with 5 mg of prednisone per day.

Diagnostic Studies Colonoscopy showed mild colitis with three areas of dysplasia (see Fig. 13.1b).

Surgical Findings Mild chronic colitis with multiple pseudopolyps. No tumor seen. She underwent a total proctocolectomy and ileostomy (see Fig. 13.1a).

Pathology Mildly active chronic proctosigmoiditis with sessile villous dysplastic lesion in the cecum. Multiple areas of focal hyperplasia. No areas of dysplasia in the hepatic flexure and rectosigmoid seen.

Follow-Up She did well after surgery. The perineal wound healed without any difficulty.

Comment This patient had a long-standing history of colitis and findings of dysplasia on surveillance colonoscopy. The lesion in the cecum was a premalignant villous lesion. The areas of low-grade dysplasia in the hepatic flexure and rectosigmoid could not be confirmed on the colectomy specimen. This patient had a proctocolectomy and ileostomy since at her age an ileoanal pull-through operation is not always a good choice. Fortunately, there was no invasive carcinoma and she is doing well 2 years later (Fig. 13.1).

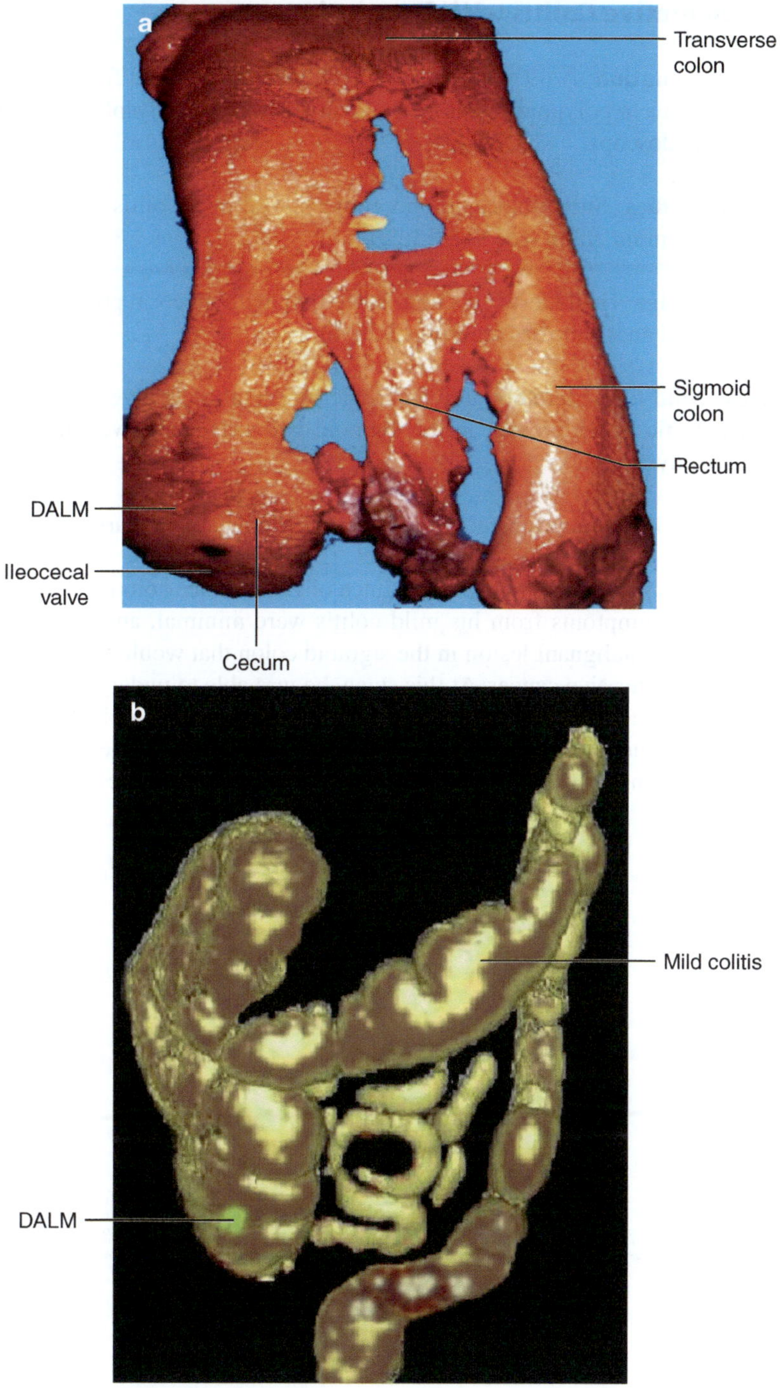

Fig. 13.1 (**a** and **b**) Ulcerative colitis with dysplasia

13.2 Ulcerative Colitis with Dysplasia

Clinical Presentation A 39-year-old man with ulcerative colitis for 22 years. He was found to have a polypoid lesion in the rectosigmoid with dysplasia on routine surveillance endoscopy.

Diagnostic Studies Surveillance colonoscopy showed mild colitis and a polypoid lesion in the sigmoid colon (see Fig. 13.2c).

Surgical Findings He underwent a total colectomy with mucosal proctectomy and J-pouch ileoanal anastomosis (see Fig. 13.2a, b).

Pathology Mild to moderately active chronic universal ulcerative colitis. Sessile villous dysplastic polyp present in the sigmoid colon. No invasive carcinoma or other areas of dysplasia.

Follow-Up He had an uneventful recovery and is doing well 2 years later.

Comment This patient shows the importance of surveillance colonoscopy. He was doing well, the symptoms from his mild colitis were minimal, and yet he had an asymptomatic premalignant lesion in the sigmoid colon that would have eventually progressed to an invasive cancer. At this stage, he was able to undergo total proctocolectomy with ileoanal anastomosis and has done well. Once an invasive cancer develops, the surgical treatment is more complicated because of the possible need for chemoradiation and the risk of development of recurrent disease (Fig. 13.2).

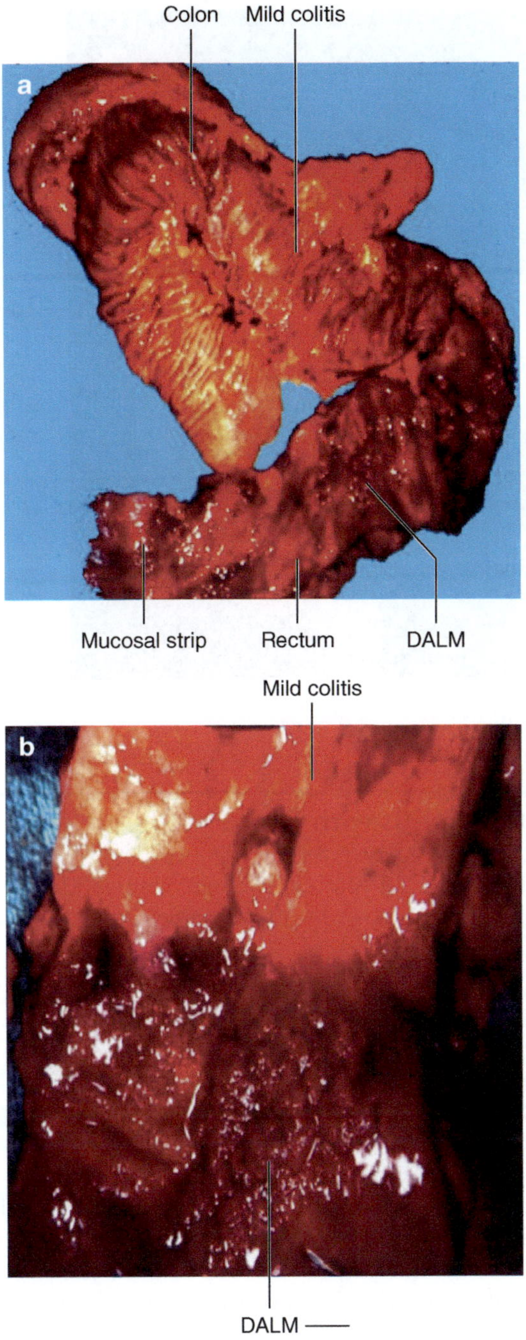

Fig. 13.2 (**a–c**) Ulcerative colitis with dysplasia

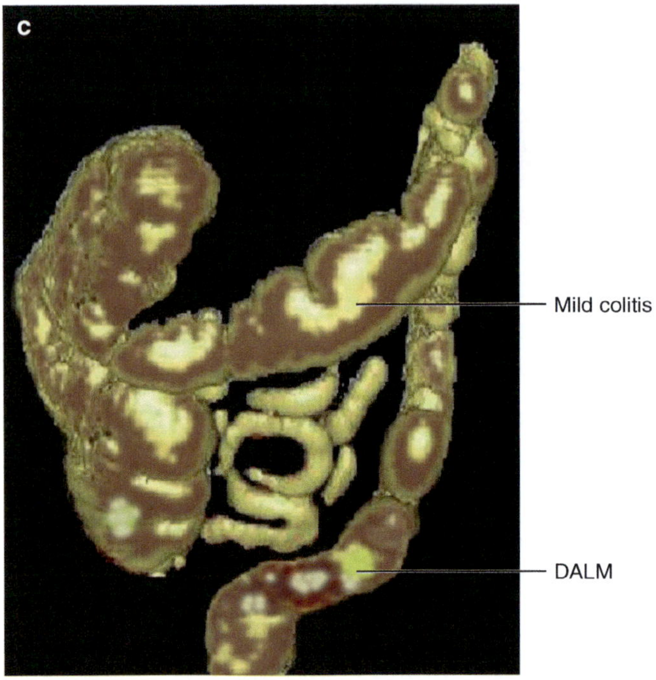

Fig. 13.2 (continued)

13.3 Ulcerative Colitis with Cancer

Clinical Presentation A 46-year-old woman with mild ulcerative colitis for 15 years. She had recent colonoscopy after developing rectal bleeding.

Diagnostic Studies Endoscopy showed mild colitis with rectal cancer present at 12 cm from the anal verge (see Fig. 13.3b).

Surgical Findings This patient underwent a colectomy with mucosal proctectomy, sphincter preservation, and Brooke ileostomy. Three months later, she had an ileo-anal pull-through (see Fig. 13.3a).

Pathology Inactive chronic ulcerative colitis with moderately differentiated rectal adenocarcinoma invading the submucosa. Lymph nodes are negative for tumor.

Follow-Up She had an uneventful recovery after surgery and is well 4 years later.

Comment This patient was fortunate that this was a distal lesion and that she had mild colitis. The presence of blood with bowel movements was a new symptom and prompted her to undergo a colonoscopy. This tumor was large at 5 cm in diameter but had only submucosal invasion. She initially underwent proctocolectomy with mucosectomy and sphincter preservation because the stage of the tumor was unknown and there was a possibility that she would require radiation. Once it became evident that the tumor was only superficially invasive and that chemoradiation would not be required, she was able to undergo a J-pouch anal anastomosis (Fig. 13.3).

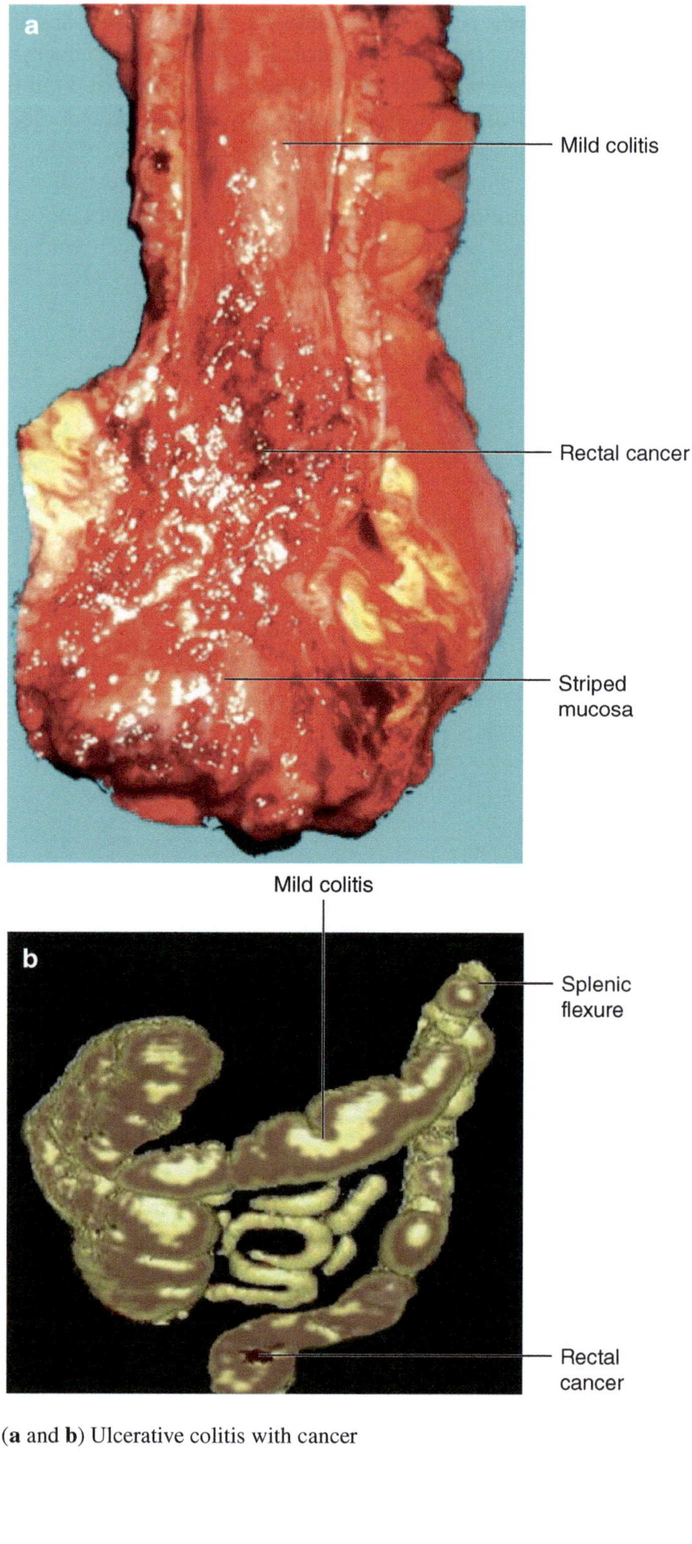

Fig. 13.3 (**a** and **b**) Ulcerative colitis with cancer

13.4 Ulcerative Colitis with Cancer

Clinical Presentation A 40-year-old man with mild ulcerative colitis present for 20 years was found to have cancer of the sigmoid colon on colonoscopy.

Diagnostic Studies Colonoscopy showed universal colitis with an ulcerated lesion in the sigmoid colon (see Fig. 13.4c).

Surgical Findings Superficial tumor at the sigmoid colon with chronic ulcerative colitis. The patient underwent total proctocolectomy with mucosectomy and ileo-anal anastomosis (see Fig. 13.4a, b).

Pathology Inactive chronic universal colitis with moderately differentiated adenocarcinoma of the sigmoid colon invading the muscularis propria. Foci of flat low-grade dysplasia are present in the transverse and sigmoid colon. Forty lymph nodes showed no evidence of metastasis.

Follow-Up He did well after surgery. The loop ileostomy was closed 3 months later.

Comment This patient was found to have a relatively early lesion at the rectosigmoid. Since the rectum was normal and there was no evidence of metastatic disease, he underwent proctocolectomy with mucosectomy and ileoanal anastomosis. At this location, had there been nodal metastasis, he would not have required radiation to the pelvis, and therefore, there was no contraindication to performing an ileoanal pull-through. Since the lesion was superficial, chemotherapy was also not indicated. The multicentric nature of the process is underscored by the presence of two areas of dysplasia in the transverse and sigmoid colon (Fig. 13.4).

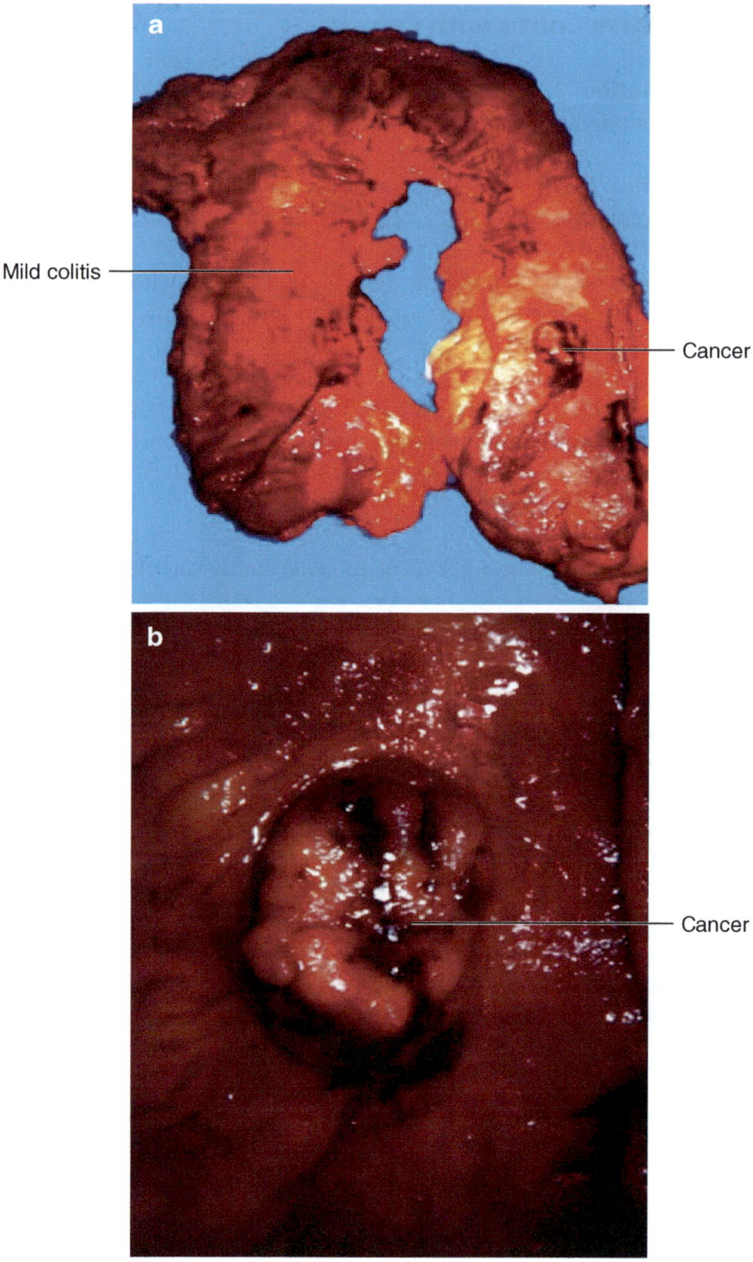

Fig. 13.4 (**a–c**) Ulcerative colitis with cancer

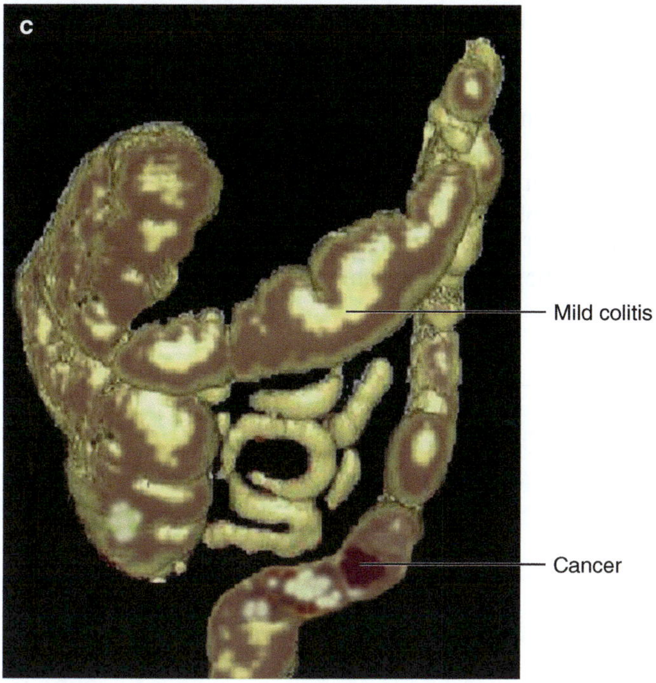

Fig. 13.4 (continued)

13.5 Ulcerative Colitis with Cancer

Clinical Presentation A 33-year-old man with ulcerative colitis for 12 years admitted with intestinal obstruction caused by a rectal cancer. He was initially treated with an ileostomy.

Diagnostic Studies Distal rectal cancer palpable on digital exam. Examination under anesthesia showed a circumferential tumor extending to 2 cm from the dentate line with complete obstruction of the rectum (see Fig. 13.5c).

Surgical Findings Ulcerative colitis with obstructing distal rectal cancer. The patient underwent a total proctocolectomy with ileostomy (see Fig. 13.5a, b).

Pathology Mildly active universal chronic ulcerative colitis with well-differentiated rectal adenocarcinoma infiltrating into the perirectal fat. Dysplasia is present only in the mucosa adjacent to the tumor. One of the 57 examined lymph nodes contains a micrometastasis.

Follow-Up He did well following surgery. He required chemoradiation and is well 4 years later.

Comment This patient had advanced rectal cancer at 33 years of age. It underscores the importance of surveillance colonoscopy in any patient with a 10-year or more history of ulcerative colitis. Since the symptoms of the tumor are masked by the symptoms of the colitis, periodic colonoscopy is essential to make an early diagnosis. The mean age of patients with colitis and cancer is 55 years, but cancer, such as in this case, can often occur in much younger patients (Fig. 13.5).

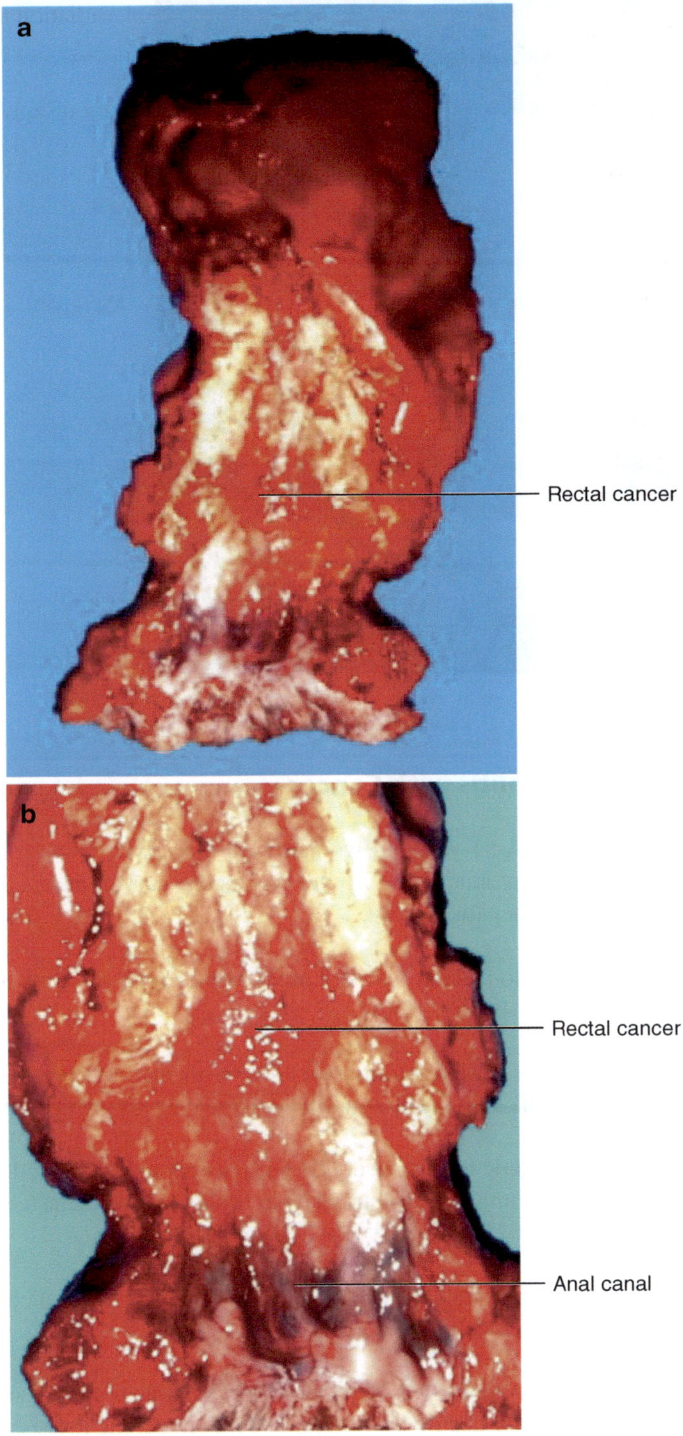

Fig. 13.5 (**a–c**) Ulcerative colitis with cancer

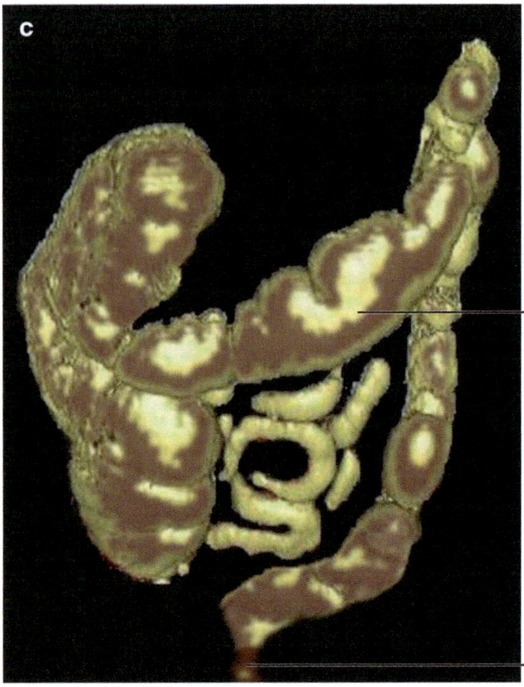

Fig. 13.5 (continued)

13.6 Ulcerative Colitis with Cancer

Clinical Presentation A 51-year-old woman with ulcerative colitis for 27 years. Disease has been asymptomatic for 21 years. Recent surveillance colonoscopy showed cancer near the hepatic flexure.

Diagnostic Studies Colonoscopy showed mild colitis with an ulcerated cancer near the hepatic flexure (see Fig. 13.6c).

Surgical Findings This patient had a colectomy with mucosal proctectomy and J-pouch anal anastomosis (see Fig. 13.6a, b).

Pathology Inactive chronic ulcerative colitis with deeply invasive, moderately differentiated adenocarcinoma of the transverse colon with metastasis to two lymph nodes.

Follow-Up She recovered well following surgery and was subsequently treated with chemotherapy. She is well 18 months later.

Comment Although this tumor was asymptomatic and was found on surveillance colonoscopy, it was already deeply infiltrating and had nodal metastasis. The lesion itself was less than 2 cm in diameter but was obviously an aggressive cancer. Since there was no evidence of distant metastasis and the lesion was in the colon where radiation would not be needed, she underwent a total proctocolectomy with mucosectomy and J-pouch-anal anastomosis. The loop ileostomy was kept in place for 6 months while she underwent chemotherapy (Fig. 13.6).

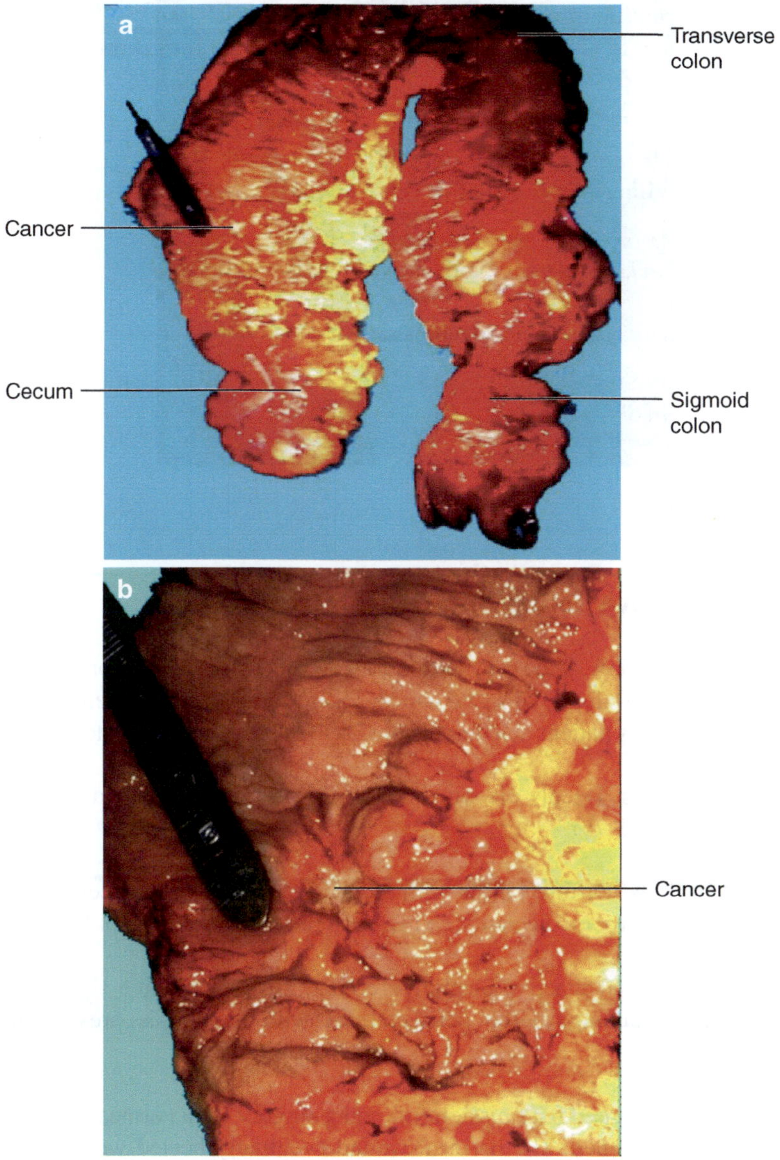

Fig. 13.6 (a–c) Ulcerative colitis with cancer

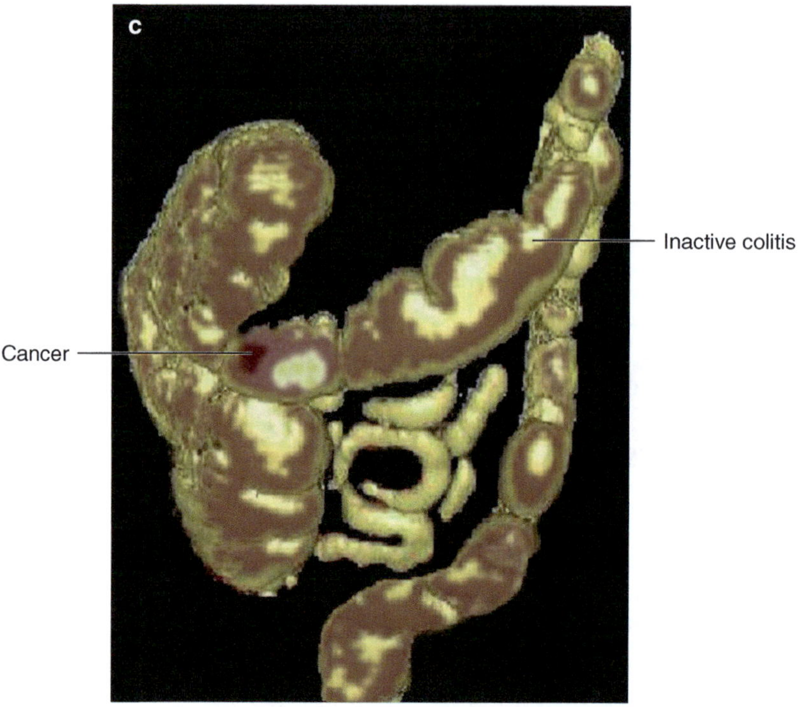

Fig. 13.6 (continued)

13.7 Ulcerative Colitis with Cancer

Clinical Presentation A 65-year-old man with ulcerative colitis for 30 years was found to have circumferential rectal cancer located just above the dentate line on a physical exam. This patient also has chronic renal disease and diabetes.

Diagnostic Studies Deeply ulcerated circumferential tumor located near the dentate line (see Fig. 13.7b).

Surgical Findings Diffuse colitis with advanced distal rectal cancer. The patient underwent a total proctocolectomy and Brooke ileostomy (see Fig. 13.7a).

Pathology Universal inactive ulcerative colitis. Deeply invasive signet ring cell rectal cancer extending to the perirectal fat with metastasis present in three lymph nodes.

Follow-Up He required readmission following surgery for a perineal wound infection, which was drained. The perineal wound eventually healed well, and he was treated with chemotherapy and radiation.

Comment This patient had mild colitis with minimal symptoms. This case is another example that severity of colitis does not correlate with cancer risk. He had colitis for over 30 years and unfortunately did not have regular surveillance colonoscopy. The diagnosis of this lesion was made only after it became symptomatic. At that point, the tumor was deeply invasive and circumferential, and there were several positive lymph nodes. At this location in the distal rectum, a total proctocolectomy with Brooke ileostomy was the only curative surgical procedure available (Fig. 13.7).

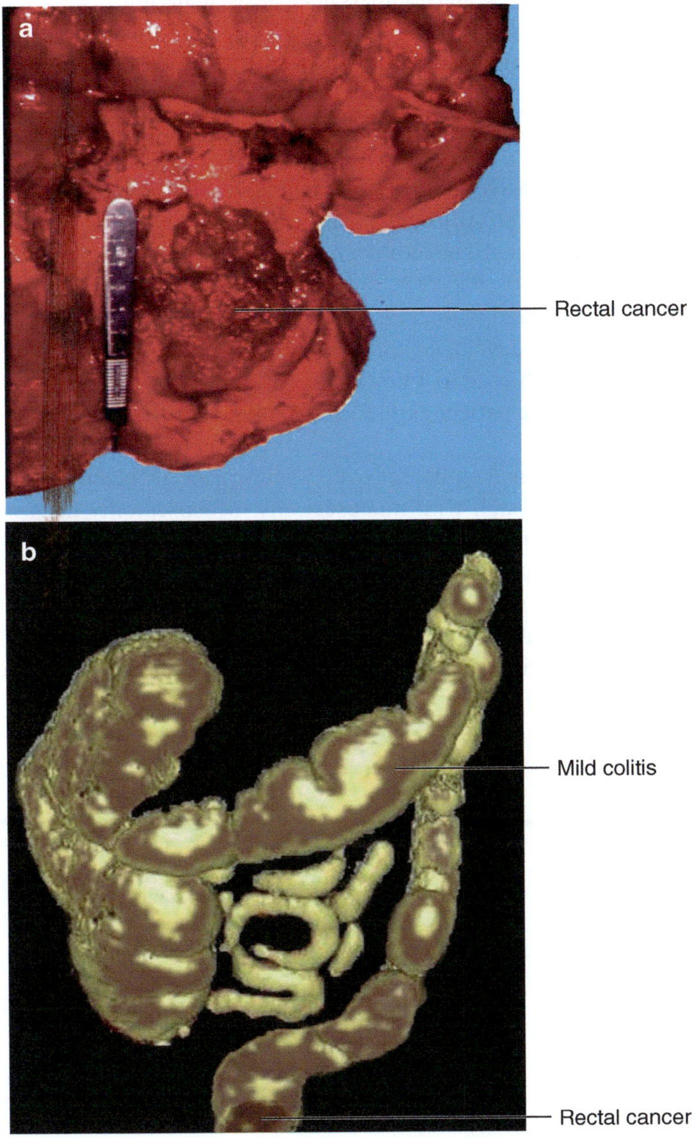

Fig. 13.7 (**a** and **b**) Ulcerative colitis with cancer

13.8 Ulcerative Colitis with Cancer in a J-Pouch

Clinical Presentation A 42-year-old patient with ulcerative colitis since age 24. Patient underwent restorative proctocolectomy at age 29 for severe disease. Sigmoidoscopy, 12 years later, for recent onset of rectal bleeding shows a large ulcerated lesion in the J-pouch.

Diagnostic Studies Deeply ulcerated nearly circumferential tumor located in the distal J-pouch just above the anastomosis near the dentate line.

Surgical Findings Advanced distal rectal cancer. The patient underwent a total proctocolectomy and Brooke ileostomy. No evidence of metastatic disease at the time of surgery (see Fig. 13.8a, b, c).

Pathology Deeply invasive poorly differentiated signet ring adenocarcinoma invading the subserosal fat. Adjacent mucosa with low- and high-grade dysplasia. Margins of resection clear, 10 negative lymph nodes.

Follow-Up He was treated with chemotherapy and pelvic radiation following surgery. Two years later, he developed recurrent disease in the pelvis and a lung nodule on a PET scan. The CEA rose to 44.5. The recurrent tumor was resistant to further systemic therapy, and the patient expired 26 months after the surgery.

Comment This patient had colitis for over 5 years prior to colectomy and 12 years after creation of the J-pouch with mucosectomy. Mucosectomy does not prevent cancer development after pouch surgery since it has been shown that there are residual microscopic islands of mucosa, which are then covered by the pouch. The diagnosis of this lesion was made only after it became symptomatic. At that point, the tumor was deeply invasive and nearly circumferential. Cancer after pouch surgery is uncommon; in our series, it occurs in only 1% of patients, and few are diagnosed at an early stage (Fig. 13.8).

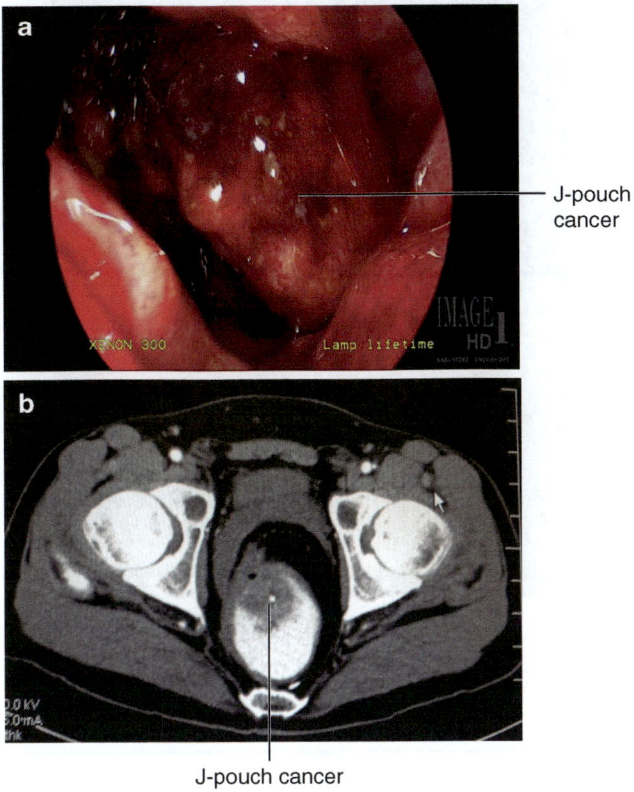

Fig. 13.8 (**a**–**c**) Ulcerative colitis with cancer in a J-pouch

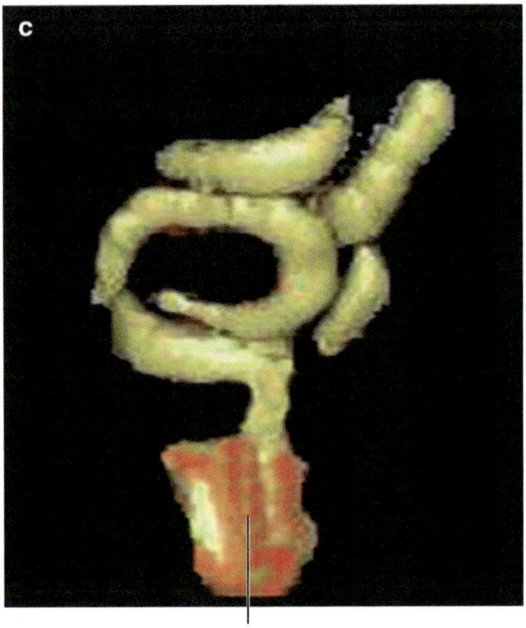

Fig. 13.8 (continued)

Further Reading

Branco BC, Sachar DB, Heimann TM, Sarpel U, Harpaz N, Greenstein AJ. Adenocarcinoma following Ileal pouch-anal anastomosis for ulcerative colitis: review of 26 cases. Inflamm Bowel Dis. 2009;15(2):295–9.

Heimann TM, Greenstein AJ, Bolnick K, Yoelson S, Aufses AH Jr. Colorectal cancer in familial polyposis coli and ulcerative colitis. Dis Colon Rectum. 1985;28:658–61.

Heimann TM, Oh SC, Martinelli G, Szporn A, Luppescu N, Lembo C, Kurtz RJ, Fasy TM, Greenstein AJ. Colorectal carcinoma associated with ulcerative colitis: a study of prognostic indicators. Am J Surg. 1992;164:13–7.

Kurtz MP, Heimann TM. Perineal adenocarcinoma thirty years after proctocolectomy. Dis Colon Rectum. 2007;50(12):2241–3.

Sugita A, Greenstein AJ, Ribeiro MB, Sachar DB, Bodian C, Panday AKN, Szporn A, Pozner J, Heimann TM, Palmer M, Aufses AH Jr. Survival with colorectal cancer in ulcerative colitis: a study of 102 cases. Ann Surg. 1993;218:189–95.

Intestinal Cancer in Crohn's Disease 14

Tomas M. Heimann and Robert J. Kurtz

Patients with Crohn's disease are prone to develop small bowel cancer in diseased segments. These tumors usually present with symptoms of obstruction due to stricture formation. Patients undergoing strictureplasty should have a biopsy of the stricture since often the malignant nature of the narrowed segment of the bowel is not always evident at the time of surgery.

The incidence of colorectal cancer is also higher in patients with Crohn's disease when compared to the general population. Although there is still some controversy over surveillance colonoscopy in patients with Crohn's colitis, there is increasing evidence that the colorectal cancer risk is similar to that seen in ulcerative colitis. Patients with Crohn's colitis and cancer should usually undergo total proctocolectomy with Brooke ileostomy since the cancer risk involves the entire colon and rectum.

14.1 Crohn's Ileitis with Cancer

Clinical Presentation A 72-year-old man with a 31-year history of Crohn's disease. He presented with obstructive symptoms manifested by abdominal pain and 20-lb weight loss.

Diagnostic Studies Small bowel series showed a dilated ileum with an area of severe narrowing (see Fig. 14.1a, e).

T. M. Heimann (✉) · R. J. Kurtz
Department of Surgery, Icahn School of Medicine at Mount Sinai, New York, NY, USA
e-mail: Tomas.Heimann@mountsinai.org; Robert.Kurtz@mountsinai.org

T. M. Heimann (ed.), *Atlas of Surgical Treatment of Inflammatory Bowel Disease*, https://doi.org/10.1007/978-3-031-62431-5_14

Surgical Treatment Massive dilatation of ileum with annular cancer causing near-complete obstruction and multiple proximal fecaliths. He had a small bowel resection with end-end anastomosis. Multiple liver metastasis were also present (Fig. 14.1b, c, d).

Pathology Crohn's disease of the ileum with moderately differentiated adenocarcinoma of the small bowel infiltrating into the mesentery. Regional lymph nodes are free of tumor.

Follow-Up He initially did well and was placed on 5-FU-based chemotherapy.

Comment Small bowel cancer in Crohn's disease is seldom diagnosed before surgery. These tumors may cause obstruction, usually appearing as recurrent Crohn's disease or may be found incidentally during resection or strictureplasty. Cancers producing symptoms of obstruction are often advanced, and the prognosis is poor. Tumors found incidentally may be resected at an earlier stage and have a better prognosis. Often these cancers appear as an area of thickening in the wall of the bowel, rather than the ulcerated appearance seen in de novo small bowel cancers (Fig. 14.1).

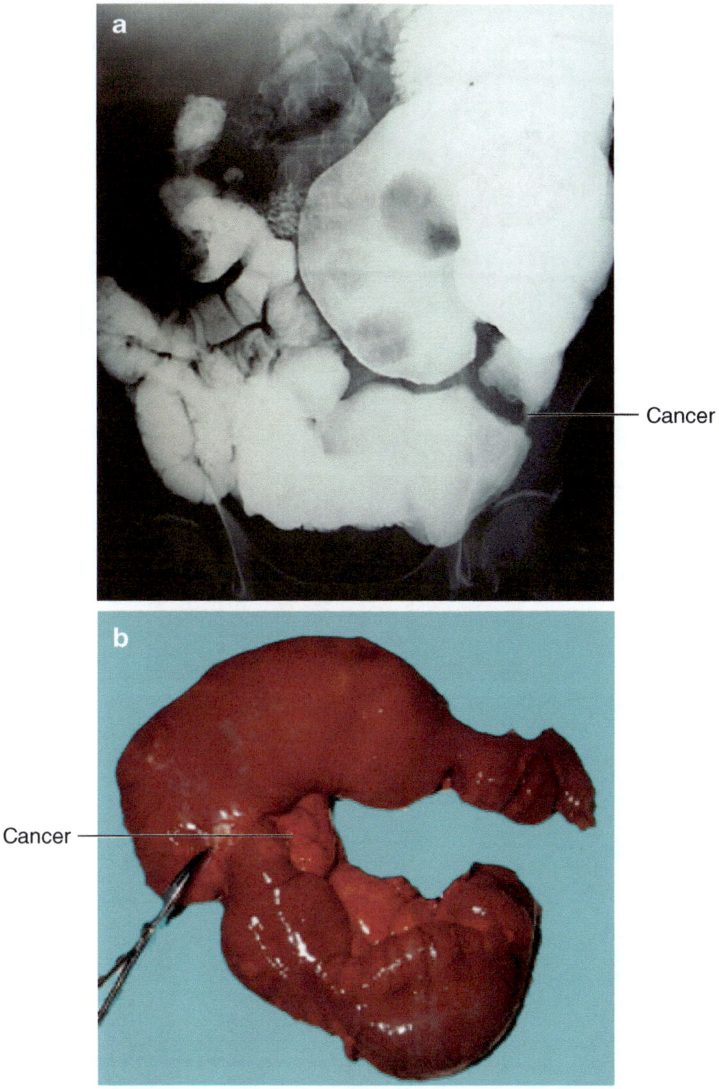

Fig. 14.1 Crohn's ileitis with cancer

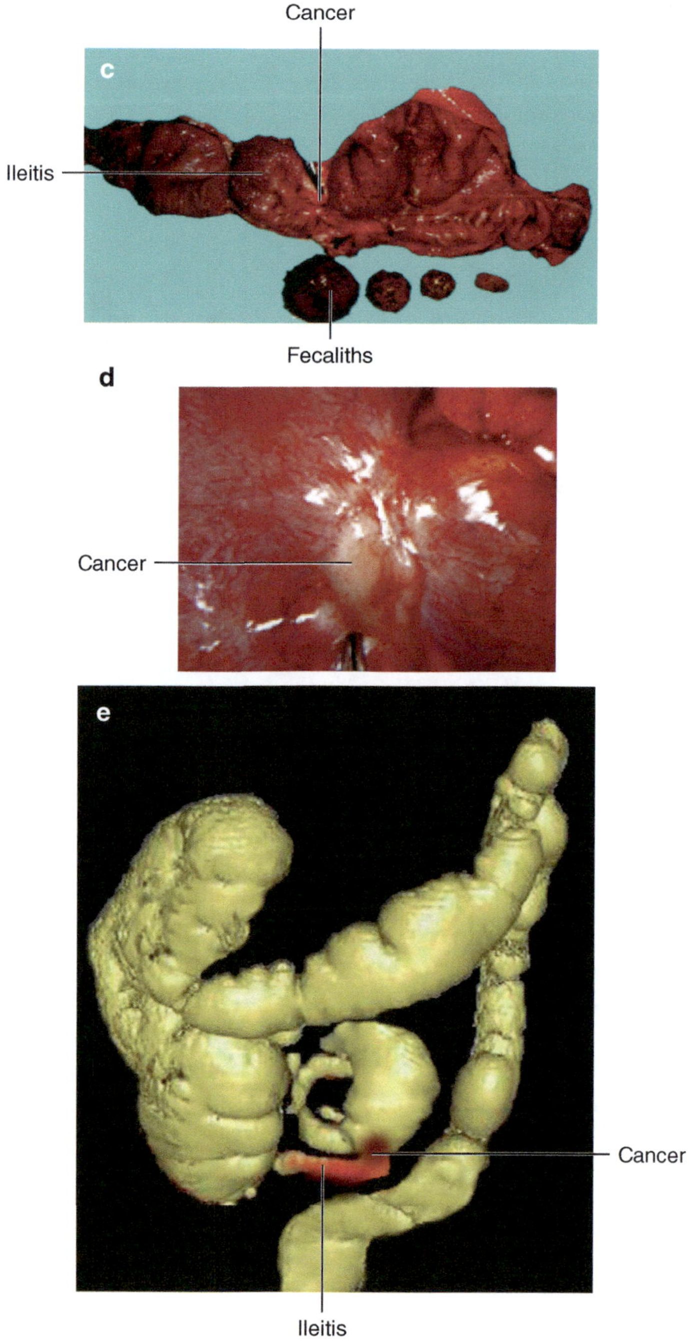

Fig. 14.1 (continued)

14.2 Granulomatous Colitis with Cancer

Clinical Presentation A 21-year-old woman with a 13-year history of colitis. This patient is moderately symptomatic requiring 30 mg of prednisone daily to control her symptoms. Recent colonoscopy showed an area of dysplasia in the sigmoid colon.

Diagnostic Studies Colonoscopy revealed universal colitis with sigmoid lesion (see Fig. 14.2b).

Surgical Treatment At surgery, the patient had universal colitis with Crohn's disease of the terminal ileum and an indurated area in the sigmoid colon. She underwent a subtotal colectomy and ileostomy (see Fig. 14.2a).

Pathology Active Crohn's ileocolitis with well-differentiated adenocarcinoma of the sigmoid colon invading the serosa. The surrounding mucosa shows severe dysplasia. Forty-eight lymph nodes are negative for tumor.

Follow-Up She did well after surgery. She completed a course of chemotherapy and 1 year later underwent completion proctectomy with abdominoperineal resection of the rectum.

Comment This patient was young at the age of diagnosis of colon cancer but already had a 13-year history of colitis. Biopsies of the area with a polypoid lesion in the sigmoid colon showed severe dysplasia. The malignant lesion was not seen until the time of surgery when a small area of induration in the sigmoid colon was palpated and biopsy confirmed the presence of a small deeply invasive carcinoma. The area with severe dysplasia in this patient was a marker of high cancer risk and was adjacent to an area of invasive cancer, which was not visible on surveillance colonoscopy (Fig. 14.2).

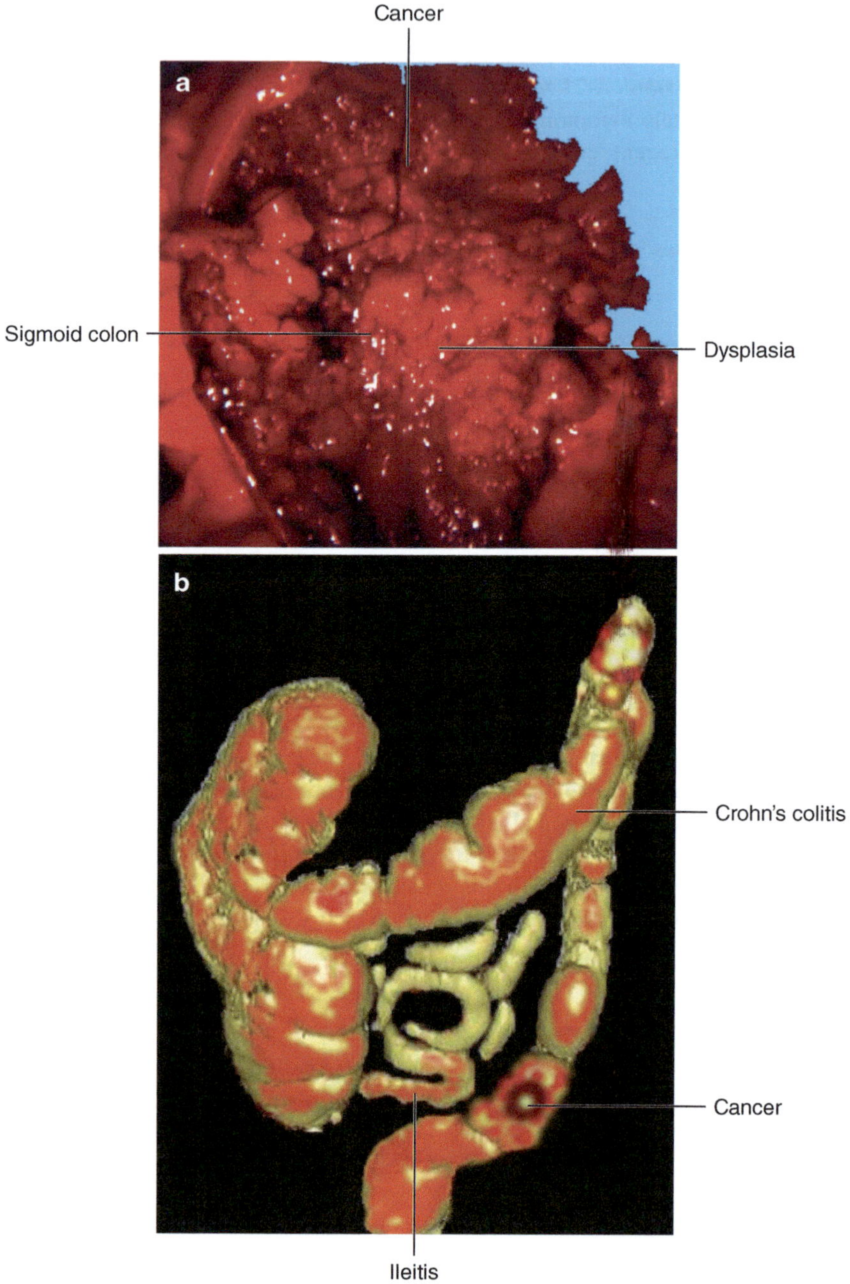

Fig. 14.2 Granulomatous colitis with cancer

14.3 Recurrent Ileocolitis with Cancer

Clinical Presentation A 59-year-old woman with a 40-year history of Crohn's colitis. She had a previous ileocolic resection for ileocolitis at age 17 and now comes in with a recent onset of anemia and left lower quadrant pain.

Diagnostic Studies Colonoscopy showed an adenocarcinoma in the descending colon. No evidence of metastatic disease on the CT scan (see Fig. 14.3c).

Surgical Treatment This patient underwent a proctocolectomy with Brooke ileostomy (see Fig. 14.3a, b).

Pathology Inactive Crohn's ileocolitis with adenocarcinoma of the descending colon invading the perirectal fat. Lymph nodes are negative for tumor.

Follow-Up This patient received adjuvant chemotherapy following surgery and is well 3 years later.

Comment This patient presented with anemia probably secondary to chronic blood loss from this ulcerated tumor. She also had pain caused by the narrowing of the colonic lumen. The tumor was deeply invasive but free of metastasis. This case underscores the need for yearly surveillance colonoscopy in Crohn's colitis. When symptoms develop, the tumor is usually advanced, and the cure rate is much lower than when asymptomatic tumors are found on yearly endoscopy. This patient did well after proctocolectomy and ileostomy, and there is no evidence of recurrence at this time (Fig. 14.3).

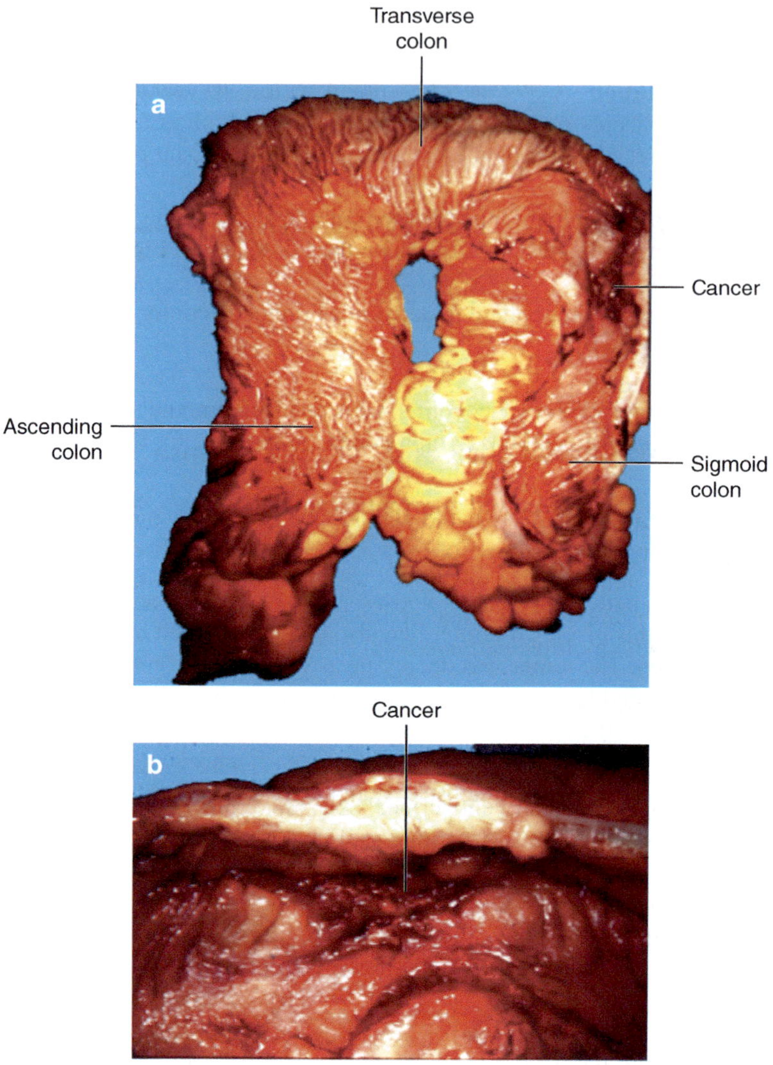

Fig. 14.3 Recurrent ileocolitis with cancer

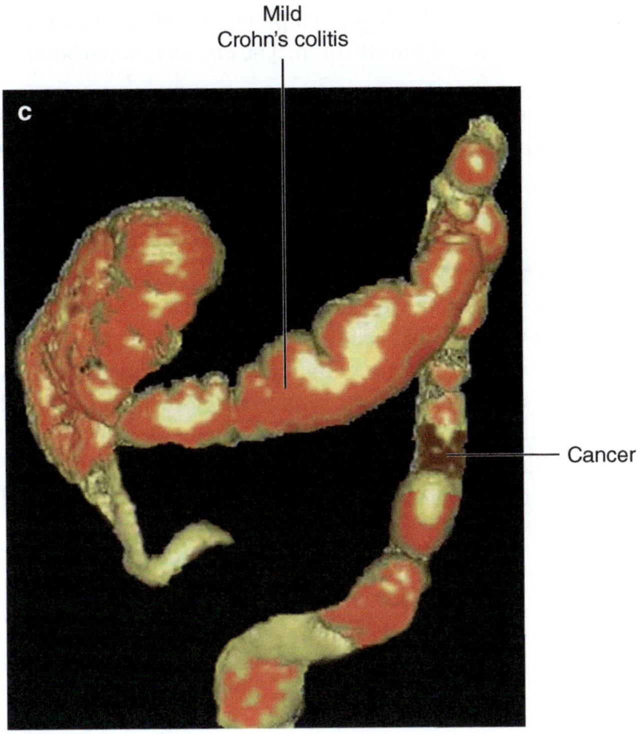

Fig. 14.3 (continued)

14.4 Ileocolitis with Cancer

Clinical Presentation A 59-year-old woman with a 33-year history of Crohn's colitis. She has been known to have a sigmoid stricture for 6 years. Found to have a colonic adenocarcinoma of the splenic flexure on surveillance colonoscopy (see Fig. 14.4b). Previous colonoscopy was 2 years before and did not show this lesion. Physical exam showed no abdominal masses, liver was normal in size, and rigid sigmoidoscopy showed minimal rectal inflammation.

Diagnostic Studies CT scan of the abdomen showed no evidence of metastatic disease.

Surgical Treatment This patient underwent a total proctocolectomy with Brooke ileostomy (see Fig. 14.4a).

Pathology Crohn's ileocolitis with mucin-secreting signet ring adenocarcinoma of the splenic flexure, invading the pericolonic fat. Small metastatic nodules are present in the serosal surfaces. Multiple lymph nodes contain metastatic carcinoma. Inflammatory stricture in the sigmoid colon. The colitis is superficial and quiescent.

Follow-Up This patient had an uneventful postoperative recovery, she received chemotherapy following surgery and developed recurrent disease in the peritoneal surfaces 1 year later.

Comment Strictures in ulcerative colitis are more likely to be malignant than colonic strictures in Crohn's disease. This patient is an example that cancer may be responsible for the development of a new stricture in Crohn's disease. This lesion was not seen at a previous colonoscopy 2 years ago, nevertheless, at the time of resection, the tumor was advanced with nodal and small peritoneal metastasis. Signet ring cell tumors, such as this one, tend to be more aggressive and more likely to metastasize. She initially did well following proctocolectomy and ileostomy but developed recurrent disease 1 year later. This case demonstrates that 2 years between colonoscopy is too long an interval to find these tumors before they become advanced (Fig. 14.4).

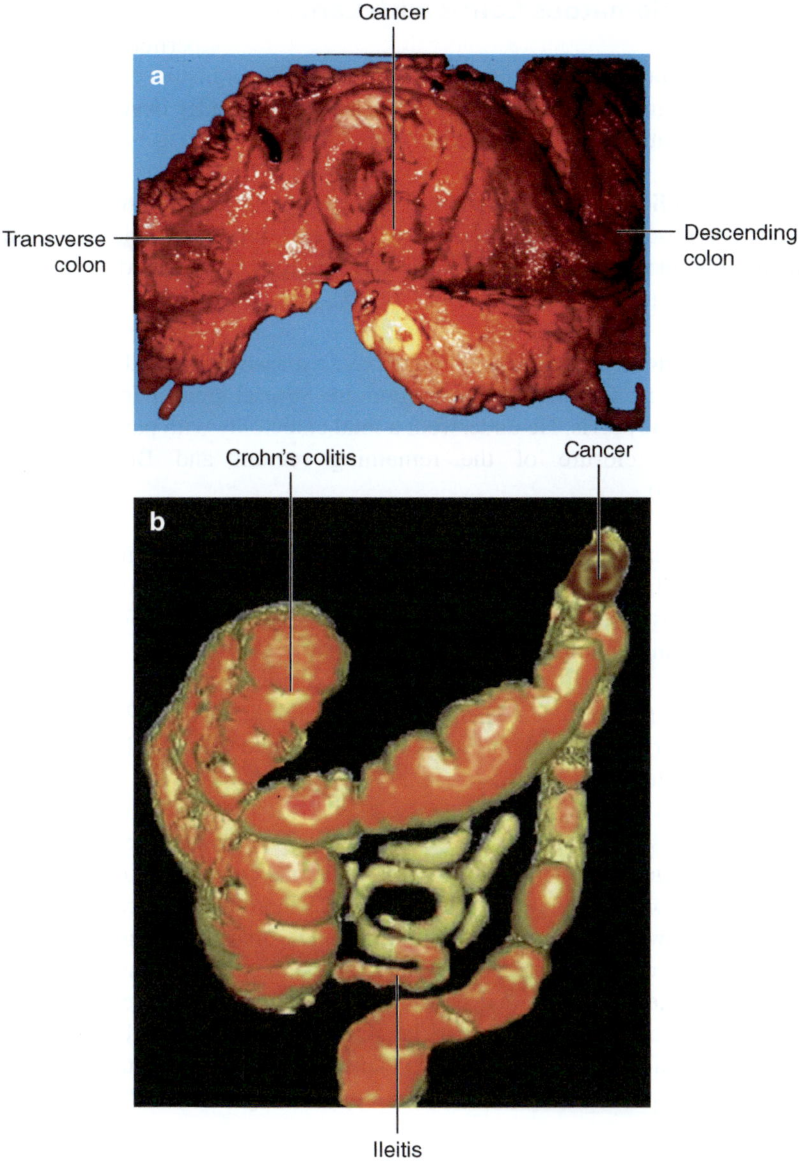

Fig. 14.4 Ileocolitis with cancer

14.5 Granulomatous Colitis with Cancer

Clinical Presentation A 48-year-old man with a 30-year history of Crohn's colitis. He has had a sigmoid stricture for several years but recently developed increased abdominal distention and vomiting.

Diagnostic Studies Endoscopy showed an obstructing lesion in the rectosigmoid. Previous colonoscopies showed pancolitis. CT scan showed colonic dilatation with a transition point in the distal sigmoid colon. Previous barium studies showed normal small bowel (see Fig. 14.5c).

Surgical Treatment Patient was found to have a massively dilated colon at surgery with an obstructing tumor at the rectosigmoid. Several small peritoneal implants were present in the pelvis. He underwent a total colectomy with partial proctectomy and Hartmann's closure of the remaining rectum and Brooke ileostomy (see Fig. 14.5a, b).

Pathology Extensive Crohn's colitis with mucinous adenocarcinoma of the sigmoid colon infiltrating the pericolonic fat. Four lymph nodes contain metastatic carcinoma. Biopsy of pelvic nodule also contains metastatic adenocarcinoma. The ileum shows minimal nonspecific inflammation.

Follow-Up The patient received chemotherapy and did well for 2 years following surgery. He then returned with intestinal obstruction and was found to have multiple peritoneal metastases.

Comment The stricture in the area of the rectosigmoid was due to an advanced tumor in this patient. At the time of resection, he had colonic obstruction, and several pelvic peritoneal implants were present. He therefore underwent a palliative total colectomy with resection of the tumor and Hartmann's closure of the rectum. He subsequently did well for 2 years until a metastatic deposit obstructed the distal ileum and he required a proximal ileostomy. The malignant nature of the rectosigmoid stricture was not initially appreciated, and biopsies showed only inflammation. As the tumor progressed and the patient became obstructed, preoperative colonoscopic biopsies were positive for carcinoma (Fig. 14.5).

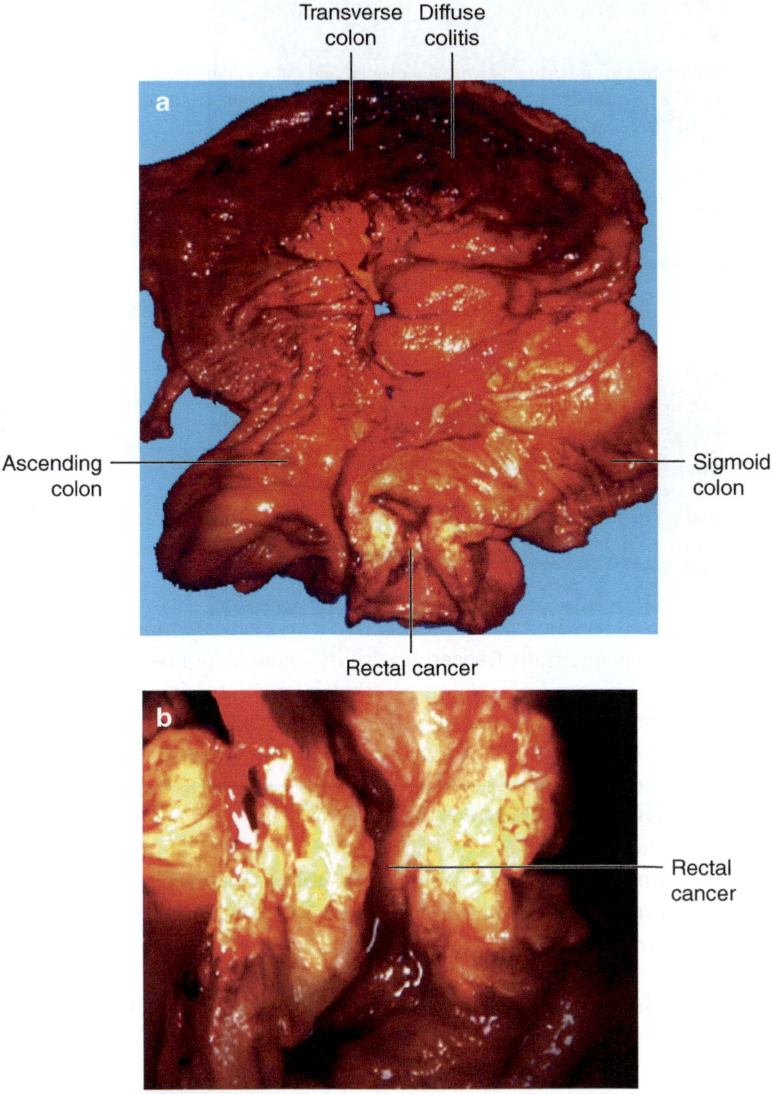

Fig. 14.5 Granulomatous colitis with cancer

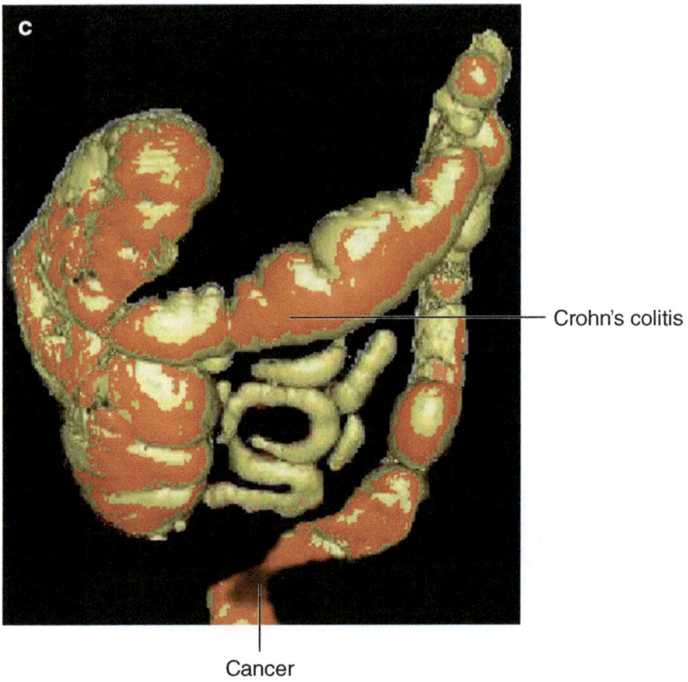

Fig. 14.5 (continued)

14.6 Ileocolitis with Cancer

Clinical Presentation A 28-year-old woman with a 12-year history of colitis. She was found to have a lesion in the rectum at 8 cm from the anal verge, which on biopsy was an adenocarcinoma.

Diagnostic Studies Colonoscopy showed mild diffuse colitis with a 2 cm lesion in the mid-rectum (see Fig. 14.6b).

Surgical Findings Diffuse colitis with ileitis of the terminal ileum. This patient underwent total proctocolectomy with Brooke ileostomy (see Fig. 14.6a).

Pathology Ileum with chronic ileitis. The colon showed chronic colitis with four independent carcinomas. Two cancers are located in the rectum, one in the sigmoid, and another in the descending colon. All four cancers invade the muscularis propria. A metastatic subserosal nodule was present in the rectosigmoid. The lymph nodes were negative for tumor.

Follow-Up She had an uneventful recovery after surgery and is well 6 years later.

Comment This patient demonstrates the multicentric nature of colorectal cancer in Crohn's colitis. Statistically, the cancer risk increases with duration of the disease, and most patients with cancer are older. However, colorectal cancer can occur in younger patients such as this 28-year-old woman. It is possible that patients with early-onset cancer may have another genetic predisposition that makes them more cancer-prone. Total proctocolectomy is essential in these patients since any residual colorectal mucosa would have a very high risk of further cancer formation (Fig. 14.6).

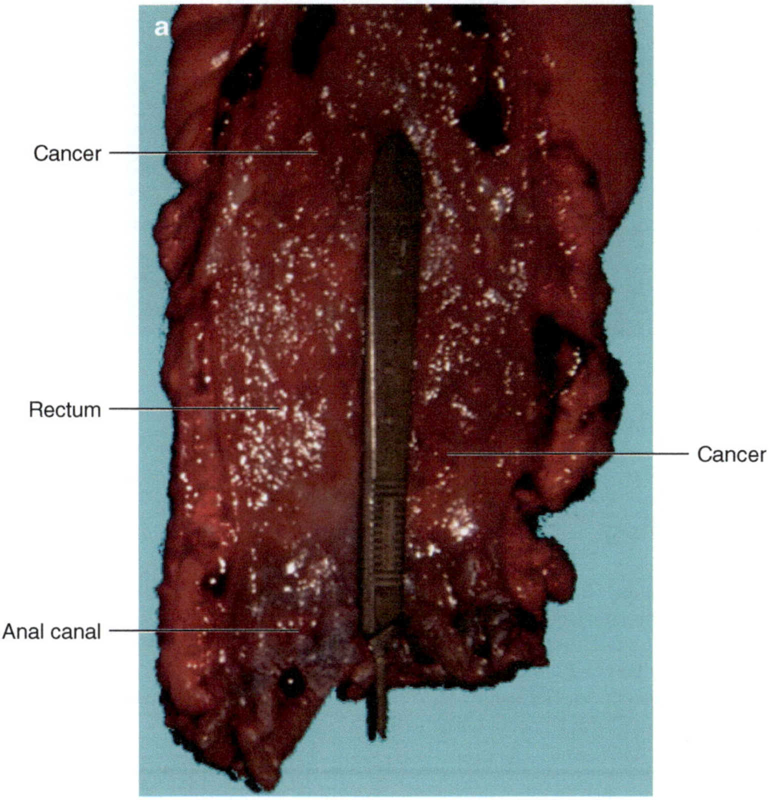

Fig. 14.6 Ileocolitis with cancer

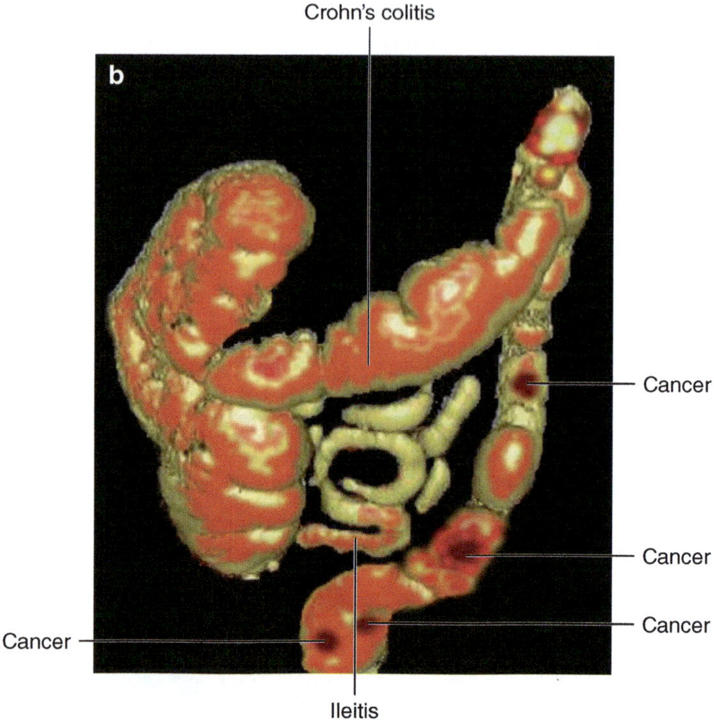

Fig. 14.6 (continued)

Further Reading

Greenstein AJ, Gennuso R, Sachar DB, Heimann TM, Smith H, Janowitz HD, et al. Extraintestinal cancers in inflammatory bowel disease. Cancer. 1985;56:2914–21.

Greenstein AJ, Mullin GE, Strauchen JA, Heimann TM, Janowitz HD, Aufses AH, et al. Lymphoma in inflammatory bowel disease. Cancer. 1992;69:1119–23.

Ribeiro MB, Greenstein AJ, Heimann TM, Aufses AH Jr. Adenocarcinoma of the small intestine in Crohn's disease. Surg Gynecol Obstet. 1991;173:343–9.

Index

T. M. Heimann (ed.), *Atlas of Surgical Treatment of Inflammatory Bowel Disease*, https://doi.org/10.1007/978-3-031-62431-5

GPSR Compliance

The European Union's (EU) General Product Safety Regulation (GPSR) is a set of rules that requires consumer products to be safe and our obligations to ensure this.

If you have any concerns about our products, you can contact us on ProductSafety@springernature.com

In case Publisher is established outside the EU, the EU authorized representative is:

Springer Nature Customer Service Center GmbH
Europaplatz 3
69115 Heidelberg, Germany

Batch number: 10739801

Printed by Printforce, the Netherlands